RECENT ADVANCES IN THE BIOLOGY, THERAPY AND MANAGEMENT OF MELANOMA

Edited by **Lester M. Davids**

Recent Advances in the Biology, Therapy and Management of Melanoma

http://dx.doi.org/10.5772/46052

Edited by Lester M. Davids

Contributors

Pu Wang, Peipei Guan, Sadako Yamagata, Tatsuya Yamagata, Shawn M. Swavey, John D'Orazio, James Lagrew, Amanda Marsch, Stuart Jarrett, Laura Cleary, Norma E. Herrera, Jianli Dong, Gengming Huang, Rasheen Imtiaz, Fangling Xu, Randy Burd, Erin Mendoza, Nicholas Panayi, Elliot Breshears, Paola Savoia, Paolo Fava, Pietro Quaglino, Maria Grazia Bernengo, Jung-Feng Hsieh, Wen-Tai Li, Hsiang-Wen Tseng, Isabel Pires, Justina Prada, Felisbina Luisa Queiroga, Joana Almeida Gomes, Dinora Pereira, Miriam Jasiulionis, Fabiana Melo, Fernanda Molognoni, Bryan E. Strauss, Eugenia Costanzi-Strauss, Małgorzata Latocha, Aleksandra Zielińska, Magdalena Jurzak, Dariusz Kuśmierz, Jiri Vachtenheim, Brian Wall, Tania Creczynski-Pasa

Published by InTech

Janeza Trdine 9, 51000 Rijeka, Croatia

Publishing Process Manager Ana Pantar
Technical Editor InTech DTP team
Cover InTech Design team

Additional hard copies can be obtained from orders@intechopen.com

Recent Advances in the Biology, Therapy and Management of Melanoma, Edited by Lester M. Davids
p. cm.
ISBN 978-953-51-0976-1

For EU product safety concerns:
IN TECH d.o.o., Prolaz Marije Krucifikse Kozulić 3, 51000 Rijeka, Croatia, info@intechopen.com or visit our website at intechopen.com.

Meet the editor

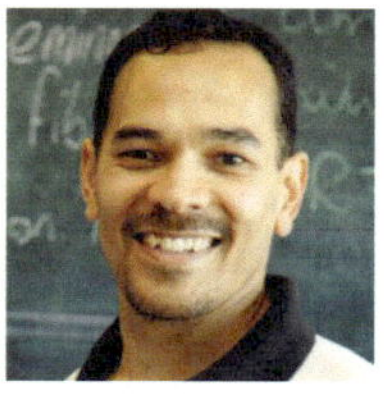

Dr Lester M. Davids completed his under- and post-graduate studies at the University of Cape Town. His PhD was completed in the Department of Medicine in 2003 studying the heme disorder, porphyria. Four years of postdoctoral work under the mentorship of Prof Sue Kidson led to him joining the academic staff of the Dept of Human Biology in 2010, where he is currently a Senior Academic Lecturer. He established the Redox Laboratory Research Group (http://redoxlab.uct.ac.za) in 2010 which uses human skin as a model to study the biological effectiveness of photodynamic therapy as an adjuvant form of melanoma skin cancer therapy. Thus far 10 postgraduate students have graduated under his mentorship and since 2008 he has published 8 peer-reviewed international publications.

Contents

Preface

The book Recent Advances in the Biology, Therapy and Management of Melanoma brings the latest, up-to-date information regarding the biological mechanisms underlying melanoma epidemiology, molecular mechanisms and the therapeutic options that are employed in combating this dreaded disease. The first section covers the genetics of melanoma development with associated risk factors. Understanding the underlying molecular mechanisms of melanomagenesis, the biomarkers, and the proteins that contribute to melanoma, all lead to illuminating potential targets in the fight against this disease. This section is comprehensively reviewed and is essential to be interweaved and translated with the final section which culminates in current treatment options and clinically relevant regimes. The novelty of new treatment options are further highlighted in this section.

This book is intended to be a reference book for both the scientific and clinical communities. It is not often easy to interweave these two disciplines but this book brings both of these together in an easy, readable way. The fact that there is so much ongoing scientific and clinical research in the field of melanoma is an indicator of the importance and relevance attached to understanding the human melanocyte and the factors that cause it to go awry. This fundamental scientific understanding has to then be translated to the clinic in order for us to make significant strides in eradicating this dreaded disease.

It is hoped that scientists, clinicians, students and residents find this book useful in their studies on melanoma and that it not only expands their perspectives and views on the field, but challenges them to forge ahead towards discovering the ultimate cure.

Lester M. Davids
Redox Laboratory, Department of Human Biology, Faculty of Health Sciences
University of Cape Town, South Africa

Section 1

Melanoma Epidemiology

Chapter 1

Melanoma — Epidemiology, Genetics and Risk Factors

John A. D'Orazio, Stuart Jarrett, Amanda Marsch,
James Lagrew and Laura Cleary

Additional information is available at the end of the chapter

http://dx.doi.org/10.5772/55172

1. Introduction

1.1. Melanoma a growing problem

The U.S. National Cancer Institute's Surveillance Epidemiology and End Results (SEER) Cancer Statistics Review estimates over 70,000 people will be diagnosed and 9,000 will die from melanoma in the United States in 2012. Though melanoma can affect persons of essentially any age, it is mainly a disease of adulthood, with median ages of diagnosis and death between 61 and 68 years, respectively (Weinstock, 2012). Nonetheless, melanoma incidence is increasing across age groups, over the past several decades in the United States (Fig. 1) (Ekwueme et al., 2011). In 1935, the average American individual had a 1 in 1,500 lifetime risk of developing melanoma. In 2002, the approximate risk of developing melanoma increased to 1 in 68 individuals (Rigel, 2002). Globally, Australia and New Zealand have the highest incidence rate of melanoma, an abundance of fair-skinned residents living in a UV-rich geography widely believed to be a major factor (Lens and Dawes, 2004). The current melanoma risk for Australian and New Zealander populations may be as high as 1 in 50 (Rigel, 2010). Considering melanoma is being diagnosed more often in young adults, could be prevented by UV-avoiding behaviors, and can be associated with extensive morbidity and mortality, it is truly an emerging public health concern. Part of the apparent increase in melanoma incidence may be due to better surveillance and earlier detection (Erdmann et al., 2012) however, even with heightened melanoma awareness and screening, there seems to have been a real increase in melanoma incidence over the past several decades.

1.2. The ultraviolet connection

Historically, humans have been exposed to UV radiation primarily as a consequence of unprotected exposure to sunlight (Holman et al., 1983; Holman et al., 1986;Woodward and

Boffetta, 1997). Since the early 20th century, a tanned appearance has been culturally associated with health and well-being in Western civilizations. The desire to sport a dark tan has been matched by increased opportunities for sunbathing outdoors as well as proliferation of indoor tanning salons. UV radiation has many deleterious effects on cells (Zaidi et al., 2012), producing both direct and indirect DNA damage, resulting in mutations that can contributed to carcinogenesis in skin cells. Direct damage occurs when DNA absorbs UV photons and undergoes cleavage of the 5-6 double bond of pyrimidines. When two adjacent pyrimidines undergo this 5-6 double bond opening, a covalent ring structure referred to as a cyclobutane pyrimidine dimer (thymine dimer) can be formed. Alternatively, a pyrimidine 6-4 pyrimidone (6,4)-photoproduct can result when a 5-6 double bond in a pyrimidine opens and reacts with the exocyclic moiety of the adjacent 3' pyrimidine to form a covalent 6-4 linkage (Kadekaro et al., 2003; Pfeifer et al., 2005; Maddodi and Setaluri, 2008). Both (6,4)-photoproducts and cyclobutane dimers can result in characteristic transition mutations between adjacent pyrimidines. "UV signature mutations" involving T-to-C or C-to-T changes are a common feature of UV-induced malignancies such as skin cancers (Kanjilal et al., 1993; Nataraj et al., 1996; Soehnge et al., 1997; Sarasin, 1999). UV radiation also damages cellular macromolecules indirectly, through production of oxidative free radicals [20]. Several DNA modifications can result from oxidative injury, including 7,8-dihydro-8-oxoguanine (8-oxoguanine; 8-OH-dG), which promotes mutagenesis (specifically GC-TA transversion mutations) (Kino and Sugiyama, 2005). Both direct and indirect DNA changes interfere with transcription and replication, and render skin cells susceptible to mutagenesis. It is estimated that one day's worth of sun exposure can cause up to 100,000 potentially mutagenic UV-induced photolesions in each skin cell (Nakabeppu et al., 2006).

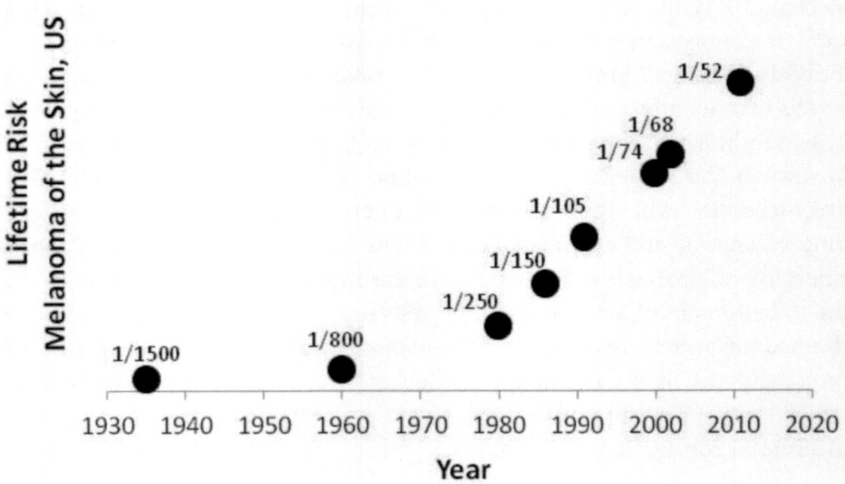

Figure 1. Increasing incidence of melanoma of the skin, US. Data are reported as lifetime risk and are taken from NCI SEER reports.

Much of solar UV energy is absorbed by stratospheric ozone, and gradual depletion of stratospheric ozone over the last several decades has resulted in higher levels of solar UV radiation striking Earth's surface (van der Leun et al., 2008). Increased ambient UV radiation from global climate change may be an important factor to explain the burgeoning prevalence of melanoma (Schmalwieser et al., 2005). Increased exposure to ambient UV radiation is a feature of global climate change because of thinning of atmospheric ozone and increased outdoor occupational and recreational activities associated with a warming climate (de Gruijl et al., 2003; van der Leun et al., 2008; Andrady et al., 2010; Makin, 2011; McKenzie et al., 2011; Norval et al., 2011). UV exposure in youth seems particularly important, affording the longest amount of time for the gradual accumulation of mutagenic UV lesions. Thus, high UV exposures in childhood, adolescence and young adulthood are strongly linked to risk of skin cancer later in life. For example, first exposure to indoor tanning before the age of 35 years raises lifetime risk of melanoma by seventy five percent (Schulman and Fisher, 2009).

1.3. Geographic location

UV radiation varies with altitude and with proximity to the equator. Since UV radiation can be absorbed, reflected back into space or scattered by particles in the atmosphere, ambient UV doses on the surface of the Earth vary according to the amount of atmosphere solar radiation must pass through. The more atmosphere solar radiation passing through, the weaker the corresponding UV content of the sunlight realized on the surface of the Earth. Sunlight strikes Earth most directly at the equator and more tangentially toward the poles. The more direct the sunlight's path, the less atmosphere radiation has to traverse and the more powerful the UV component will be (Fig. 2). Thus, UV content of sunlight is most powerful in equatorial locations and weakest in polar extremes. Equatorial locations are also typically the hottest environments, therefore people living in such places tend to wear lesser amounts of clothing. Fabrics and other materials used for clothing typically block large amounts of UV radiation, as evidenced by the pattern of "farmer tans" among people who wear short sleeve tee shirts. Persons living in cold, polar climates would be expected to realize far less UV radiation from sunlight both because the UV dosage in ambient sunlight is weaker in such locations and because people living there probably are covered with more clothing. Thus in general, individuals living in equatorial locations typically receive much higher ambient UV doses than persons inhabiting temperate climates (Lee and Scotto, 1993). In the United States, risk of melanoma is higher in the South than in the North (Crombie, 1979). Worldwide, melanoma rates are highest in UV-rich environments such as Australia (Franceschi and Cristofolini, 1992; Elwood and Koh, 1994; Marks, 1995). One study examining the low rates of melanoma in Scandinavia pointed to data showing that ambient UV levels in Norway were significantly lower than most of the world because of its high latitude (Moan et al., 2009). Altitude and the amount of particulate matter in the atmosphere also influence the amount of UV found in a particular geographic location. The higher the altitude, the nearer the location to the sun and the more powerful the sunlight's UV dose will be. Similarly, the more particles in the atmosphere, the higher the likelihood of interference with UV and the weaker the UV energy at the earth's surface (Atkinson et al., 2011).

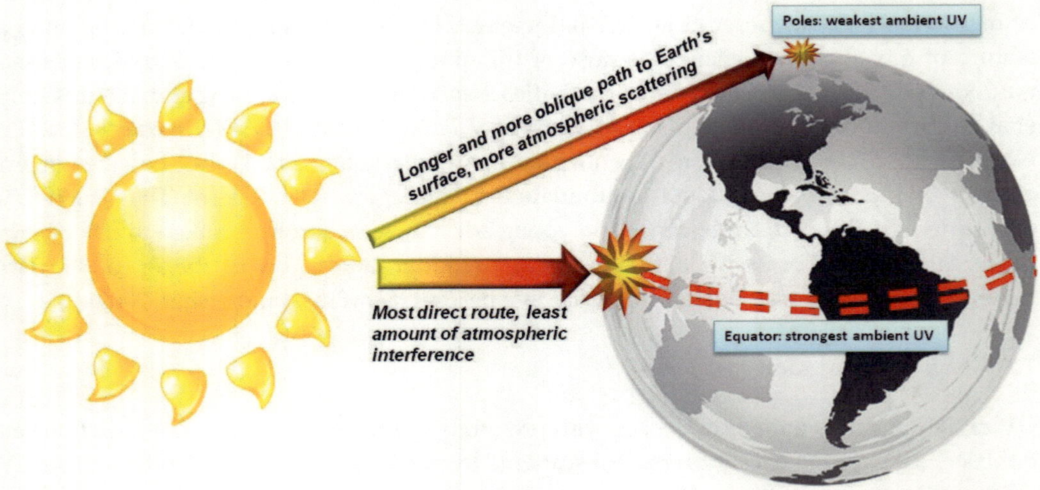

Figure 2. Strength of ambient UV varies with geographic location. UV radiation in sunlight can be blocked by the atmosphere. Consequently, the longer the distance sunlight must travel, the weaker the UV component hitting Earth will be. The highest UV doses in sunlight are found at the equator, where the sun hits the Earth at a direct angle.

2. Risk factors

2.1. Older age

Melanoma incidence increases markedly with advancing age (Fig. 3), presumably because of the time it takes to accumulate mutations in melanocyte-relevant genes that drive carcinogenesis (Gilchrest et al., 1999). However other factors may also be relevant, including a more permissive environment for tumors to develop because of the natural age-related decline in cellular immunity (Weiskopf et al., 2009; Malaguarnera et al., 2010). According to the SEER data, from 2005-2009, the median age of melanoma diagnosis was 61 years. Nonetheless, although older adults are more at risk for melanoma, the incidence of melanoma in young adults, especially in young adult women, is increasing at a faster rate (Reed et al., 2012). For women and men between the ages of 20-29, melanoma is the second and third most commonly diagnosed cancer respectively (Siegel et al., 2012).

2.2. Solar UV exposure

Decreasing UV radiation exposure, from both sun exposure and artificial UV light, may be the single best preventable factor for decreasing the incidence rate of melanoma (Lucas et al.,

2008). The ultraviolet portion of sunlight is divided into UVC (<280 nm), UVB (280-315 nm) and UVA (315-400 nm), with wavelengths below 290 nm being absorbed by stratospheric ozone (Fig. 4). UVB constitutes 5 -10% of solar UV irradiation and is mainly absorbed by the epidermal layer of the skin. The most frequent form of DNA damage induced by UVB are molecular rearrangements resulting in the dimerization of pyrimidines, generating 2 classes of mutagenic lesions, cyclobutane pyrimidine dimers (CPDs) and pyrimidine (6-4) pyrimidone photoproducts (6-4 PP) through direct absorption by DNA. CPDs are formed through a ring structure involving C5 and C6 of neighboring bases whereas 6-4 PP are formed with a non-cyclic bond between C6 and C4 (Budiyanto et al., 2002). These photoproducts promote cytosines (C)- thymines (T) and CC-TT transitions, with regions of DNA containing 5-methylocytosine being hot spots for UVB-induced mutations. Radiation in UVA range is associated with lower energy but has the ability to penetrate deeper into the dermis. In contrast to UVB, UVA is poorly absorbed by DNA, but excites numerous endogenous chromophores, generating reactive oxygen species (ROS) e.g. singlet oxygen and hydroxyl radicals. The predominant ROS-induced lesions formed are oxidized bases, such as 8-oxo-dG with DNA single and double strand breaks (Mouret et al., 2006). Both ultraviolet A radiation (320 to 400 nm) and ultraviolet B radiation (290 to 320 nm) contribute to the development of melanoma (Gilchrest et al., 1999).

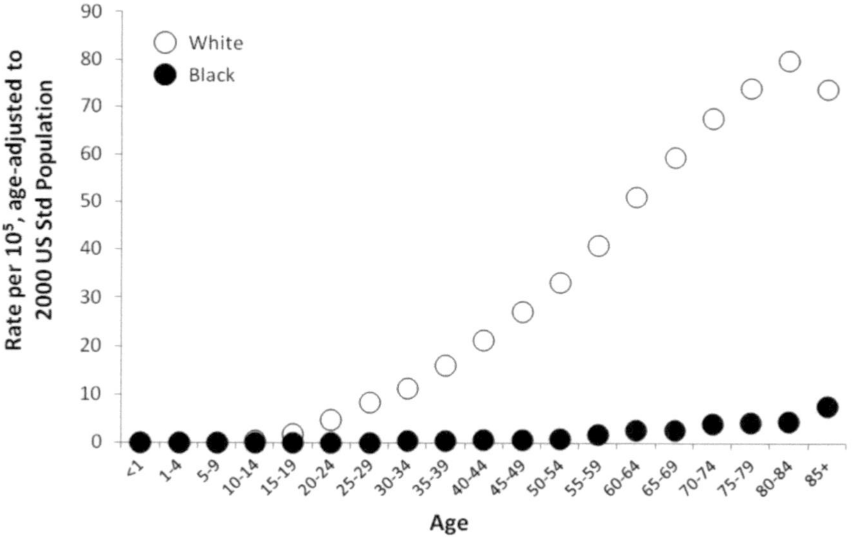

Figure 3. Melanoma incidence by age, US. Incidence rates (per 100,000 individuals) are based on NCI SEER data. Note the marked increase in melanoma incidence with increasing age. Also evident is the tremendous discrepancy in melanoma incidence between persons of fair- and dark-skinned complexions.

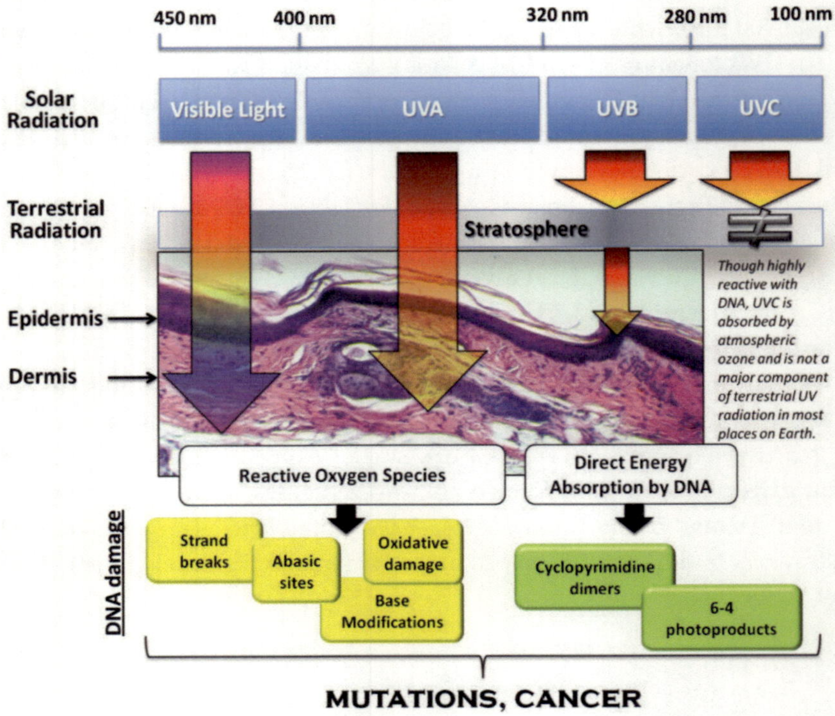

Figure 4. Electromagnetic spectrum of visible and UV radiation and biologic effects on the skin. The diagram shows the subdivision of the solar UV spectrum with the shorter UV wavelengths (i.e. UVC) being entirely absorbed by stratospheric oxygen, and the majority of UVB (> 90 %) being absorbed by ozone. UV light penetrates the skin and is absorbed by different layers in a wavelength- dependent manner. The visible and UVA components of solar radiation penetrates deeply into the dermis reaching the dermal stratum papillare. In contrast, UVB is almost completely absorbed by the epidermis, with only ~20 % reaching the epidermal stratum basale. UVA and visible light make up the majority of the total terrestrial solar energy and are able to generate reactive oxygen species that can damage DNA via indirect photosensitizing reactions. UVB is directly absorbed by DNA which causes molecular rearrangements forming the specific photoproducts CPD and 6-4 PP. Mutations and cancer can result from a variety of modifications to DNA.

2.3. Sunburns

While squamous cell carcinoma of the skin has been closely associated with long term occupational exposure to the sun, risk of developing melanoma seems to be more associated with intermittent, high intensity sun exposure (MacKie and Aitchison, 1982; Lew et al., 1983). Prevalence of sunburns among children is high, with one study finding that approximately 69% of adolescents experienced sunburn the previous summer and only 40% used sun protection methods (Buller et al., 2011). Positive association between severe, painful sunburn and the development of melanoma and a negative association between Early found a positive melanoma and long-term recreational/occupational sun exposure (MacKie and Aitchison, 1982; Lew et al., 1983). Sunburn represents an inflammatory response of the skin to a significant amount of acute UV damage. It is mediated by a complex series of cellular and hormonal events, including the generation of cytokines and mediators of vasodilatation. Risk of sunburn is related not only to UV exposure, but also to innate melanin content of the skin. Thus, sunburn mostly occurs in fair skinned people without sun protection exposed to high intensities of UV radiation, for example in equatorial or high altitude locations. Various epidemiologic studies support the finding that the number of severe sunburns and total childhood sun exposure are positively associated with the development of melanoma (Holman et al., 1986; Scotto and Fears, 1987; Cust et al., 2011; Newton-Bishop et al., 2011; Volkovova et al., 2012). The carcinogenic effects of sunburn have also been demonstrated experimentally using transgenic mice forcing overexpression of the hepatocyte growth/scatter factor (HGF/SF) in melanocytes. In these mice, HGF over-expression altered the distribution of melanocytes to create a "humanized" model, which mimics human skin with melanocytes located in the basal layer of the epidermis, rendering them more susceptible to DNA damaging effects of UVR. Remarkably, a single erythemal UV dose to neonatal mice caused the development of melanomas in roughly half of animals at one year of age (Noonan et al., 2001). This animal model has been used by several laboratories to study a variety of melanoma susceptibility genes in context of UV-induced childhood sunburn and melanoma initiation and metastasis (Recio et al., 2002).

2.4. Indoor tanning

Whereas only one percent of Americans ever used a tanning bed in 1988, now more than twenty five percent have participated in indoor tanning. With more than 25,000 facilities in the US alone, indoor tanning represents a multi-billion dollar industry. Employing over 160,000 people, the tanning industry has a customer base of nearly thirty million people and exerts political influence through powerful lobbying efforts. Nonetheless, there are clear health risks associated with indoor tanning. UV radiation emitted by tanning lamps is typically more powerful than direct ambient sunlight. It is estimated that half an hour in a tanning booth yields the same UV damage to skin as much as 300 minutes in unprotected sun. Levels of UVA/UVB emitted by tanning beds are unpredictable, widely unregulated, and much higher than environmental exposure. A study of 62 tanning salons in North Carolina found that the average UVA output of a tanning bed was 192.1 W/m^2 (vs. average UVA summer solar output at noon in Washington D.C. of 48 W/m^2) and the average UVB output of a tanning bed was 0.35 W/m^2 (vs. average UVB summer solar output at noon in Washington D.C. of 0.18 W/m^2) (Hornung et al., 2003). Tanning bed use is clearly associated with skin cancers of all varieties. Persons who have ever used a tanning bed have a 50% increased risk of basal cell carcinoma and more than a 100% increased risk of squamous cell carcinoma (Karagas et al., 2002).

The risk association between melanoma development and indoor tanning has been well substantiated (Autier, 2004; Rados, 2005; Han et al., 2006). Data accumulated from several studies suggest that the use of a tanning salon before the age of 35 is associated with a 75% increased lifetime risk of melanoma, while over-use of tanning salons was associated with a 15% increased risk of melanoma (Fig. 5) (Schulman and Fisher, 2009). Risk of carcinogenesis is enhanced for all types of tanning beds (UVA, UVB and mixed output) and increases with years of use, number of sessions, and hours exposed (Lazovich et al., 2010). There currently is no "safe" way to tan by UV without the inherent risk of photodamage and malignancy. The use of tanning salons despite the established risks, however, remains popular, especially in female young adults and adolescents. A recent survey found that 18.1% of female and 6.3% of male Caucasian adults reported using a tanning salon in the past 12 months (Choi et al., 2010). Among 10,000 adolescents across the 50 states, 24.6% of girls under 18 reported tanning, with prevalence of use steadily increasing from age 12 to 18 years (Geller et al., 2002). California and Vermont have recently banned (January 2012 and July 2012 respectively) use of indoor tanning beds for minors, while many other states require parental permission or have proposed legislation for restricting the use of tanning beds for minors. The use of tanning salons by adolescents did not decline from 1998 to 2004, even though more states restricted use by minors (Cokkinides et al., 2009), which suggests that these partial restrictions may not be effective. Predictors of using tanning salons for women were residing in the Midwest and the South and using spray tan products, while men who lived in metropolitan areas were more likely to visit tanning salons.

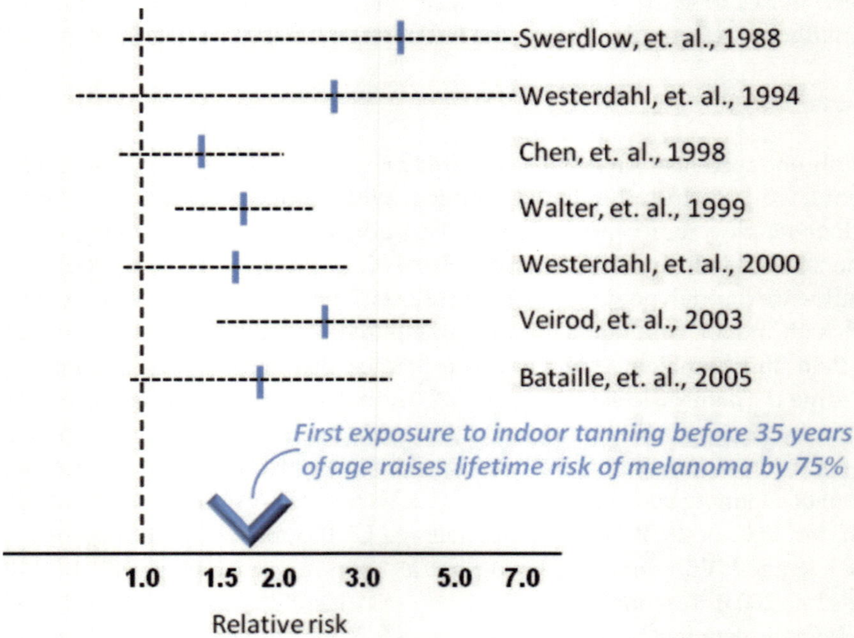

Figure 5. Relative risk of melanoma associated with exposure to indoor tanning. Results of seven studies and overall estimate. Values higher than 1.0 indicate heightened risk of melanoma. Modified from (Schulman and Fisher, 2009).

2.5. PUVA therapy

Ultraviolet A radiation therapy (PUVA) is a common and effective treatment for psoriasis that was first introduced in the 1970s. Since UVA exposure from the sun and artificial sources like tanning beds is a clear risk for melanoma, there is concern that PUVA therapy may predispose to malignancies including melanoma. One large cohort study that followed patients for 20 years found that there was a 10-fold increase in the incidence of invasive melanoma in patients who had received PUVA therapy versus age matched controls (Stern, 2001). Increased risk began at 15 years post-PUVA therapy exposure, and there was a stronger association with patients exposed to higher doses of PUVA therapy, more treatments (greater than 250), and in patients with fair skin. Thus, limiting exposure to PUVA to minimal doses and carefully selecting appropriate patients for the treatment can maximize the effectiveness of this treatment and minimize the risks. Patients who receive PUVA therapy should be carefully followed to facilitate early detection of melanoma and other skin cancers.

2.6. Skin pigmentation

Although individuals from any race or skin pigmentation group can be affected by melanoma, risk of disease is much higher in fair-skinned persons (Fig. 6) (Beral et al., 1983; Rees and Healy, 1997; Sturm, 2002). Created by Dr. Thomas Fitzpatrick in 1975, the Fitzpatrick scale is commonly used to describe skin tone and resultant UV sensitivity (Draelos, 2011). Skin complexion is mainly determined by the amount of black melanin in the epidermis. This pigment, called eumelanin, is a potent blocker of UV radiation. Thus the more eumelanin in the skin, the less UV penetrates into the deep layers of the epidermis, and the less UV-mediated mutagenesis will occur. Risk of sunburn is also heavily influenced by epidermal eumelanin content. In fair-skinned individuals with low Fitzpatrick skin types, it takes a much lower dose of UV to induce inflammation. The amount of UV needed to cause a sunburn is termed the "minimal erythematous dose" (MED), and a lower MED correlates with low levels of epidermal eumelanin and a higher risk of melanoma (Ravnbak et al., 2010) (Fig. 7). Thus, risk of melanoma for Caucasian males and females is 31.6 and 19.9 per 100,000 respectively, while risk for African American males and females is only 1.1 and 0.9 per 100,000 in comparison (Ekwueme et al., 2011; Park et al., 2012).

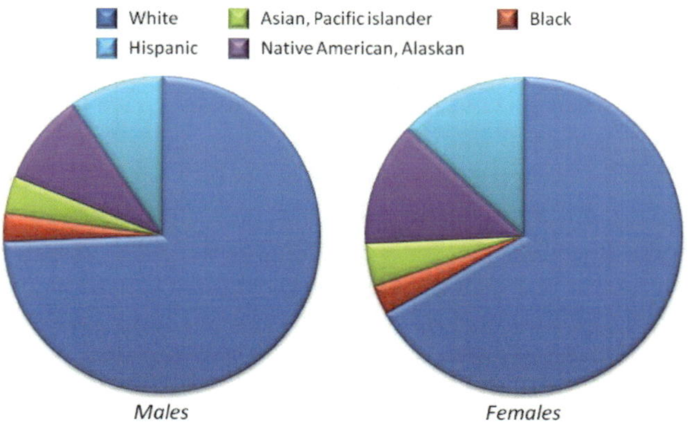

Figure 6. Racial Disparity in Melanoma Incidence (US). Incidence rates based on NCI SEER data. Note that in general, the darker a race's average skin tone, the lower their incidence of melanoma, irrespective of gender.

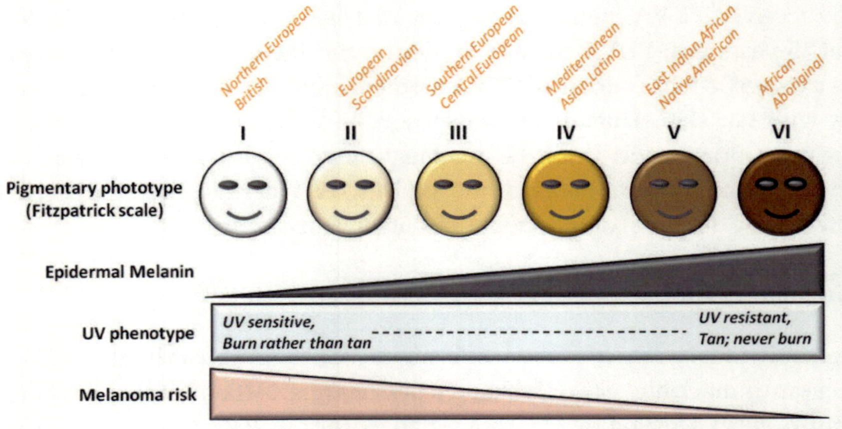

Figure 7. Melanoma risk varies according to skin complexion. Skin complexion can be estimated by the Fitzpatrick scale wherein the higher the number, the more deeply melanized and pigmented the skin is. Fair-skinned individuals are much more UV sensitive and tend to burn rather than tan after UV exposure. Melanoma risk is highest in fair-skinned individuals.

2.7. Nevi

The majority of melanomas arise out of pre-existing moles (nevi), therefore the more nevi a person has, the higher the likelihood that a melanoma may develop (Grob et al., 1990; Newton-Bishop et al., 2010). One study found a seven-fold increased relative risk for melanoma if a patient has more than one hundred nevi (Gandini et al., 2005). Most patients, however, do a poor job in estimating their own mole counts (Melia et al., 2001), and a patient's self assessment of nevus count should not be relied upon in lieu of a full skin exam for melanoma screening (Psaty et al., 2010). Despite the link between nevi and melanoma, risk of any given mole progressing to malignancy is very low (Metcalf and Maize, 1985; Halpern et al., 1993). One study estimated the 60 year risk of malignant transformation to be 1:11,000 for an individual nevus on a 20 year-old woman (Tsao et al., 2003).

A molecular link between benign nevi and malignant melanoma was established in 2003 when Pollock and coworkers reported that a gain of function mutation in the BRAF gene was common to the majority of benign nevi and melanomas (Pollock et al., 2003). Specifically, the V599E amino-acid substitution in BRAF results in enhanced MAPkinase signaling which stimulates melanocytes to proliferate. Clearly other genetic and/or epigenetic cellular events, such as loss of the tumor suppressor p16, are required for full malignant transformation, as BRAF mutation is sufficient for nevi formation but not melanomagenesis.

Congenital melanocytic nevi are pigmented lesions found on individuals at birth (Zaal et al., 2005; Krengel et al., 2006). Those that are particularly large (>20 cm in diameter) seem particularly prone to malignant transformation, and are associated with a lifetime melanoma risk of approximately 10% (Krengel et al., 2006). Smaller congenital melanocytic nevi have a significantly lower risk of malignant degeneration. Given their relatively high malignant potential, large congenital melanocytic nevi warrant consideration for prophylactic excision (Psaty et al., 2010) preferably during childhood, since up to 70% of melanomas associated with congenital melanocytic nevi occur by the individual's tenth year (Marghoob et al., 2006).

Atypical Mole Syndrome (also referred to as Dysplastic Nevus Syndrome or Familial Atypical Multiple-Mole Melanoma Syndrome) has emerged as one of the most significant risk factors for the development of melanoma (Carey et al., 1994; Slade et al., 1995; Seykora and Elder, 1996). In the general population, dysplastic nevi are relatively common: found on 2-8% of Caucasians especially among those under 30 (Naeyaert and Brochez, 2003). A combination of both UV exposure and genetic susceptibility is believed to contribute to dysplastic nevi formation (Naeyaert and Brochez, 2003). Atypical Mole Syndrome is an important melanoma risk factor (Halpern et al., 1993); individual melanoma risk approaches 82% in affected individuals by the age of 72 (Tucker et al., 1993).

2.8. Chemical exposure and occupational risk

Geographic discrepancy in melanoma incidence may be influenced by factors other than UV exposure and skin pigmentation (Fortes and de Vries, 2008). A number of environmental and occupational substances have been linked to development of malignant melanoma including heavy metals, polycyclic aromatic hydrocarbons (PAHs) and benzene (Ingram, 1992; Vinceti et al., 2005; Meyskens and Yang, 2011). As a result of working around many of these chemicals, petroleum workers, for example, have been reported to have up to an eight-fold increased risk of melanoma (Magnani et al., 1987). Polyvinyl chloride (PVC), a substance used widely in the clothing and chemical industries, is also linked to increased risk of melanoma (Lundberg et al., 1993; Langard et al., 2000). Printers and lithographers, through their exposure to PAH and benzene solvents, have up to a 4.6-fold increased risk of disease (McLaughlin et al., 1988). Ionizing radiation exposure, as might occur from medical radiation exposure or atomic energy occupational exposure has also been linked to melanoma risk (Fink and Bates, 2005; Lie et al., 2008; Korcum et al., 2009). Pesticide exposure was reported to almost triple melanoma risk (Burkhart and Burkhart, 2000). Clearly a better understanding of occupational risk factors, especially when coupled to UV risk, is needed to guide more targeted public health efforts for the prevention of melanoma (Fortes and de Vries, 2008).

2.9. Immunodeficiency

Immunodeficiency, either from inherited defects in cell-mediated immunity or from infection-associated immunosuppression (e.g. AIDS) clearly predisposes individuals for the development of melanoma (Silverberg et al., 2011). Furthermore, with the increasing prevalence of autoimmune disorders and solid organ transplantation requiring medical restraint of native immune function, iatrogenic immunosupression is becoming an increasingly important risk factor for malignancy (DePry et al., 2011). The number of individuals in the US living with solid organ transplant has more than doubled since 1998 to more than 225,000 individuals (Sullivan et al., 2012). Although immunosuppressive agents expose patients to increased risk for a large number of malignancies, cutaneous cancer risk is particularly affected (Engels et al., 2011), and skin cancers in immunsuppressed patients may behave more aggressively than those in immunocompetent persons (Brewer et al., 2011). Cancer patients treated with chemotherapy also have a higher incidence of melanoma, presumably either because of the mutagenic effects of chemotherapy on melanocytes or perhaps through immunosuppression (Smith et al., 1993). Therefore, solid tumor transplant patients, persons with inborn or acquired deficiencies of T cell function and anyone with a current or past pharmacologic history of chemotherapy or immunosuppressive medications should be advised to practice UV-avoiding strategies and be regularly screened for cutaneous malignancies.

3. Genetic factors

While UV exposure is the most significant environmental risk factor for melanoma, there are several genes that when mutated clearly influence melanoma risk (Meyle and Guldberg, 2009; Nelson and Tsao, 2009; Ward et al., 2012). These genes have been identified largely through studying melanoma-prone families or individuals with extraordinary UV sensitivity or melanoma predisposition. Some of these genetic defects cause bone fide familial cancer syndromes, characterized by heritable predisposition to one or more types of malignancy. Each cancer syndrome is associated with unique cancer risk. Clinical "clues" to melanoma familial cancer syndromes include: melanomas diagnosed at a young age (e.g. below forty years of age), multiple primary melanomas diagnosed in the same person over time, multiple family members affected by melanoma, and extreme UV sensitivity (D'Orazio 2010). It is estimated that up to twelve percent of patients diagnosed with melanoma will have a positive family history of melanoma, yet even among this group, there is often no identifiable melanoma susceptibility gene (Gandini et al., 2005). Many of these melanoma susceptibility genes can portend risk vastly exceeding that of the general population (Udayakumar and Tsao, 2009).

3.1. Cyclin-Dependent Kinase Inhibitor 2A (CDKN2A)

The familial atypical multiple mole and melanoma (FAMMM) syndrome was first described in two families in which affected individuals harbored more than one hundred dysplastic nevi and had a lifetime cumulative incidence of melanoma approaching one hundred percent (Clark et al., 1978; Lynch et al., 1978). This syndrome, also called "dysplastic nevus syndrome" was associated with many of the features of a familial cancer syndrome, including melanomas at young ages (median age of 33 years in one study) (Goldstein et al., 1994). Heterozygous loss of CDKN2A function is associated with roughly 40% of cases of familial melanoma (Kamb et al., 1994; Holland et al., 1995)

Linkage studies performed in melanoma pedigrees identified loss of heterozygosity in the chromosome 9p21 region (Fountain et al., 1992). Later, the cyclin-dependent kinase inhibitor 2A gene was identified through positional cloning to be the tumor suppressor on 9p21 that was mutated in many melanoma-prone families (Kamb et al., 1994; Weaver-Feldhaus et al., 1994). Interestingly, affected individuals were not only at higher risk of malignant melanoma of the skin, but also for central nervous system gliomas, lung cancers and leukemias (Nobori et al., 1994). CDKN2A actually encodes two distinct tumor suppressor proteins- p16 and p14ARF that are transcribed in alternate reading frames directed through the use of alternative first exons (Chin et al., 1998; Sharpless and DePinho, 1999; Sharpless and Chin, 2003). p16/INK4a is produced from a transcript generated from exons 1α, 2 and 3, and p14/Arf is generated in an alternative reading frame, from a transcript of exons 1β, 2 and 3 (Udayakumar and Tsao, 2009). The majority of melanoma-associated mutations impacting exon 1β, which is specific for p16INK4a. Most germline mutations in CDKN2A found to contribute to melanoma susceptibility are loss-of-function missense or nonsense mutations of p16 (Goldstein et al., 2006; Goldstein et al., 2007).

The p16 tumor suppressor protein acts to regulate cell proliferation at the G1/S cell cycle checkpoint by inhibiting the cyclin-dependent kinases CDK4 and CDK6 to prevent entry into S-phase of the cell cycle (Serrano et al., 1993; Ohtani et al., 2001). Cyclin-dependent kinases in complex with cyclin D function jointly to inactivate the retinoblastoma (RB1) by phosphorylation. Once phosphorylated, RB1 is released from the transcription factor E2F-1, thereby permitting E2F-dependent transcription of genes that propel cells into proliferation. By binding to and inhibiting CDK4, p16 acts to prevent cell cycle progression, and when p16 function is lost, cells lose regulatory control over CDK/cyclin activity and proceed into unregulated cell division (Bartkova et al., 1996; Chin et al., 1998; Liggett and Sidransky, 1998). As with many other tumor suppressor genes, it is thought that inactivation or underexpression of both alleles of CDKN2A may be required for a cancer phenotype to emerge (the "two-hit" hypothesis) (Knudson, 1996; Tomlinson et al., 2001; Payne and Kemp, 2005). Thus individuals with inherited loss of one copy of p16 are at risk for p16-dependent malignancies such as melanoma (Ranade et al., 1995), with cancers developing only if the remaining p16 allele is inactivated to a sufficient extent either through mutation or epigenetic inactivation (Berger et al., 2011).

3.2. Cyclin-Dependent Kinase 4 (CDK4)

Several melanoma-prone kindreds have been discovered who carry mutations not in CDKN2A, but in its target- cyclin-dependent kinase 4 (CDK4) (Zuo et al., 1996; Soufir et al., 1998; Goldstein et al., 2000). Unlike CDKN2A whose p16 protein product acts as a tumor suppressor by negatively regulating melanocyte proliferation, CDK4 is an oncogene whose activity enhances cell division. The gain-of-function mutations in CDK4 melanoma-prone families typically result in amino acid changes that render the CDK4 enzyme insensitive to p16 inhibition, thereby resulting in a functional p16 null phenotype (Zuo et al., 1996; Newton Bishop et al., 1999; Goldstein et al., 2000).

3.3. Xeroderma Pigmentosum (XP) genes

Xeroderma pigmentosum (XP) is a rare autosomal recessive disorder of the nucleotide excision DNA repair (NER) pathway caused by homozygous deficiency of any one of at least eight genes (XPA, XPB, XPC, XPD, XPE, XPF, XPG and XPV) that work in complex to repair bulky DNA lesions such as mutagenic DNA photoproducts caused by UV radiation (Leibeling et al., 2006) (Fig. 8). NER functions by recruiting a protein complex known as XPC-hHR23B to UV-induced photoproducts in the DNA, with XPE aiding lesion verification. TFIIH, a transcription factor containing multiple enzymes including XPA, XPB and XPD then unwind the DNA in the vicinity of the damaged bases, and then two endonucleases XPF-ERCC1 and XPG incise the lesion on either side of the photodamage to release the damaged DNA section. Finally, using the undamaged strand as a template to ensure fidelity, DNA polymerase, PCNA, RFC and DNA ligase I act in concert to synthesize and ligate the new DNA fragment. In this manner, the NER pathway is the cell's major defense against DNA damage and if defective, UV-induced mutations accumulate in the genome.

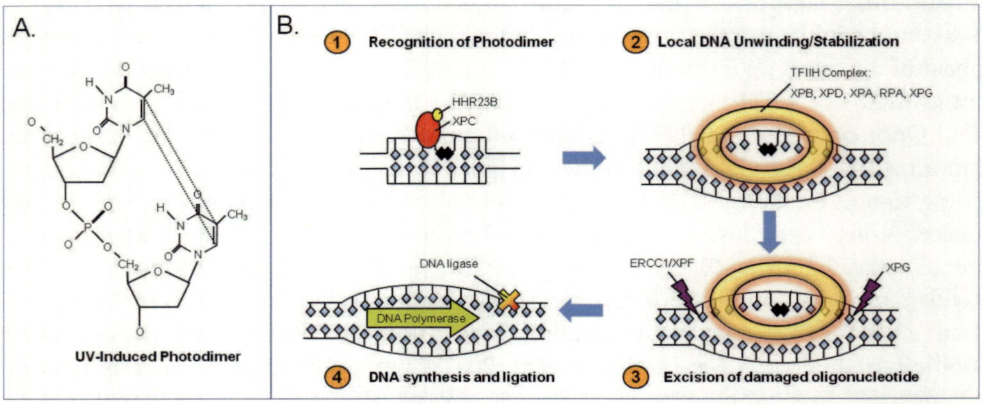

Figure 8. UV-induced cyclobutane dimers- structure (A) and repair by the Nucleotide Excision DNA Repair (NER) pathway (B). The NER pathway is mediated by at least eight enzymes that work together to identify bulky DNA lesions that distort the structure of the double helix, excise the damaged portion and replace the excised region by DNA synthesis directed by the complementary strand. Homozygous deficiency in any one of the NER enzymes leads to the clinical condition known as Xeroderma Pigmentosum (XP). Please note that although not shown, NER can also be initiated in actively transcribed regions of the genome by involvement of the Cockayne syndrome proteins A and B.

As a result of the inability of the skin to recover after UV exposure, intense sun sensitivity is one of the first manifestations of XP. Estimated incidences vary from 1 in 20,000 in Japan to 1 in 250,000 in the US (Robbins et al., 1974). Beginning in the first or second year of life, UV-exposed skin (e.g. on the face and arms) develops areas of hypo- or hyper-pigmented macules, telangiectasias and atrophy, all signs of chronic sun exposure that normally take decades to develop. Premalignant lesions such as actinic keratoses develop, and typically malignancies such as basal cell carcinomas, squamous cell carcinomas and melanomas start appearing by the age of ten years. XP patients have more than a thousand-fold increased risk of skin cancer and develop malignancies decades earlier than unaffected patients (Van Patter and Drummond, 1953; Lynch et al., 1981; Cleaver, 2005; Jen et al., 2009; Rao et al., 2009; Wang et al., 2009). Melanomas isolated from XP patients clearly bear evidence of "UV signature mutations", lending support to the concept that defective repair of UV-induced photodimers underlies carcinogenesis of melanocytes (Takebe et al., 1989; Sato et al., 1993). Beside skin cancer, XP patients suffer a 20-fold increased risk of other malignancies including lung cancer, gastric carcinoma and brain cancer, perhaps reflecting the importance of NER in the repair of damage produced by agents other than UV. Overall, approximately 70% of persons with XP die by the age of 40 years from cancer. Currently there is no accepted therapy for treating XP other than avoidance of sunlight and careful surveillance and local control of pre-malignant or malignant lesions as they appear. The use of topical DNA repair enzymes such asT4 endonuclease V which cleaves UV-induced photolesions(Cafardi and Elmets, 2008) and novel UV-protective strategies such as the pharmacologic induction of cutaneous melanin levels which block penetration of UV radiation (D'Orazio et al., 2006) are being developed and may hold great promise for these exceptionally UV-sensitive individuals.

Intriguingly, although the homozygous condition known as XP reveals much about the importance of the NER pathway in melanoma resistance and ability of UV radiation to fuel melanomagenesis, evidence is accumulating that polymorphisms in NER enzymes in the general (non-XP) population may influence melanoma risk. For example, several studies have found an association between polymorphisms in certain NER enzymes and melanoma including XPD (Tomescu et al., 2001; Mocellin et al., 2009), XPC and XPF (Winsey et al., 2000; Baccarelli et al., 2004; Blankenburg et al., 2005; Debniak et al., 2006). Some groups have posited that multiple NER variants in a single individual may be required to influence melanoma susceptibility (Li et al., 2006).

3.4. Melanocortin 1 Receptor (MC1R)

The MC1R is a seven transmembrane G_s-coupled protein that, when bound by melanocyte stimulating hormone (MSH), activates adenylyl cyclase and cAMP generation (Fig. 9). This cAMP second messenger signaling leads to activation of the protein kinase A (PKA) cascade which, in turn, leads to up-regulation of the MITF and CREB transcription factors that together induce expression of melanin biosynthetic enzymes such as tyrosinase and dopachrome tautomerase (Yasumoto et al., 1994; Bertolotto et al., 1996; Fang and Setaluri, 1999). In this manner, MC1R signaling enhances the production and export of melanin by melanocytes to maturing epidermal keratinocytes, thereby controlling the melanin levels and innate UV resistance of the skin (Fig. 9). When MC1R signaling is defective, then melanocytes alter the type and amount of melanin they manufacture. Specifically, a red/blonde sulfated pigment known as pheomelanin is produced rather than the brown/black eumelanin species. Pheomelanin is a much poorer blocker of UV photons and may even contribute to oxidative damage within melanocytes, itself a possible mutagenic mechanism.

Loss-of-function polymorphisms have been identified in MC1R, with the vast majority of allelic variation occurring in European and Asian populations. The most prevalent MC1R mutations (D84E, R142H, R151C, R160W, and D294H) are known as the "RHC" (red hair color) alleles because of the association with a blonde/red hair color, freckling and tendency to burn rather than tan after UV exposure (Scherer and Kumar, 2010). RHC MC1R alleles are also associated with a relatively high lifetime risk of melanoma (increased odds ratio of 2.40 in one study) (Williams et al., 2011). MC1R variants may also modify other melanoma-relevant alleles (van der Velden et al., 2001; Demenais et al., 2010; Kanetsky et al., 2010; Kricker et al., 2010). In a Australian cohort, for example, co-inheritance of either the MC1R variants R151C, R160W or D294H with CDKN2A mutations and decreased latency for melanoma by approximately 20 years (Box et al., 2001). A more recent study found that MC1R variants significantly increased penetrance and lowered the age of melanoma diagnosis in people with CDKN2A mutations, (Fargnoli et al., 2010).

In addition to its role in skin melanization, MC1R may influence melanoma development by non-pigmentary pathways as well (Matichard et al., 2004; Goldstein et al., 2005). Specifically, we and others have found that MC1R signaling influences the ability of melanocytes to recover from UV-induced DNA damage (Hauser et al., 2006; Abdel-Malek et al., 2009; Song et al., 2009). MC1R signaling directly enhances NER in melanocytes, and studies are underway to discover the molecular mechanisms linking MC1R signaling to the NER DNA damage repair pathway. Overall, there is much evidence placing MC1R as a "master regulator" of melanocyte UV physiologic responses.

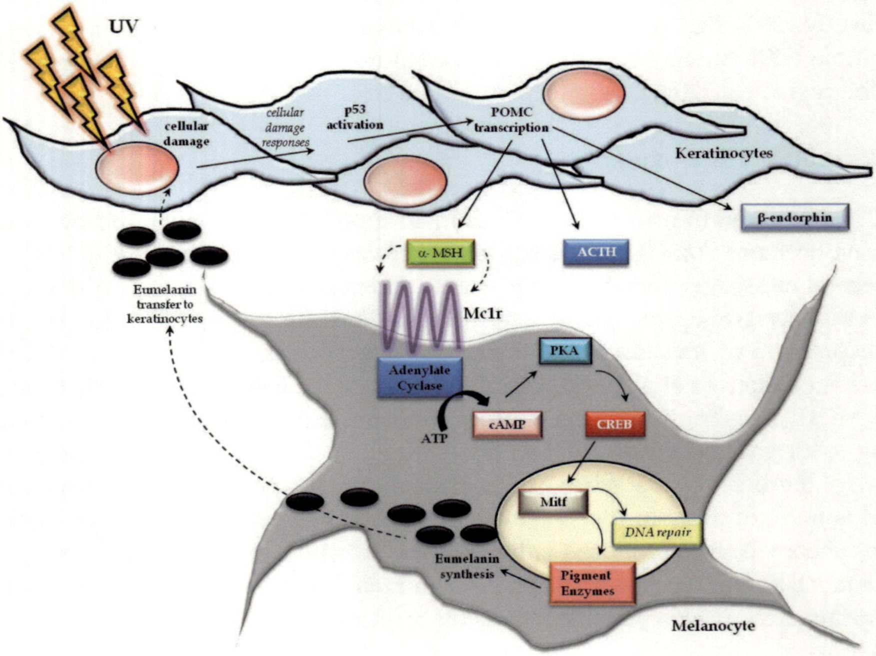

Figure 9. The central role of the melanocortin 1 receptor (MC1R) in the epidermal response to UV radiation. UV-induced cellular and DNA damage to epidermal keratinocytes induces activation of the global damage response protein p53, which mediates transcriptional activation of the pro-opiomelanocortin (POMC) gene. The POMC gene encodes a propeptide that is cleaved into melanocyte stimulating hormone (MSH) along with β-endorphin and adrenocorticotropic hormone (ACTH). MSH secreted from UV-exposed keratinocytes then is hypothesized to bind melanocortin 1 receptors (MC1R) on melanocytes in the basal epidermis. MSH binding induces generation of the second messenger cAMP via MC1R-mediated activation of adenylate cyclase in melanocytes. Generation of cAMP triggers a number of downstream events including activation of the protein kinase A signaling pathway and up-regulation of the cAMP responsive binding element (CREB) and microphthalmia (Mitf) transcription factors. CREB and Mitf induce melanin production through transcriptional up-regulation of melanin biosynthetic enzymes. Thus, MSH-MC1R signaling leads to enhanced pigment synthesis and subsequent transfer of melanin to epidermal keratinocytes. In this manner, the skin is more protected against subsequent UV exposure. MSH-MC1R signaling may also enhance nucleotide excision repair (NER) in melanocytes, which would enhance recovery from UV damage.

http://dx.doi.org/10.5772/55172

3.5. Microphthalmia (MITF)

Mitf is a myc-like transcription factor that is critical to melanocyte development and survival (Levy et al., 2006). Defective Mitf leads to disorders of melanocyte function and pigmentation (Fisher, 2000; Goding, 2000; Widlund and Fisher, 2003; Steingrimsson et al., 2004). In humans, for example, Waardenburg syndrome type 2 is caused by inactivating mutations of Mitf, and is characterized by pigmentary defects due to the congenital absence of melanocytes in distinct anatomic locations (hair, skin eyes) (Hughes et al., 1994; Tassabehji et al., 1994). Mitf Immunohistochemical staining has long been used to identify surgical tumor isolates as melanomas (King et al., 1999; Salti et al., 2000), but its oncogenic contribution to melanoma wasn't realized until Garraway and colleagues reported Mitf to be amplified in a subset of melanomas, particularly in aggressive disease (Garraway et al., 2005). Mitf may be amplified in up to 20% of metastatic melanomas and is associated with activation of the hypoxia inducible factor (HIF1A) pathway (Busca et al., 2005; Cheli et al., 2012) and reduced patient survival (Ugurel et al., 2007).

More recently, melanoma predisposition due to point mutations of Mitf (rather than gene amplification) were described. The E318K Mitf variant correlated with a positive melanoma family history, multiple primary melanomas or risk of melanoma and renal cell carcinoma in the same patient. Mechanistically, it is thought that the E318K Mitf variant leads to gain-of-function in Mitf by impairing its SUMO-mediated clearance (Bertolotto et al., 2011; Yokoyama et al., 2011). Thus whether by increased gene doseage or increased protein stability, Mitf seems to be a relevant melanoma oncogene, and current research efforts are attempting to devise pharmacologic targeting of MITF (Flaherty et al., 2010).

4. Conclusions

An explosion of information regarding the molecular pathways involved in melanoma development has been witnessed in the last several years. The MAPkinase cascade, for example, has emerged as a critical oncogenic pathway that drives the majority of cases of melanoma. Gain of function mutations in BRAF, most notably the V600E point mutation that results in unregulated BRAF signaling, have been described in at least half of all cutaneous melanomas (Davies et al., 2002; Pollock and Meltzer, 2002; Pollock et al., 2003). Oncogenic BRAF mutations lead to constitutive activation of kinase activity of BRAF, providing continuous growth signals in the absence of extracellular stimuli (Nikolaou et al., 2012). In many melanomas in which BRAF has not been mutated or in melanomas treated with BRAF inhibitors, N-Ras oncogene upregulation has been observed, leading again to increased signaling through the MAPkinase cascade (Padua et al., 1984; van 't Veer et al., 1989; Ball et al., 1994; Carr and Mackie, 1994; Wagner et al., 1995; Goydos et al., 2005; Nazarian et al., 2010). Though targeted inhibition of the MAPkinase signaling pathway has led to significant advances in the treatment of melanoma (Flaherty et al., 2010; Falchook et al., 2012), to date, somatic inheritance of MAPkinase activating mutations leading to melanoma predisposition, have not been reported.

The incidence of melanoma has risen at an alarming rate over the last several decades. The reasons for this increase are unclear, but probably represent the confluence of a variety of environmental and inherited risk factors. Though significant progress has been made over the last several years in immunotherapy (Hodi et al., 2010; Kaplan, 2011; Wilson, 2011) and targeted kinase inhibition against melanoma (Flaherty et al., 2010; Chapman et al., 2011; Flaherty et al., 2012; Sosman et al., 2012), clearly it would be better to prevent development of disease in the first place. As our understanding of the molecular mechanisms that underlie the malignant degeneration of melanocytes expands, so hopefully will our ability to develop rational interventions to prevent the development of melanoma.

Acknowledgements

The authors thank Miss Hope D. Johnson, Markey Cancer Center Research Communications Office, for critically editing this chapter.

Author details

John A. D'Orazio*, Stuart Jarrett, Amanda Marsch, James Lagrew and Laura Cleary

*Address all correspondence to: jdorazio@uky.edu

University of Kentucky College of Medicine, Markey Cancer Center, Department of Pediatrics, and Department of Molecular and Biomedical Pharmacology, Lexington, USA

References

[1] Abdel-malek, Z. A, Ruwe, A, Kavanagh-starner, R, Kadekaro, A. L, Swope, V, et al. (2009). alpha-MSH tripeptide analogs activate the melanocortin 1 receptor and reduce UV-induced DNA damage in human melanocytes." *Pigment Cell Melanoma Res.*

[2] Andrady, A, Aucamp, P. J, Bais, A. F, Ballare, C. L, Bjorn, L. O, et al. (2010). Environmental effects of ozone depletion and its interactions with climate change: progress report, 2009." *Photochem Photobiol Sci* , 9(3), 275-294.

[3] Atkinson, S. K, Marlatt, V. L, Kimpe, L. E, Lean, D. R, Trudeau, V. L, et al. (2011). Environmental factors affecting ultraviolet photodegradation rates and estrogenicity of estrone and ethinylestradiol in natural waters." *Arch Environ Contam Toxicol* , 60(1), 1-7.

[4] Autier, P. (2004). Perspectives in melanoma prevention: the case of sunbeds." *Eur J Cancer* , 40(16), 2367-2376.

[5] Baccarelli, A, Calista, D, Minghetti, P, Marinelli, B, Albetti, B, et al. (2004). XPD gene polymorphism and host characteristics in the association with cutaneous malignant melanoma risk." *Br J Cancer* , 90(2), 497-502.

[6] Ball, N. J, Yohn, J. J, Morelli, J. G, Norris, D. A, Golitz, L. E, et al. (1994). Ras mutations in human melanoma: a marker of malignant progression." *J Invest Dermatol* , 102(3), 285-290.

[7] Bartkova, J, Lukas, J, Guldberg, P, Alsner, J, Kirkin, A. F, et al. (1996). The p16–cyclin D/Cdk4-pRb pathway as a functional unit frequently altered in melanoma pathogenesis." *Cancer Res* 56(23): 5475-5483.

[8] Beral, V, Evans, S, Shaw, H, & Milton, G. (1983). Cutaneous factors related to the risk of malignant melanoma." *Br J Dermatol* , 109(2), 165-172.

[9] Berger, A. H, Knudson, A. G, & Pandolfi, P. P. (2011). A continuum model for tumour suppression." *Nature* , 476(7359), 163-169.

[10] Bertolotto, C, Bille, K, Ortonne, J. P, & Ballotti, R. (1996). Regulation of tyrosinase gene expression by cAMP in B16 melanoma cells involves two CATGTG motifs surrounding the TATA box: implication of the microphthalmia gene product." *J Cell Biol* , 134(3), 747-755.

[11] Bertolotto, C, Lesueur, F, Giuliano, S, Strub, T, De Lichy, M, et al. (2011). A SUMOylation-defective MITF germline mutation predisposes to melanoma and renal carcinoma." *Nature* , 480(7375), 94-98.

[12] Blankenburg, S, Konig, I. R, Moessner, R, Laspe, P, Thoms, K. M, et al. (2005). Assessment of 3 xeroderma pigmentosum group C gene polymorphisms and risk of cutaneous melanoma: a case-control study." *Carcinogenesis* , 26(6), 1085-1090.

[13] Bohm, M, Wolff, I, Scholzen, T. E, Robinson, S. J, Healy, E, et al. (2005). alpha-Melanocyte-stimulating hormone protects from ultraviolet radiation-induced apoptosis and DNA damage." *J Biol Chem* , 280(7), 5795-5802.

[14] Box, N. F, Duffy, D. L, Chen, W, Stark, M, Martin, N. G, et al. (2001). MC1R genotype modifies risk of melanoma in families segregating CDKN2A mutations." *Am J Hum Genet* , 69(4), 765-773.

[15] Brewer, J. D, Christenson, L. J, Weaver, A. L, Dapprich, D. C, Weenig, R. H, et al. (2011). Malignant melanoma in solid transplant recipients: collection of database cases and comparison with surveillance, epidemiology, and end results data for outcome analysis." *Arch Dermatol* , 147(7), 790-796.

[16] Budiyanto, A, Ueda, M, Ueda, T, & Ichihashi, M. (2002). Formation of cyclobutane pyrimidine dimers and 8-oxo-7,8-dihydro-2′-deoxyguanosine in mouse and organ-cultured human skin by irradiation with broadband or with narrowband UVB." *Photochem Photobiol* , 76(4), 397-400.

[17] Buller, D. B, Cokkinides, V, Hall, H. I, Hartman, A. M, Saraiya, M, et al. (2011). Prevalence of sunburn, sun protection, and indoor tanning behaviors among Americans: review from national surveys and case studies of 3 states." *J Am Acad Dermatol* 65(5 Suppl 1): S, 114-123.

[18] Burkhart, C. G, & Burkhart, C. N. (2000). Melanoma and insecticides: is there a connection?" *J Am Acad Dermatol* 42(2 Pt 1): 302-303.

[19] Busca, R, Berra, E, Gaggioli, C, Khaled, M, Bille, K, et al. (2005). Hypoxia-inducible factor 1{alpha} is a new target of microphthalmia-associated transcription factor (MITF) in melanoma cells." *J Cell Biol* , 170(1), 49-59.

[20] Cafardi, J. A, & Elmets, C. A. T4 Endonuclease V: Review and application to dermatology." *Expert Opin Biol Ther* , 8(6), 829-838.

[21] Carey, W. P, Jr, C. J, Thompson, M, Synnestvedt, D. t, Guerry, A, et al. (1994). Dysplastic nevi as a melanoma risk factor in patients with familial melanoma." *Cancer* , 74(12), 3118-3125.

[22] Carr, J, & Mackie, R. M. (1994). Point mutations in the N-ras oncogene in malignant melanoma and congenital naevi." *Br J Dermatol* , 131(1), 72-77.

[23] Chapman, P. B, Hauschild, A, Robert, C, Haanen, J. B, Ascierto, P, et al. (2011). Improved survival with vemurafenib in melanoma with BRAF mutation." *N Engl J Med* 364(26): 2507-2516., 600E

[24] Cheli, Y, Giuliano, S, Fenouille, N, Allegra, M, Hofman, V, et al. (2012). Hypoxia and MITF control metastatic behaviour in mouse and human melanoma cells." *Oncogene* , 31(19), 2461-2470.

[25] Chin, L, Pomerantz, J, & Depinho, R. A. (1998). The INK4a/ARF tumor suppressor: one gene--two products--two pathways." *Trends Biochem Sci* , 23(8), 291-296.

[26] Choi, K, Lazovich, D, Southwell, B, Forster, J, Rolnick, S. J, et al. (2010). Prevalence and characteristics of indoor tanning use among men and women in the United States." *Arch Dermatol* , 146(12), 1356-1361.

[27] Clark, W. H, Jr, R. R, Reimer, M, Greene, A. M, & Ainsworth, M. J. Mastrangelo. ((1978). Origin of familial malignant melanomas from heritable melanocytic lesions.'The B-K mole syndrome'." *Arch Dermatol* , 114(5), 732-738.

[28] Cleaver, J. E. (2005). Cancer in xeroderma pigmentosum and related disorders of DNA repair." *Nat Rev Cancer* , 5(7), 564-573.

[29] Cokkinides, V, Weinstock, M, Lazovich, D, Ward, E, & Thun, M. (2009). Indoor tanning use among adolescents in the US, 1998 to 2004." *Cancer* , 115(1), 190-198.

[30] Crombie, I. K. (1979). Variation of melanoma incidence with latitude in North America and Europe." *Br J Cancer* , 40(5), 774-781.

[31] Cust, A. E, Jenkins, M. A, Goumas, C, Armstrong, B. K, Schmid, H, et al. (2011). Early-life sun exposure and risk of melanoma before age 40 years." *Cancer Causes Control* , 22(6), 885-897.

[32] Orazio, D, Nobuhisa, J. A. , T, Cui, R, Arya, M, Spry, M, et al. (2006). Topical drug rescue strategy and skin protection based on the role of Mc1r in UV-induced tanning." *Nature* , 443(7109), 340-344.

[33] Davies, H, Bignell, G. R, Cox, C, Stephens, P, Edkins, S, et al. (2002). Mutations of the BRAF gene in human cancer." *Nature* , 417(6892), 949-954.

[34] De Gruijl, F. R, Longstreth, J, Norval, M, Cullen, A. P, Slaper, H, et al. (2003). Health effects from stratospheric ozone depletion and interactions with climate change." *Photochem Photobiol Sci* , 2(1), 16-28.

[35] Debniak, T, Scott, R. J, Huzarski, T, Byrski, T, Masojc, B, et al. (2006). XPD common variants and their association with melanoma and breast cancer risk." *Breast Cancer Res Treat* , 98(2), 209-215.

[36] Demenais, F, Mohamdi, H, Chaudru, V, Goldstein, A. M, Newton Bishop, et al., J. A. ((2010). Association of MC1R variants and host phenotypes with melanoma risk in CDKN2A mutation carriers: a GenoMEL study." *J Natl Cancer Inst* , 102(20), 1568-1583.

[37] Depry, J. L, Reed, K. B, Cook-norris, R. H, & Brewer, J. D. (2011). Iatrogenic immunosuppression and cutaneous malignancy." *Clin Dermatol* , 29(6), 602-613.

[38] Draelos, Z. D. (2011). Genetic mosaicism and Fitzpatrick skin type." *J Cosmet Dermatol* , 10(3), 169-170.

[39] Ekwueme, D. U, Guy, G. P, Jr, C, Li, S. H, Rim, P, et al. (2011). The health burden and economic costs of cutaneous melanoma mortality by race/ethnicity-United States, 2000 to 2006." *J Am Acad Dermatol* 65(5 Suppl 1): S, 133-143.

[40] Elwood, J. M, & Koh, H. K. (1994). Etiology, epidemiology, risk factors, and public health issues of melanoma." *Curr Opin Oncol* , 6(2), 179-187.

[41] Engels, E. A, Pfeiffer, R. M, Fraumeni, J. F, Jr, B. L, Kasiske, A. K, et al. (2011). Spectrum of cancer risk among US solid organ transplant recipients." *JAMA* , 306(17), 1891-1901.

[42] Erdmann, F, Lortet-tieulent, J, Schuz, J, Zeeb, H, Greinert, R, et al. (2012). International trends in the incidence of malignant melanoma 1953-2008-are recent generations at higher or lower risk?" *Int J Cancer*.

[43] Falchook, G. S, Lewis, K. D, Infante, J. R, Gordon, M. S, Vogelzang, N. J, et al. (2012). Activity of the oral MEK inhibitor trametinib in patients with advanced melanoma: a phase 1 dose-escalation trial." *Lancet Oncol* , 13(8), 782-789.

[44] Fang, D, & Setaluri, V. (1999). Role of microphthalmia transcription factor in regulation of melanocyte differentiation marker TRP-1." *Biochem Biophys Res Commun* , 256(3), 657-663.

[45] Fargnoli, M. C, Gandini, S, Peris, K, Maisonneuve, P, & Raimondi, S. (2010). MC1R variants increase melanoma risk in families with CDKN2A mutations: a meta-analysis." *Eur J Cancer* , 46(8), 1413-1420.

[46] Fink, C. A, & Bates, M. N. (2005). Melanoma and ionizing radiation: is there a causal relationship?" *Radiat Res* , 164(5), 701-710.

[47] Fisher, D. E. (2000). Microphthalmia: a signal responsive transcriptional regulator in development." *Pigment Cell Res* 13 Suppl , 8, 145-149.

[48] Flaherty, K. T, Hodi, F. S, & Bastian, B. C. (2010). Mutation-driven drug development in melanoma." *Curr Opin Oncol* , 22(3), 178-183.

[49] Flaherty, K. T, Puzanov, I, Kim, K. B, Ribas, A, Mcarthur, G. A, et al. (2010). Inhibition of mutated, activated BRAF in metastatic melanoma." *N Engl J Med* , 363(9), 809-819.

[50] Flaherty, K. T, Robert, C, Hersey, P, Nathan, P, Garbe, C, et al. (2012). Improved survival with MEK inhibition in BRAF-mutated melanoma." *N Engl J Med* , 367(2), 107-114.

[51] Fortes, C, & De Vries, E. (2008). Nonsolar occupational risk factors for cutaneous melanoma." *Int J Dermatol* , 47(4), 319-328.

[52] Fountain, J. W, Karayiorgou, M, Ernstoff, M. S, Kirkwood, J. M, Vlock, D. R, et al. (1992). Homozygous deletions within human chromosome band 9in melanoma." *Proc Natl Acad Sci U S A* 89(21): 10557-10561., 21.

[53] Franceschi, S, & Cristofolini, M. (1992). Cutaneous malignant melanoma: epidemiological considerations." *Semin Surg Oncol* , 8(6), 345-352.

[54] Gandini, S, Sera, F, Cattaruzza, M. S, Pasquini, P, Abeni, D, et al. (2005). Meta-analysis of risk factors for cutaneous melanoma: I. Common and atypical naevi." *Eur J Cancer* , 41(1), 28-44.

[55] Gandini, S, Sera, F, Cattaruzza, M. S, Pasquini, P, Zanetti, R, et al. (2005). Meta-analysis of risk factors for cutaneous melanoma: III. Family history, actinic damage and phenotypic factors." *Eur J Cancer* , 41(14), 2040-2059.

[56] Garraway, L. A, Widlund, H. R, Rubin, M. A, Getz, G, Berger, A. J, et al. (2005). Integrative genomic analyses identify MITF as a lineage survival oncogene amplified in malignant melanoma." *Nature* , 436(7047), 117-122.

[57] Geller, A. C, Colditz, G, Oliveria, S, Emmons, K, Jorgensen, C, et al. (2002). Use of sunscreen, sunburning rates, and tanning bed use among more than 10 000 US children and adolescents." *Pediatrics* , 109(6), 1009-1014.

[58] Gilchrest, B. A, Eller, M. S, Geller, A. C, & Yaar, M. (1999). The pathogenesis of melanoma induced by ultraviolet radiation." *N Engl J Med* , 340(17), 1341-1348.

[59] Goding, C. R. (2000). Mitf from neural crest to melanoma: signal transduction and transcription in the melanocyte lineage." *Genes Dev* , 14(14), 1712-1728.

[60] Goldstein, A. M, Chan, M, Harland, M, Gillanders, E. M, Hayward, N. K, et al. (2006). High-risk melanoma susceptibility genes and pancreatic cancer, neural system tumors, and uveal melanoma across GenoMEL." *Cancer Res* , 66(20), 9818-9828.

[61] Goldstein, A. M, Chan, M, Harland, M, Hayward, N. K, Demenais, F, et al. (2007). Features associated with germline CDKN2A mutations: a GenoMEL study of melanoma-prone families from three continents." *J Med Genet* , 44(2), 99-106.

[62] Goldstein, A. M, Fraser, M. C, Clark, W. H, & Jr, M. A. Tucker. ((1994). Age at diagnosis and transmission of invasive melanoma in 23 families with cutaneous malignant melanoma/dysplastic nevi." *J Natl Cancer Inst* , 86(18), 1385-1390.

[63] Goldstein, A. M, Landi, M. T, Tsang, S, Fraser, M. C, Munroe, D. J, et al. (2005). Association of MC1R variants and risk of melanoma in melanoma-prone families with CDKN2A mutations." *Cancer Epidemiol Biomarkers Prev* , 14(9), 2208-2212.

[64] Goldstein, A. M, Struewing, J. P, Chidambaram, A, Fraser, M. C, & Tucker, M. A. (2000). Genotype-phenotype relationships in U.S. melanoma-prone families with CDKN2A and CDK4 mutations." *J Natl Cancer Inst* , 92(12), 1006-1010.

[65] Goydos, J. S, Mann, B, Kim, H. J, Gabriel, E. M, Alsina, J, et al. (2005). Detection of B-RAF and N-RAS mutations in human melanoma." *J Am Coll Surg* , 200(3), 362-370.

[66] Grob, J. J, Gouvernet, J, Aymar, D, Mostaque, A, Romano, M. H, et al. (1990). Count of benign melanocytic nevi as a major indicator of risk for nonfamilial nodular and superficial spreading melanoma." *Cancer* , 66(2), 387-395.

[67] Halpern, A. C, Guerry, D. t, Elder, D. E, Trock, B, Synnestvedt, M, et al. (1993). Natural history of dysplastic nevi." *J Am Acad Dermatol* , 29(1), 51-57.

[68] Han, J, Colditz, G. A, & Hunter, D. J. (2006). Risk factors for skin cancers: a nested case-control study within the Nurses' Health Study." *Int J Epidemiol* , 35(6), 1514-1521.

[69] Hauser, J. E, Kadekaro, A. L, Kavanagh, R. J, Wakamatsu, K, Terzieva, S, et al. (2006). Melanin content and MC1R function independently affect UVR-induced DNA damage in cultured human melanocytes." *Pigment Cell Res* , 19(4), 303-314.

[70] Healy, E, Flannagan, N, Ray, A, Todd, C, Jackson, I. J, et al. (2000). Melanocortin-1-receptor gene and sun sensitivity in individuals without red hair." *Lancet* , 355(9209), 1072-1073.

[71] Hodi, F. S, Day, S. J. O, Mcdermott, D. F, Weber, R. W, Sosman, J. A, et al. (2010). Improved survival with ipilimumab in patients with metastatic melanoma." *N Engl J Med* , 363(8), 711-723.

[72] Holland, E. A, Beaton, S. C, Becker, T. M, Grulet, O. M, Peters, B. A, et al. (1995). Analysis of the gene, CDKN2, in 17 Australian melanoma kindreds." *Oncogene* 11(11): 2289-2294., 16.

[73] Holman, C. D, Armstrong, B. K, & Heenan, P. J. (1986). Relationship of cutaneous malignant melanoma to individual sunlight-exposure habits." *J Natl Cancer Inst* , 76(3), 403-414.

[74] Holman, C. D, Gibson, I. M, Stephenson, M, & Armstrong, B. K. (1983). Ultraviolet irradiation of human body sites in relation to occupation and outdoor activity: field studies using personal UVR dosimeters." *Clin Exp Dermatol* , 8(3), 269-277.

[75] Hornung, R. L, Magee, K. H, Lee, W. J, Hansen, L. A, & Hsieh, Y. C. (2003). Tanning facility use: are we exceeding Food and Drug Administration limits?" *J Am Acad Dermatol* , 49(4), 655-661.

[76] Hughes, A. E, Newton, V. E, Liu, X. Z, & Read, A. P. (1994). A gene for Waardenburg syndrome type 2 maps close to the human homologue of the microphthalmia gene at chromosome 3*Nat Genet* 7(4): 509-512., 12-p14.

[77] Ingram, A. J. (1992). Review of chemical and UV light-induced melanomas in experimental animals in relation to human melanoma incidence." *J Appl Toxicol* , 12(1), 39-43.

[78] Jen, M, Murphy, M, & Grant-kels, J. M. (2009). Childhood melanoma." *Clin Dermatol* , 27(6), 529-536.

[79] Kadekaro, A. L, Kavanagh, R. J, Wakamatsu, K, Ito, S, Pipitone, M. A, et al. (2003). Cutaneous photobiology. The melanocyte vs. the sun: who will win the final round?" *Pigment Cell Res* , 16(5), 434-447.

[80] Kamb, A, Gruis, N. A, Weaver-feldhaus, J, Liu, Q, Harshman, K, et al. (1994). A cell cycle regulator potentially involved in genesis of many tumor types." *Science* , 264(5157), 436-440.

[81] Kamb, A, Shattuck-eidens, D, Eeles, R, Liu, Q, Gruis, N. A, et al. (1994). Analysis of the gene (CDKN2) as a candidate for the chromosome 9p melanoma susceptibility locus." *Nat Genet* 8(1): 23-26., 16.

[82] Kanetsky, P. A, Panossian, S, Elder, D. E, Guerry, D, Ming, M. E, et al. (2010). Does MC1R genotype convey information about melanoma risk beyond risk phenotypes?" *Cancer* , 116(10), 2416-2428.

[83] Kanjilal, S, Pierceall, W. E, Cummings, K. K, Kripke, M. L, & Ananthaswamy, H. N. (1993). High frequency of mutations in ultraviolet radiation-induced murine skin tumors: evidence for strand bias and tumor heterogeneity." *Cancer Res* 53(13): 2961-2964., 53.

[84] Kaplan, M. G. (2011). Ipilimumab plus dacarbazine in melanoma." *N Engl J Med* author reply 1257-1258., 365(13), 1256-1257.

[85] Karagas, M. R, Stannard, V. A, Mott, L. A, Slattery, M. J, Spencer, S. K, et al. (2002). Use of tanning devices and risk of basal cell and squamous cell skin cancers." *J Natl Cancer Inst* , 94(3), 224-226.

[86] King, R, Weilbaecher, K. N, Mcgill, G, Cooley, E, Mihm, M, et al. (1999). Microphthalmia transcription factor. A sensitive and specific melanocyte marker for Melanoma-Diagnosis." *Am J Pathol* , 155(3), 731-738.

[87] Kino, K, & Sugiyama, H. (2005). UVR-induced G-C to C-G transversions from oxidative DNA damage." *Mutat Res* 571(1-2): 33-42.

[88] Knudson, A. G. (1996). Hereditary cancer: two hits revisited." *J Cancer Res Clin Oncol* , 122(3), 135-140.

[89] Korcum, A. F, Sanlioglu, S, Aksu, G, Tuncel, N, & Erin, N. (2009). Radiotherapy-induced decreases in substance P levels may potentiate melanoma growth." *Mol Med Report* , 2(2), 319-326.

[90] Krengel, S, Hauschild, A, & Schafer, T. (2006). Melanoma risk in congenital melanocytic naevi: a systematic review." *Br J Dermatol* , 155(1), 1-8.

[91] Kricker, A, Armstrong, B. K, Goumas, C, Kanetsky, P, Gallagher, R. P, et al. (2010). MC1R genotype may modify the effect of sun exposure on melanoma risk in the GEM study." *Cancer Causes Control*.

[92] Langard, S, Rosenberg, J, Andersen, A, & Heldaas, S. S. (2000). Incidence of cancer among workers exposed to vinyl chloride in polyvinyl chloride manufacture." *Occup Environ Med* , 57(1), 65-68.

[93] Lazovich, D, Vogel, R. I, Berwick, M, Weinstock, M. A, Anderson, K. E, et al. (2010). Indoor tanning and risk of melanoma: a case-control study in a highly exposed population." *Cancer Epidemiol Biomarkers Prev* , 19(6), 1557-1568.

[94] Lee, J. A, & Scotto, J. (1993). Melanoma: linked temporal and latitude changes in the United States." *Cancer Causes Control* , 4(5), 413-418.

[95] Leibeling, D, Laspe, P, & Emmert, S. (2006). Nucleotide excision repair and cancer." *J Mol Histol* 37(5-7): 225-238.

[96] Lens, M. B, & Dawes, M. (2004). Global perspectives of contemporary epidemiological trends of cutaneous malignant melanoma." *Br J Dermatol* , 150(2), 179-185.

[97] Levy, C, Khaled, M, & Fisher, D. E. (2006). MITF: master regulator of melanocyte development and melanoma oncogene." *Trends Mol Med* , 12(9), 406-414.

[98] Lew, R. A, Sober, A. J, Cook, N, Marvell, R, & Fitzpatrick, T. B. (1983). Sun exposure habits in patients with cutaneous melanoma: a case control study." *J Dermatol Surg Oncol* , 9(12), 981-986.

[99] Li, C, Hu, Z, Liu, Z, Wang, L. E, Strom, S. S, et al. (2006). Polymorphisms in the DNA repair genes XPC, XPD, and XPG and risk of cutaneous melanoma: a case-control analysis." *Cancer Epidemiol Biomarkers Prev* , 15(12), 2526-2532.

[100] Lie, J. A, Kjaerheim, K, & Tynes, T. (2008). Ionizing radiation exposure and cancer risk among Norwegian nurses." *Eur J Cancer Prev* , 17(4), 369-375.

[101] Liggett, W. H, & Jr, D. Sidransky. ((1998). Role of the tumor suppressor gene in cancer." *J Clin Oncol* 16(3): 1197-1206., 16.

[102] Lucas, R. M, Mcmichael, A. J, Armstrong, B. K, & Smith, W. T. (2008). Estimating the global disease burden due to ultraviolet radiation exposure." *Int J Epidemiol* , 37(3), 654-667.

[103] Lundberg, I, Gustavsson, A, Holmberg, B, Molina, G, & Westerholm, P. (1993). Mortality and cancer incidence among PVC-processing workers in Sweden." *Am J Ind Med* , 23(2), 313-319.

[104] Lynch, H. T, Frichot, B. C, & Rd, J. F. Lynch. ((1978). Familial atypical multiple mole-melanoma syndrome." *J Med Genet* , 15(5), 352-356.

[105] Lynch, H. T, Fusaro, R, Edlund, J, Albano, W, & Lynch, J. (1981). Skin cancer developing in xeroderma pigmentosum patient relaxing sunlight avoidance." *Lancet* 2(8257): 1230.

[106] MacKie R. M. and T. Aitchison ((1982). Severe sunburn and subsequent risk of primary cutaneous malignant melanoma in scotland." *Br J Cancer* , 46(6), 955-960.

[107] Maddodi, N, & Setaluri, V. (2008). Role of UV in cutaneous melanoma." *Photochem Photobiol* , 84(2), 528-536.

[108] Magnani, C, Coggon, D, Osmond, C, & Acheson, E. D. (1987). Occupation and five cancers: a case-control study using death certificates." *Br J Ind Med* , 44(11), 769-776.

[109] Makin, J. (2011). Implications of climate change for skin cancer prevention in Australia." *Health Promot J Austr* 22 Spec (S39-41), 39-41.

[110] Malaguarnera, L, Cristaldi, E, & Malaguarnera, M. (2010). The role of immunity in elderly cancer." *Crit Rev Oncol Hematol* , 74(1), 40-60.

[111] Marghoob, A. A, Agero, A. L, Benvenuto-andrade, C, & Dusza, S. W. (2006). Large congenital melanocytic nevi, risk of cutaneous melanoma, and prophylactic surgery." *J Am Acad Dermatol* discussion 871-863., 54(5), 868-870.

[112] Marks, R. (1995). The epidemiology of non-melanoma skin cancer: who, why and what can we do about it." *J Dermatol* , 22(11), 853-857.

[113] Matichard, E, Verpillat, P, Meziani, R, Gerard, B, Descamps, V, et al. (2004). Melanocortin 1 receptor (MC1R) gene variants may increase the risk of melanoma in France independently of clinical risk factors and UV exposure." *J Med Genet* 41(2): e13.

[114] Mckenzie, R. L, Aucamp, P. J, Bais, A. F, Bjorn, L. O, Ilyas, M, et al. (2011). Ozone depletion and climate change: impacts on UV radiation." *Photochem Photobiol Sci* , 10(2), 182-198.

[115] Mclaughlin, J. K, Malker, H. S, Blot, W. J, Ericsson, J. L, Gemne, G, et al. (1988). Malignant melanoma in the printing industry." *Am J Ind Med* , 13(2), 301-304.

[116] Melia, J, Moss, S, Coleman, D, Frost, T, Graham-brown, R, et al. (2001). The relation between mortality from malignant melanoma and early detection in the Cancer Research Campaign Mole Watcher Study." *Br J Cancer* , 85(6), 803-807.

[117] Metcalf, J. S, & Maize, J. C. (1985). Melanocytic nevi and malignant melanoma." *Dermatol Clin* , 3(2), 217-224.

[118] Meyle, K. D, & Guldberg, P. (2009). Genetic risk factors for melanoma." *Hum Genet* , 126(4), 499-510.

[119] Meyskens, F. L, & Yang, S. (2011). Thinking about the role (largely ignored) of heavy metals in cancer prevention: hexavalent chromium and melanoma as a case in point." *Recent Results Cancer Res* , 188, 65-74.

[120] Moan, J, Dahlback, A, Lagunova, Z, Cicarma, E, & Porojnicu, A. C. (2009). Solar radiation, vitamin D and cancer incidence and mortality in Norway." *Anticancer Res* , 29(9), 3501-3509.

[121] Mocellin, S, Verdi, D, & Nitti, D. (2009). DNA repair gene polymorphisms and risk of cutaneous melanoma: a systematic review and meta-analysis." *Carcinogenesis* , 30(10), 1735-1743.

[122] Mouret, S, Baudouin, C, Charveron, M, Favier, A, Cadet, J, et al. (2006). Cyclobutane pyrimidine dimers are predominant DNA lesions in whole human skin exposed to UVA radiation." *Proc Natl Acad Sci U S A* , 103(37), 13765-13770.

[123] Naeyaert, J. M, & Brochez, L. (2003). Clinical practice. Dysplastic nevi." *N Engl J Med* , 349(23), 2233-2240.

[124] Nakabeppu, Y, Sakumi, K, Sakamoto, K, Tsuchimoto, D, Tsuzuki, T, et al. (2006). Mutagenesis and carcinogenesis caused by the oxidation of nucleic acids." *Biol Chem* , 387(4), 373-379.

[125] Nataraj, A. J, Black, H. S, & Ananthaswamy, H. N. Signature p53 mutation at DNA cross-linking sites in 8-methoxypsoralen and ultraviolet A (PUVA)-induced murine skin cancers." *Proc Natl Acad Sci U S A* , 93(15), 7961-7965.

[126] Nazarian, R, Shi, H, Wang, Q, Kong, X, Koya, R. C, et al. (2010). Melanomas acquire resistance to B-RAF(inhibition by RTK or N-RAS upregulation." *Nature* 468(7326): 973-977., 600E

[127] Nelson, A. A, & Tsao, H. (2009). Melanoma and genetics." *Clin Dermatol* , 27(1), 46-52.

[128] Newton-bishop, J. A, Chang, Y. M, Elliott, F, Chan, M, Leake, S, et al. (2011). Relationship between sun exposure and melanoma risk for tumours in different body sites in a large case-control study in a temperate climate." *Eur J Cancer* , 47(5), 732-741.

[129] Newton-bishop, J. A, Chang, Y. M, Iles, M. M, Taylor, J. C, Bakker, B, et al. (2010). Melanocytic nevi, nevus genes, and melanoma risk in a large case-control study in the United Kingdom." *Cancer Epidemiol Biomarkers Prev* , 19(8), 2043-2054.

[130] Newton BishopJ. A., M. Harland, D. C. Bennett, V. Bataille, A. M. Goldstein, et al. ((1999). Mutation testing in melanoma families: INK4A, CDK4 and INK4D." *Br J Cancer* 80(1-2): 295-300.

[131] Nikolaou, V. A, Stratigos, A. J, Flaherty, K. T, & Tsao, H. (2012). Melanoma: new insights and new therapies." *J Invest Dermatol* 132(3 Pt 2): 854-863.

[132] Nobori, T, Miura, K, Wu, D. J, Lois, A, Takabayashi, K, et al. (1994). Deletions of the cyclin-dependent kinase-4 inhibitor gene in multiple human cancers." *Nature* , 368(6473), 753-756.

[133] Noonan, F. P, Recio, J. A, Takayama, H, Duray, P, Anver, M. R, et al. (2001). Neonatal sunburn and melanoma in mice." *Nature* , 413(6853), 271-272.

[134] Norval, M, Lucas, R. M, Cullen, A. P, De Gruijl, F. R, Longstreth, J, et al. (2011). The human health effects of ozone depletion and interactions with climate change." *Photochem Photobiol Sci* , 10(2), 199-225.

[135] Ohtani, N, Zebedee, Z, Huot, T. J, Stinson, J. A, Sugimoto, M, et al. (2001). Opposing effects of Ets and Id proteins on expression during cellular senescence." *Nature* 409(6823): 1067-1070., 16INK4a.

[136] Padua, R. A, Barrass, N, & Currie, G. A. (1984). A novel transforming gene in a human malignant melanoma cell line." *Nature* , 311(5987), 671-673.

[137] Palmer, J. S, Duffy, D. L, Box, N. F, Aitken, J. F, Gorman, L. E. O, et al. (2000). Melanocortin-1 receptor polymorphisms and risk of melanoma: is the association explained solely by pigmentation phenotype?" *Am J Hum Genet* , 66(1), 176-186.

[138] Park, S. L, Le, L, Marchand, L. R, Wilkens, L. N, Kolonel, B. E. Henderson, et al. ((2012). Risk factors for malignant melanoma in white and non-white/non-African American populations: the multiethnic cohort." *Cancer Prev Res (Phila)* , 5(3), 423-434.

[139] Payne, S. R, & Kemp, C. J. (2005). Tumor suppressor genetics." *Carcinogenesis* , 26(12), 2031-2045.

[140] Pfeifer, G. P, You, Y. H, & Besaratinia, A. (2005). Mutations induced by ultraviolet light." *Mutat Res* 571(1-2): 19-31.

[141] Pollock, P. M, Harper, U. L, Hansen, K. S, Yudt, L. M, Stark, M, et al. (2003). High frequency of BRAF mutations in nevi." *Nat Genet* , 33(1), 19-20.

[142] Pollock, P. M, & Meltzer, P. S. A Genome-based strategy uncovers frequent BRAF mutations in melanoma." *Cancer Cell* , 2(1), 5-7.

[143] Psaty, E. L, Scope, A, Halpern, A. C, & Marghoob, A. A. (2010). Defining the patient at high risk for melanoma." *Int J Dermatol* , 49(4), 362-376.

[144] Rados, C. (2005). Teen tanning hazards." *FDA Consum* , 39(2), 8-9.

[145] Ranade, K, Hussussian, C. J, Sikorski, R. S, Varmus, H. E, Goldstein, A. M, et al. (1995). Mutations associated with familial melanoma impair function." *Nat Genet* 10(1): 114-116., 16INK4.

[146] Rao, T. N, Bhagyalaxmi, A, Ahmed, K, & Mohana Rao and K. Venkatachalam, T. S. ((2009). A case of melanoma in xeroderma pigmentosum." *Indian J Pathol Microbiol* , 52(4), 524-526.

[147] Ravnbak, M. H, Philipsen, P. A, & Wulf, H. C. (2010). The minimal melanogenesis dose/minimal erythema dose ratio declines with increasing skin pigmentation using solar simulator and narrowband ultraviolet B exposure." *Photodermatol Photoimmunol Photomed* , 26(3), 133-137.

[148] Recio, J. A, Noonan, F. P, Takayama, H, Anver, M. R, Duray, P, et al. (2002). Ink4a/arf deficiency promotes ultraviolet radiation-induced melanomagenesis." *Cancer Res* , 62(22), 6724-6730.

[149] Reed, K. B, Brewer, J. D, Lohse, C. M, Bringe, K. E, Pruitt, C. N, et al. (2012). Increasing incidence of melanoma among young adults: an epidemiological study in Olmsted County, Minnesota." *Mayo Clin Proc* , 87(4), 328-334.

[150] Rees, J. L. (2000). The melanocortin 1 receptor (MC1R): more than just red hair." *Pigment Cell Res* , 13(3), 135-140.

[151] Rees, J. L, & Healy, E. (1997). Melanocortin receptors, red hair, and skin cancer." *J Investig Dermatol Symp Proc* , 2(1), 94-98.

[152] Rigel, D. S. (2002). The effect of sunscreen on melanoma risk." *Dermatol Clin* , 20(4), 601-606.

[153] Rigel, D. S. (2010). Trends in dermatology: melanoma incidence." *Arch Dermatol* 146(3): 318.

[154] Robbins, J. H, Kraemer, K. H, Lutzner, M. A, Festoff, B. W, & Coon, H. G. (1974). Xeroderma pigmentosum. An inherited diseases with sun sensitivity, multiple cutaneous neoplasms, and abnormal DNA repair." *Ann Intern Med* , 80(2), 221-248.

[155] Robinson, S, Dixon, S, August, S, Diffey, B, Wakamatsu, K, et al. (2010). Protection against UVR involves MC1R-mediated non-pigmentary and pigmentary mechanisms in vivo." *J Invest Dermatol* , 130(7), 1904-1913.

[156] Salti, G. I, Manougian, T, Farolan, M, Shilkaitis, A, Majumdar, D, et al. (2000). Micropthalmia transcription factor: a new prognostic marker in intermediate-thickness cutaneous malignant melanoma." *Cancer Res* , 60(18), 5012-5016.

[157] Sarasin, A. (1999). The molecular pathways of ultraviolet-induced carcinogenesis." *Mutat Res* 428(1-2): 5-10.

[158] Sato, M, Nishigori, C, Zghal, M, Yagi, T, & Takebe, H. (1993). Ultraviolet-specific mutations in gene in skin tumors in xeroderma pigmentosum patients." *Cancer Res* 53(13): 2944-2946., 53.

[159] Scherer, D, & Kumar, R. (2010). Genetics of pigmentation in skin cancer--a review." *Mutat Res* , 705(2), 141-153.

[160] Schmalwieser, A. W, Schauberger, G, Janouch, M, Nunez, M, Koskela, T, et al. (2005). Global forecast model to predict the daily dose of the solar erythemally effective UV radiation." *Photochem Photobiol* , 81(1), 154-162.

[161] Schulman, J. M, & Fisher, D. E. (2009). Indoor ultraviolet tanning and skin cancer: health risks and opportunities." *Curr Opin Oncol* , 21(2), 144-149.

[162] Scotto, J, & Fears, T. R. (1987). The association of solar ultraviolet and skin melanoma incidence among caucasians in the United States." *Cancer Invest* , 5(4), 275-283.

[163] Serrano, M, Hannon, G. J, & Beach, D. (1993). A new regulatory motif in cell-cycle control causing specific inhibition of cyclin D/CDK4." *Nature* , 366(6456), 704-707.

[164] Seykora, J, & Elder, D. (1996). Dysplastic nevi and other risk markers for melanoma." *Semin Oncol* , 23(6), 682-687.

[165] Sharpless, E, & Chin, L. (2003). The INK4a/ARF locus and melanoma." *Oncogene* , 22(20), 3092-3098.

[166] Sharpless, N. E, & Depinho, R. A. (1999). The INK4A/ARF locus and its two gene products." *Curr Opin Genet Dev* , 9(1), 22-30.

[167] Siegel, R, Desantis, C, Virgo, K, Stein, K, Mariotto, A, et al. (2012). Cancer treatment and survivorship statistics, 2012." *CA Cancer J Clin* , 62(4), 220-241.

[168] Silverberg, M. J, Chao, C, Leyden, W. A, Xu, L, Horberg, M. A, et al. (2011). HIV infection, immunodeficiency, viral replication, and the risk of cancer." *Cancer Epidemiol Biomarkers Prev* , 20(12), 2551-2559.

[169] Slade, J, Marghoob, A. A, Salopek, T. G, Rigel, D. S, Kopf, A. W, et al. (1995). Atypical mole syndrome: risk factor for cutaneous malignant melanoma and implications for management." *J Am Acad Dermatol* , 32(3), 479-494.

[170] Smith, M. B, Xue, H, Strong, L, Takahashi, H, Jaffe, N, et al. (1993). Forty-year experience with second malignancies after treatment of childhood cancer: analysis of outcome following the development of the second malignancy." *J Pediatr Surg* discussion 1348-1349., 28(10), 1342-1348.

[171] Soehnge, H, Ouhtit, A, & Ananthaswamy, O. N. (1997). Mechanisms of induction of skin cancer by UV radiation." *Front Biosci* 2: d, 538-551.

[172] Song, X, Mosby, N, Yang, J, Xu, A, Abdel-malek, Z, et al. (2009). alpha-MSH activates immediate defense responses to UV-induced oxidative stress in human melanocytes." *Pigment Cell Melanoma Res* , 22(6), 809-818.

[173] Sosman, J. A, Kim, K. B, Schuchter, L, Gonzalez, R, Pavlick, A. C, et al. (2012). Survival in BRAF advanced melanoma treated with vemurafenib." *N Engl J Med* 366(8): 707-714., 600-mutant

[174] Soufir, N, Avril, M. F, Chompret, A, Demenais, F, Bombled, J, et al. (1998). Prevalence of and CDK4 germline mutations in 48 melanoma-prone families in France. The French Familial Melanoma Study Group." *Hum Mol Genet* 7(2): 209-216., 16.

[175] Steingrimsson, E, Copeland, N. G, & Jenkins, N. A. (2004). Melanocytes and the microphthalmia transcription factor network." *Annu Rev Genet* , 38, 365-411.

[176] Stern, R. S. (2001). The risk of melanoma in association with long-term exposure to PUVA." *J Am Acad Dermatol* , 44(5), 755-761.

[177] Sturm, R. A. (2002). Skin colour and skin cancer- MC1R, the genetic link." *Melanoma Res* , 12(5), 405-416.

[178] Sullivan, A. N, Bryant, E. A, & Mark, L. A. (2012). Malignant melanoma in transplant patients: a case report and review of the literature." *Cutis* , 89(3), 133-136.

[179] Takebe, H, Nishigori, C, & Tatsumi, K. (1989). Melanoma and other skin cancers in xeroderma pigmentosum patients and mutation in their cells." *J Invest Dermatol* 92(5 Suppl): 236S-238S.

[180] Tassabehji, M, Newton, V. E, & Read, A. P. (1994). Waardenburg syndrome type 2 caused by mutations in the human microphthalmia (MITF) gene." *Nat Genet* , 8(3), 251-255.

[181] Tomescu, D, Kavanagh, G, Ha, T, Campbell, H, & Melton, D. W. (2001). Nucleotide excision repair gene XPD polymorphisms and genetic predisposition to melanoma." *Carcinogenesis* , 22(3), 403-408.

[182] Tomlinson, I. P, Roylance, R, & Houlston, R. S. (2001). Two hits revisited again." *J Med Genet* , 38(2), 81-85.

[183] Tsao, H, Bevona, C, Goggins, W, & Quinn, T. (2003). The transformation rate of moles (melanocytic nevi) into cutaneous melanoma: a population-based estimate." *Arch Dermatol* , 139(3), 282-288.

[184] Tucker, M. A, Crutcher, W. A, Hartge, P, & Sagebiel, R. W. (1993). Familial and cutaneous features of dysplastic nevi: a case-control study." *J Am Acad Dermatol* , 28(4), 558-564.

[185] Udayakumar, D, & Tsao, H. (2009). Melanoma genetics: an update on risk-associated genes." *Hematol Oncol Clin North Am* vii., 23(3), 415-429.

[186] Ugurel, S, Houben, R, Schrama, D, Voigt, H, Zapatka, M, et al. (2007). Microphthalmia-associated transcription factor gene amplification in metastatic melanoma is a prognostic marker for patient survival, but not a predictive marker for chemosensitivity and chemotherapy response." *Clin Cancer Res* , 13(21), 6344-6350.

[187] Valverde, P, Healy, E, Sikkink, S, Haldane, F, Thody, A. J, et al. (1996). The Asp84Glu variant of the melanocortin 1 receptor (MC1R) is associated with melanoma." *Hum Mol Genet* , 5(10), 1663-1666.

[188] van'Veer, t, Burgering, L. J. , B. M, Versteeg, R, Boot, A. J, Ruiter, D. J, et al. (1989). N-ras mutations in human cutaneous melanoma from sun-exposed body sites." *Mol Cell Biol* , 9(7), 3114-3116.

[189] Van Der Leun, J. C, Piacentini, R. D, & De Gruijl, F. R. (2008). Climate change and human skin cancer." *Photochem Photobiol Sci* , 7(6), 730-733.

[190] Van Der Velden, P. A, Sandkuijl, L. A, Bergman, W, Pavel, S, Van Mourik, L, et al. (2001). Melanocortin-1 receptor variant R151C modifies melanoma risk in Dutch families with melanoma." *Am J Hum Genet* , 69(4), 774-779.

[191] Van Patter, H. T, & Drummond, J. A. (1953). Malignant melanoma occurring in xeroderma pigmentosum; report of a case." *Cancer* , 6(5), 942-947.

[192] Vinceti, M, Bassissi, S, Malagoli, C, Pellacani, G, Alber, D, et al. (2005). Environmental exposure to trace elements and risk of cutaneous melanoma." *J Expo Anal Environ Epidemiol* , 15(5), 458-462.

[193] Volkovova, K, Bilanicova, D, Bartonova, A, Letasiova, S, & Dusinska, M. (2012). Associations between environmental factors and incidence of cutaneous melanoma. Review." *Environ Health* 11 Suppl 1: S12.

[194] Wagner, S. N, Ockenfels, H. M, Wagner, C, Hofler, H, & Goos, M. (1995). Ras gene mutations: a rare event in nonmetastatic primary malignant melanoma." *J Invest Dermatol* , 104(5), 868-871.

[195] Wang, Y, Digiovanna, J. J, Stern, J. B, Hornyak, T. J, Raffeld, M, et al. (2009). Evidence of ultraviolet type mutations in xeroderma pigmentosum melanomas." *Proc Natl Acad Sci U S A* , 106(15), 6279-6284.

[196] Ward, K. A, Lazovich, D, & Hordinsky, M. K. (2012). Germline melanoma susceptibility and prognostic genes: A review of the literature." *J Am Acad Dermatol.*

[197] Weaver-feldhaus, J, Gruis, N. A, Neuhausen, S, Le, D, & Paslier, E. Stockert, et al. ((1994). Localization of a putative tumor suppressor gene by using homozygous deletions in melanomas." *Proc Natl Acad Sci U S A* , 91(16), 7563-7567.

[198] Weinstock, M. A. (2012). Reducing death from melanoma and standards of evidence." *J Invest Dermatol* , 132(5), 1311-1312.

[199] Weiskopf, D, Weinberger, B, & Grubeck-loebenstein, B. (2009). The aging of the immune system." *Transpl Int* , 22(11), 1041-1050.

[200] Widlund, H. R, & Fisher, D. E. (2003). Microphthalamia-associated transcription factor: a critical regulator of pigment cell development and survival." *Oncogene* , 22(20), 3035-3041.

[201] Williams, P. F, Olsen, C. M, Hayward, N. K, & Whiteman, D. C. (2011). Melanocortin 1 receptor and risk of cutaneous melanoma: a meta-analysis and estimates of population burden." *Int J Cancer* , 129(7), 1730-1740.

[202] Wilson, K. S. (2011). Ipilimumab plus dacarbazine in melanoma." *N Engl J Med* 365(13): 1256; author reply , 1257-1258.

[203] Winsey, S. L, Haldar, N. A, Marsh, H. P, Bunce, M, Marshall, S. E, et al. (2000). A variant within the DNA repair gene XRCC3 is associated with the development of melanoma skin cancer." *Cancer Res* , 60(20), 5612-5616.

[204] Woodward, A, & Boffetta, P. (1997). Environmental exposure, social class, and cancer risk." *IARC Sci Publ*(138): 361-367.

[205] Yasumoto, K, Yokoyama, K, Shibata, K, Tomita, Y, & Shibahara, S. (1994). Microphthalmia-associated transcription factor as a regulator for melanocyte-specific transcription of the human tyrosinase gene." *Mol Cell Biol* , 14(12), 8058-8070.

[206] Yokoyama, S, Woods, S. L, Boyle, G. M, Aoude, L. G, & Mac, S. Gregor, et al. ((2011). A novel recurrent mutation in MITF predisposes to familial and sporadic melanoma." *Nature* , 480(7375), 99-103.

[207] Zaidi, M. R, De Fabo, E. C, Noonan, F. P, & Merlino, G. (2012). Shedding light on melanocyte pathobiology in vivo." *Cancer Res* , 72(7), 1591-1595.

[208] Zuo, L, Weger, J, Yang, Q, Goldstein, A. M, Tucker, M. A, et al. (1996). Germline mutations in the binding domain of CDK4 in familial melanoma." *Nat Genet* 12(1): 97-99., 16INK4a.

Section 2

Molecular Mechanisms

Chapter 2

Aberrant Death Pathways in Melanoma

Nicholas D. Panayi, Erin E. Mendoza,
Elliot S. Breshears and Randy Burd

Additional information is available at the end of the chapter

http://dx.doi.org/10.5772/55173

1. Introduction

Melanoma is the most aggressive form of skin cancer and accounts for 4% of all skin cancers and nearly 75% of all melanoma deaths. According the National Cancer Institute, the incidence of melanoma is increasing 6-7% annually. In 2012, it is estimated that there will be 76,250 new cases of melanoma and more than 9,000 deaths. Risk factors for melanoma include one or more severe sunburns, a familial history, excessive presence of moles, and fair skin. Melanoma is unique from many cancers in that it that the tumor suppressor p53 is functional in a relatively high percentage of tumors. Despite functional p53 protein, melanoma cells evade p53-mediated apoptosis because of complex alterations in the apoptotic pathways. This chapter will discuss the aberrant apoptosis mechanisms that exist in melanoma and provide insight on to how these alterations could be therapeutically targeted.

2. P53

The tumor suppressor protein p53 has long been regarded as the guardian of the genome and is mutated in more than half of all human cancers. The functional status of p53 is of significant clinical importance because of its role in apoptosis, cell cycle arrest, and DNA repair; all cellular processes targeted by chemotherapy and radiation therapy [1]. The human p53 gene is highly conserved and consists of seven exons. The protein exists in a latent form and is activated through tetramerization, allowing p53 to then bind with high affinity to DNA. The tetramer conformation forms through interactions between regions in the C-terminus. Once activated, p53 can recognize sequence specific binding sites on target genes and stimulate their activation. p53 mutations are predominantly seen in the DNA binding domain, and very rarely occur in the oligomerization region [2]. The half-life of p53 is short and is increased acutely in response to DNA damage or changes in oxidation status. Upon activation, p53 is phosphorylated at various serine residues at the N or C terminus. The phoshorylation sites vary depending on the type of damage inflicted on the cell. Once phosphorylated, p53 acts as a transcription factor, translocating to the nucleus and binding to promoter elements of downstream target genes [3].

3. p53 and apoptosis

One of the essential roles of p53 is to maintain cellular integrity through transducing apoptosis, programmed cell death, in the event of an irreparable damage to prevent propagation of this aberrancy through uninterrupted proliferation. The mechanism of cell growth without checks and balances is the essence of malignancy; making p53 central to the governing of cell growth. Cellular damage caused by agents such as UV light, ionizing radiation, hypoxia, and oxidative stress will lead to the activation of p53, allowing for p53-dependent apoptosis to occur. The role of p53 in the mitochondrial apoptotic cascade is largely through its activities as a transcription factor for several pro-apoptotic proteins. p53 induced apoptosis can be activated via intrinsic and the extrinsic cellular pathways [4;5].

3.1. Intrinsic apoptosis

The intrinsic or mitchondrial apoptotic cascade results from genotoxic stress such as UV damage, oxidative stress, hypoxia, chemotherapy, or ionizing radiation. As depicted in Figure 1, activation of p53 from stress stimuli leads to activation of Bax and Bak. These proteins are important players in apoptosis and are members of the Bcl-2 family, which is made up of both pro and anti-apoptotic proteins. Family members are classified by structural similarity to the Bcl-2 homology (BH) domains (BH1, BH2, BH3, and BH4), as well as a transmembrane domain. The BH3 domain is referred to as the "death domain" and is the minimum requirement for the protein to have pro-apoptotic functions. Once activated, pro-apoptotic Bax and Bak lead to depoloarization of mitochondria and the release of cytochrome c, a small heme protein, which is bound loosely within the mitochondrial membrane. The pro-apoptotic functions of Bax and Bak are antagonized by the structurally similar anti-apoptotic proteins Bcl-2 and Bcl-xL. The Bcl-2 family also contains 'BH3 only' proteins that are exclusively pro-apoptotic and include Bax, PUMA, and Bid. Upon release, cytochrome c complexes with apoptosis protease activation factor (APAF-1) to form an apoptosome. The apoptosome then binds to inactivated procaspase 9, the initiating caspase. Once activated, caspase 9 goes on to cleave caspase 3, the effector caspase responsible for executing apoptosis [6-8].

3.2. Extrinsic apoptosis

Extrinsic apoptosis involves death receptor activation through activation of the TNF-R family proteins (Tumor necrosis factor receptor) including Fas, PERP, and DR5. The Fas receptor is located on the cell surface and is activated by the ligand FasL, which is largely expressed by T cells. Fas ligands, which usually exist as trimmers, bind and activate their receptors by inducing receptor trimerization. Activated receptors recruit adaptor molecules such as Fas-associating protein with death domain (FADD), which then recruit procaspase 8 to the receptor complex, where it undergoes autocatalytic activation. Activated caspase 8 activates caspase 3 through two pathways. In the more complex pathway caspase 8 activates Bcl-2 interacting protein (Bid), which interacts with Bax to promote translocation of Bax to the inner mitochondrial membrane where it triggers cytochrome c release. The released cytochrome c binds to apoptotic protease activating factor-1 (Apaf-1). As in intrinsic apoptosis, the apoptosome leads to activation of caspase 9, which is then able to cleave and activate procaspase 3, ultimately leading to DNA fragmentation [8;9]. Figure 1 depicts the intersection of intrinisic and extrinsic apoptosis and onset of extrinsic apoptosis through death receptor activation.

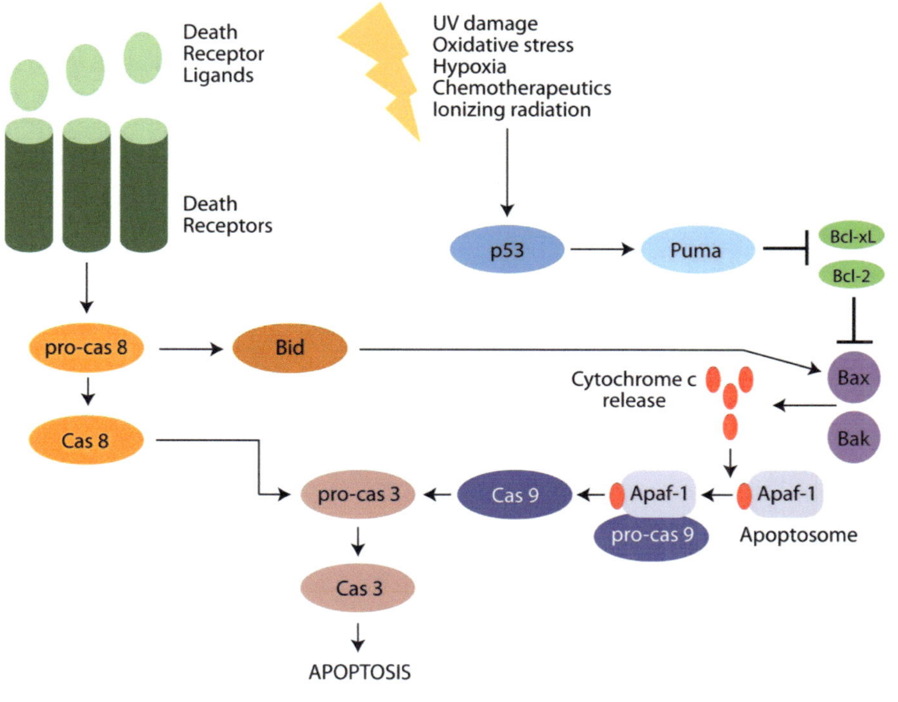

Figure 1. Intersecting intrinsic and extrinsic apoptotic pathways

4. Role of p53 in melanogenesis

4.1. Tyrosinase

The role of DNA damage and DNA repair in the stimulation of melanogenesis is corroborated by the observation that activated p53 upregulates transcription of tyrosinase, the rate-limiting enzyme involved in melanin production. Tyrosinase is a glycoprotein found in the melanosomal membrane. The protein has an inner melanosomal domain, which contains a catalytic region and a short transmembrane, and a cytoplasmic domain made up of about 30 amino acids. Histidine residues present in the catalytic domain portion of tyrosinase bind copper ions needed for tyrosinase activity. Structural studies of the tyrosinase promoter region have revealed the presence of a TATA box, CAAT box, 5 AP-1 sites, 2 AP-2, 2 glucocorticoid responsive elements, 2 UV responsive elements, and 3 Oct-1 sites [10]. The role of tyrosinase in pigmentation reactions is the result of the oxidation of phenols.Tyrosinase hydroxylates tyrosine in the first step of melanogenesis.Tyrosinase then catalyzes the hydroxylation of *L*-tyrosinse to *L*-Dopa and its subsequent oxidation to dopaquinone. Dopaquinone then undergoes a series of reactions that lead to the synthesis of melanin within the melanocyte. Tyrosinase has been studied as a prognostic marker of melanoma and has been useful in staging the disease and determining prognosis [11;12]. Pathological analysis of melanoma tissue samples have shown that tyrosinase detection is 97-100% specific to melanoma versus other tumor types. Detection of tyrosinase mRNA in peripheral blood in patients with metastatic melanoma using RT-PCR has been correlated to poor survival following immunotherapy with IL-2 [12]. It has also been observed that patients with primary lesions do not show tyrosinase mRNA in peripheral blood. Tyrosinase mRNA is not observed in peripheral blood in patients with previous metastatic disease but who are currently disease free, implicating that tyrosinase could be a useful prognostic tool [13].

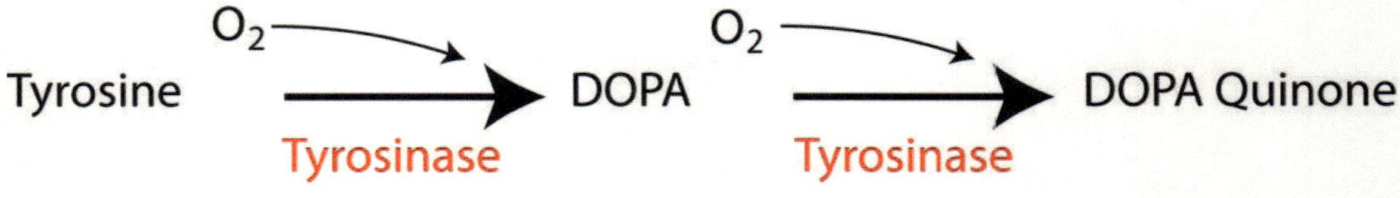

Figure 2. Tyrosinase catalyzed reactions during melanogenesis

4.2. Melanogenesis

The activities of p53 as a tranducer of melanin production was further elucidated by Cui et al. A p53 consensus sequence was discovered in the proopiomelanocortin (POMC) gene promoter, establishing a line of communication between UV-induced DNA damage and the sun tan response. The binding of p53 to the POMC promoter leads to an increase in the release of POMC-derived alpha-melanocyte stimulating hormone (alpha-MSH), an important messenger inducing melanogenesis. Once released, alpha-MSH acts as a ligand for the melanocortin-1 receptor (MC1R), and binding results in the production of eumelanin [14]. Yamaguchi et al. demonstrated that within keratinocytes, melanin acts as a native sunscreen. Melanin absorbs UV light, thus protecting DNA from damage. In dark skin, which possesses higher levels of melanin, protein levels of p53 are markedly lower following exposure to UV light compared to more fair skin when p53 is highly stabilized following the same exposure. The photo absorbent property of melanin protects from DNA damage, decreasing the activation of p53 [15]. Additionally, this observation supports that p53 is central to the UV damage response through stimulation of melanogenesis as an innate means to protect skin from damage through increased pigmentation.

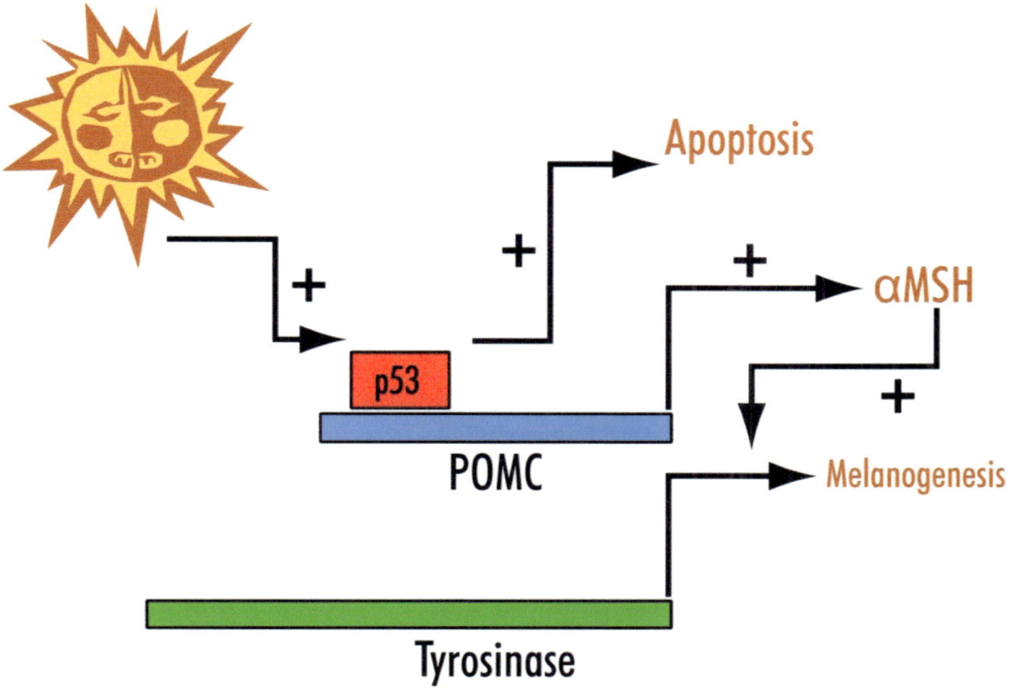

Figure 3. Role of p53 in transducing melanogenesis

5. p53 in melanoma

It has been observed that the frequency of p53 mutations in melanocytic tumors ranges from 5-25%, which is considerably lower than other types of cancers. Although mutations in p53 itself remain less frequent, the functional anti-tumor properties of p53 can be repressed by many other mechanisms [16;17]. For example, p53 may be wildtype in melanoma but its repressor, MDM2, is often overexpressed, causing p53 destabilization and a decreasing in its transcriptional activities. Furthermore, the p53 upstream protein p14ARF is responsible for the regulation of MDM2; once activated, p14ARF activates p53 through inhibition of MDM2, allowing p53 to avoid proteosomal degradation and subsequent phosphorylation. Mutations or a loss of p14ARF are frequently seen in melanoma [18]. Loss of function of one or both of the p14ARF of p16INK4a proteins is thought to lead to a compensatory increase in p53 stability as melanoma progresses [19].

In normal melanocytes, the apoptotic functions of p53 are attenuated in response to UV stress in order to facilitate a longer cell life. One way this occurs is by upregulation of the p53 responsive gene GADD45a, which inhibits intrinsic apoptosis mediated through p53. It is speculated that this alteration in the apoptotic machinery that is specific to melanocytes could be the genesis of the inherent chemoresistence of melanoma [20].

5.1. MDM2

The murine double minute protein (MDM2) functions as a negative regulator of p53. Its ability to inhibit p53 is regulated by a negative feedback loop in which activated p53 leads to the transcription and translation of MDM2, which then inhibits p53 [21]. Studies conducted in mice have shown that MDM2 knockout mice are embryonic lethal in a p53-dependent manner, where incessant p53 activity causes excessive apoptosis and ultimately death. A rescue effect was observed by p53 knockout, confirming the role of MDM2 in p53 regulation [22]. MDM2 interacts with the transactivation domain of p53 via a p53-interacting domain on the N-terminus of MDM2. This binding of MDM2 to p53 prevents p53 from binding to its transcriptional co-activators and subsequently prevents p53 from activating target genes [21]. In melanoma, MDM2 has been found to be highly expressed in half of invasive primary and metastatic melanomas. Amplification of the MDM2 locus is infrequent and over-expression is the most common occurrence. In patient follow-up studies, decreased MDM2 expression was associated with higher rates of survival. It has also been observed that both MDM2 and p53 are overexpressed in patients with melanoma [23]. This could be explained by the auto-regulatory loop between p53 and MDM2. Increased expression of MDM2 is also possible due to the loss of its repressor $p14^{ARF}$, a common mutation or deletion seen in melanoma [24]. Without its repressor, MDM2 is constitutively active. This could account for the apoptotic resistance observed in melanoma despite the largely wild-type status of p53.

5.2. INK4a/ARF locus

The INK4a/ARF locus contains the open reading frames of the proteins $p16^{INK4a}$ and $p14^{ARF}$. This locus is of particular importance in melanoma because primary melanoma tumors and nearly all melanoma cell lines carry a deletion at this locus [25]. Melanocytes have an intrinsically longer life than many other cell types in the body. The anti-proliferative properties of p53 may be attenuated in melanocytes to accommodate this longer cell life. All normal cells have a finite number of cellular divisions. After this number is reached the cells enter a phase called senescence, which is a protective cellular mechanism in cancer because it prevents aberrant cell growth. Senescence can also be triggered through tumor suppressor proteins when damage is sensed, minimizing uncontrolled cell growth and halting the path to malignancy [26]. The $p16^{INK4a}$/Rb pathway as shown in Figure 4, is a key pathway for triggering cellular senescence. The loss of this pathway in melanoma is thought to contribute to the pathogenesis of melanoma. It is likely that loss of this protective cellular pathway is more damaging than the potential loss of p53, offering an explanation as to why a p53 mutation is not required for melanocytic tumorigenesis [26]. The $p16^{INK4a}$ protein works as a tumor suppressor by binding to the cyclin-D-dependent protein kinases Cdk4 and Cdk6, preventing them from phosphorylating Rb and preventing entrance into the cell cycle. The genes that encode for both p16INK4a and Cdk4 have be identified as melanoma susceptibility genes [27]. The CdkN2A locus encodes p16INK4a as well as the tumor suppressor $p14^{ARF}$. The $p14^{ARF}$ gene is encoded by a different promoter through the use of alternative reading frames. Both p14ARF and p16I^{NK4a} share exons 2 and 3, while Exon 1B encodes p14 ^{ARF} and Exon 1A encodes for p16^{INK4a}. The two share no sequence homology and are not isoforms. The main regulatory function of p14^{ARF} is its binding to MDM2, which prevents the ubiquitination and subsequent degradation of p53 [28]. In cases of familial melanoma, either p16INK4a or both p16I^{NK4a} and p14^{ARF} are mutated or deleted. It is rare to see mutations or deletions of p14ARF alone. Germline mutations at the p16^{INK4a}/p14^{ARF} locus are observed in 20-40% of familial cases of melanoma [25]. Somatic melanomas often involve mutations, deletions, or methylation of p16INK4a. Due to a shared open reading frame, up to 40% of mutations or deletions that affect p16^{INK4a} will affect p14^{ARF} [29]. Loss of homozygousity of the p16^{INK4a}/p14^{ARF} locus is observed in half of sporadic melanomas and loss of p16^{INK4a} and p14^{ARF} expression occurs in 50-70% of invasive melanomas [30].

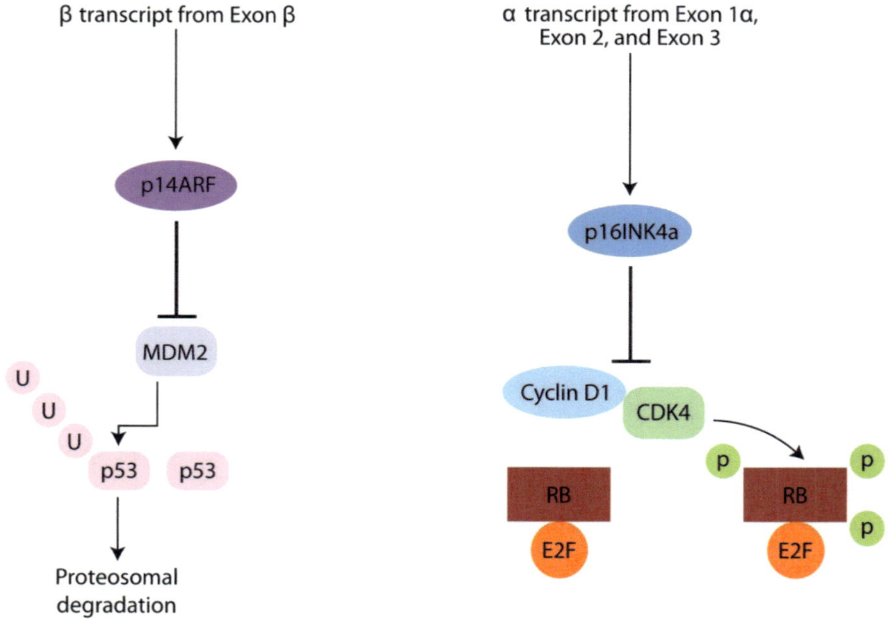

Figure 4. Gene products from the INK4a/ARF locus

5.3. APAF-1

Apoptosis protease-activating factor-1 (APAF-1) is a regulator in the intrinsic apoptosis pathway. When APAF-1 complexes with cytochome c a multimeric apoptosome is formed that recruits and activates pro-caspase 9, the initiator of the mitochondrial apoptotic cascade. Once activated, caspase 9 proceeds to activate pro-caspase 3 for the execution of apoptosis. A p53 transactivation site has been identified on APAF-1 determining that APAF-1 is a p53 responsive gene [31]. Downregulation of APAF-1 has been observed at the protein and mRNA level during melanoma progression, possibly contributing to the ability of melanoma to evade apoptosis and thus conferring chemoresistance. Noncancerous melanocytes have normal APAF-1 protein and mRNA levels. Conversely, loss of homozygousity has been detected in 42% of metastatic melanoma samples. Analysis of 19 metastatic lines revealed 10 lines with low APAF-1 staining. Other studies have demonstrated significantly higher APAF-1 staining in benign nevi compared with primary melanomas. Lower APAF-1 staining has also been associated with greater tumor thickness in primary melanocytic tumors [32;33].

5.4. Bcl-2

The proapoptotic namesake for the Bcl-2 protein family has a complicated role in melanocytes and in melanoma. Its proapoptotic role in melanocytes prevents premature cell death to allow for continued production of pigment during the long life of the melanocyte. Bcl-2 knockout studies in mice resulted in greying of the mice two weeks after birth due to melanocyte death. The prognostic role of Bcl-2 in melanocytic tumors is controversial. Some analyses have shown that melanoma primary tumors overexpressing Bcl-2 have an increased risk for invasion and are responsible for drug resistance. It has also been observed that Bcl-2 levels actually decrease in melanoma progression. Tumorigenic melanoma cells may take advantage of high endogenous Bcl-2 levels to survive under adverse environmental conditions that they may encounter during metastatic transformation and chemotherapeutic intervention [5;34].

5.5. Bax

The protein Bcl-2 associated X protein (Bax) is a pro-apoptotic Bcl-2 family member highly involved in the mitochondrial apoptotic cascade. It is a p53 target gene and in response to stress, p53 will bind to the Bax promoter leading to its transcription, making it a valuable indicator of p53 transcriptional activity as well as an indicator of intrinsic apoptosis. Bax will translocate to the inner mitochondrial membrane, facilitating the depolarization and release of cytochrome c. It has been observed that expression of Bax increases with melanoma progression, although the tumors remain largely chemoresistant. This implicates that a ratio effect is taking place; the inherent increase of Bcl-2 in melanocytes is potentially high enough to negate the increased expression of Bax, thus facilitating tumor resistance to apoptosis. An increase in Bax expression could also be a result of increased p53 stability and transcriptional activity from mutation or deletion of proteins at the INK4a/ARF locus [35;36].

5.6. PUMA

The BH3-only mitchondrial protein p53 upregulated modulator of apoptosis (PUMA) belongs to the Bcl-2 family of apoptotic regulators. The BH3 domain and its localization within the mitochondria are necessary for PUMA to induce apoptosis or decrease cell growth. Studies have not demonstrated that PUMA is post-translationally modified like other BH3 only proteins. In response to stress stimuli, PUMA is transactivated by p53 [37]. Once activated, PUMA promotes the apoptotic pathway through inhibition of the anti-apoptotic protein Bcl-2, allowing Bax and Bak to become activated and fosters cytochrome c release from the inner mitochondrial membrane to signal initiation of apoptosis. The main pro-apoptotic effect of PUMA is such that once activated by p53, it will inhibit Bcl-2 anti-apoptotic family members in order to transduce apoptosis [38]. It is possible that a loss of PUMA activity in melanoma cells could give rise to an increase in Bcl-2 activity, leading to either evasion of apoptosis by therapy or propagating transformation [39]. Complete silencing of PUMA in melanoma is not known. However, immunostaining for PUMA in benign nevi have shown increased PUMA staining in comparison to dysplastic nevi, primary melanoma, and metastatic tissues. When this data was compared to patient 5-year survival, patients exhibiting increased PUMA staining had a better prognosis and therapeutic response compared to those with little or no PUMA staining [40].

5.7. p73

The p73 protein is a p53 homolog with tumor supressor activities, but it can also demonstrate oncogenic properties, as the p73 gene can be transcribed into several different isoforms. The full length p73 (TAp73) contains a N-terminal transactivation domain, proline rich region, DNA binding domain, and C-terminal oligmerization domain. Members of the p53 family generally carry approximately 70% sequence homology to p53, primarily in the DNA binding domain. Homology in the DNA binding domain allows p73 to recognize and regulate p53 target genes. Splice variants are generated through the use of an internal promoter, the use of an alternative translation start site, or alternative splicing of the first exons. The splice variants have a truncated N-terminus and do not contain a functional DNA binding domain, resulting in a dominant negative protein with anti-apoptotic and growth promoting characteristics. These variants are referred to as delta Np73. The delta isoforms possess antagonistic properties and counteract the tumor supressor activities of TAp73.The intracellular concentration of the of the delta isoforms in relation to the concentration of TAp73 is believed to be of significance. The ratio of the delta isoforms to TAp73 levels may determine the role p73 plays in cell survival [41;42]. Loss or mutation of the p73 gene have not been determined to be major events in the development in melanoma. However, immunostaining of several of the Delta isoforms have shown increased levels of delta isoforms in metastatic melanoma, in addition to strong p73 staining. This suggests p73 may have a role as a positive regulator of tumor growth. In this situation, the ratio of the delta isoforms to TAp73 may be of importance [43]. It is important to note that the delta isoforms are markedly more stable in comparison to TA73, promoting the antagonistic effects. It has been observed that MDM2 can disrupt p73 activities through interfering with the acetyl-transferase p300/CBP. The interaction between p53 and p73 with MDM2 are similar in that they both interact with the same hydrophobic pocket of MDM2, suggests that increased MDM2 activity may decrease the actions of TAp73 as well as that of its isoforms [44].

6. p53-related targeted therapy

Targeting p53 pathways pharmacologically can serve as a very effective means of circumventing chemoresistance observed in melanoma. The use of the small molecule inhibitor nutlin-3 to inhibit MDM2 can restore the anti-tumor effects of p53. Due to the common loss of p14ARF seen in melanoma and the compensatory increase in MDM2, p53 is unable to serve as a mediator of chemosensitivity. The sequesteration of MDM2 in combination with temezolomide potentiated the effects of the drug and increased sensitivity *in vivo*. The use of nutlin-3 to reinstate p53 function was also shown to be successful with the topoisomerase inhibitor Topotecan [45]. It has also been suggested that the use of nutlin-3 could reverse inaction of p73 through MDM2 inactivation. Given the presence of antagonistic isoforms of p73, the presence of MDM2 could potentially be a defect to exploit in melanoma in order to cease the anti-apoptotic functions of the delta isoforms. Another possibility of therapeutic intervention is the combination of p73 antissense in order to reduce the antagonistic effects of p73 while restoring the native function of p53.

Along with the loss of the $p16^{INK4a}/p14^{ARF}$ locus, an overexpression of cyclin D1 can occur in melanoma, exacerbating the lack of the G1/S cell cycle checkpoint. Sauter et. al. demonstrated that cyclin D1 antisense can work to sensitize melanoma cell lines to apoptosis. The intrinsic increase of Bcl-2 in melanoma results in apoptotic resistance and a decrease in therapeutic outcomes [46]. A study of 771 patients with advanced melanoma were treated with the Bcl-2 antisense Oblimersen in combination with Dacarbazine and had improved 24-month survival and drug response, indicating a role of Bcl-2 in chemoresistence [47].

7. Conclusion

P53-mediated signaling in melanoma provides exceptional insight into the delicate signaling interplay involved in melanoma progression. The role of p53 in the compensatory responses to the infamous deletions and mutations associated with melanocytic tumors will further elucidate mechanisms involved in tumor progression. Increased understanding of these pathways will no doubt propel development of new treatment protocols forward, resulting in new and more effective means to treat this very aggressive disease.

Author details

Nicholas D. Panayi[1], Erin E. Mendoza[2], Elliot S. Breshears[2] and Randy Burd[2*]

*Address all correspondence to: rburd@u.arizona.edu

1 College of Medicine, University of Arizona, Tucson, AZ, USA

2 Department of Nutritional Sciences, University of Arizona, Tucson, AZ, USA

References

[1] Chene P. Targeting p53 in cancer. 2001 Aug.

[2] Chene P. The role of tetramerization in p53 function. Oncogene 2001 May 10;20(21): 2611-7.

[3] Gu B, Zhu WG. Surf the post-translational modification network of p53 regulation. Int J Biol Sci 2012;8(5):672-84.

[4] Haupt S, Berger M, Goldberg Z, Haupt Y. Apoptosis - the p53 network. J Cell Sci 2003 Oct 15;116(Pt 20):4077-85.

[5] Hussein MR, Haemel AK, Wood GS. p53-related pathways and the molecular pathogenesis of melanoma. Eur J Cancer Prev 2003 Apr;12(2):93-100.

[6] Shamas-Din A, Brahmbhatt H, Leber B, Andrews DW. BH3-only proteins: Orchestrators of apoptosis. Biochim Biophys Acta 2011 Apr;1813(4):508-20.

[7] Lindsay J, Esposti MD, Gilmore AP. Bcl-2 proteins and mitochondria--specificity in membrane targeting for death. Biochim Biophys Acta 2011 Apr;1813(4):532-9.

[8] Sayers TJ. Targeting the extrinsic apoptosis signaling pathway for cancer therapy. Cancer Immunol Immunother 2011 Aug;60(8):1173-80.

[9] Mackenzie SH, Clark AC. Targeting cell death in tumors by activating caspases. Curr Cancer Drug Targets 2008 Mar;8(2):98-109.

[10] Khlgatian MK, Hadshiew IM, Asawanonda P, Yaar M, Eller MS, Fujita M, et al. Tyrosinase gene expression is regulated by p53. J Invest Dermatol 2002 Jan;118(1):126-32.

[11] Gradilone A, Cigna E, Agliano AM, Frati L. Tyrosinase expression as a molecular marker for investigating the presence of circulating tumor cells in melanoma patients. Curr Cancer Drug Targets 2010 Aug;10(5):529-38.

[12] Mellado B, Del C, V, Colomer D, Gutierrez L, Castel T, Quinto L, et al. Tyrosinase mRNA in blood of patients with melanoma treated with adjuvant interferon. J Clin Oncol 2002 Oct 1;20(19):4032-9.

[13] Visus C, Andres R, Mayordomo JI, Martinez-Lorenzo MJ, Murillo L, Saez-Gutierrez B, et al. Prognostic role of circulating melanoma cells detected by reverse transcriptase-polymerase chain reaction for tyrosinase mRNA in patients with melanoma. Melanoma Res 2007 Apr;17(2):83-9.

[14] Cui R. Central role of p53 in the suntan response and pathologic hyperpigmentation. 2007 Mar 9.

[15] Yamaguchi Y, Brenner M, Hearing VJ. The regulation of skin pigmentation. J Biol Chem 2007 Sep 21;282(38):27557-61.

[16] Benjamin CL. p53 and the pathogenesis of skin cancer. 2007 Nov 1.

[17] Box NF. The role of p53 in pigmentation, tanning and melanoma. 2008 Oct.

[18] Hayward N. New developments in melanoma genetics. 2000 Jul.

[19] Meyle KD. Genetic risk factors for melanoma. 2009 Oct.

[20] Soengas MS. Apoptosis and melanoma chemoresistance. 2003 May 19.

[21] Wang X, Jiang X. Mdm2 and MdmX partner to regulate p53. FEBS Lett 2012 May 21;586(10):1390-6.

[22] Ji Z. p53 rescue through HDM2 antagonism suppresses melanoma growth and potentiates MEK inhibition. 2012 Feb.

[23] Polsky D, Bastian BC, Hazan C, Melzer K, Pack J, Houghton A, et al. HDM2 protein overexpression, but not gene amplification, is related to tumorigenesis of cutaneous melanoma. Cancer Res 2001 Oct 15;61(20):7642-6.

[24] Pho L. Melanoma genetics: a review of genetic factors and clinical phenotypes in familial melanoma. 2006 Mar.

[25] Satyamoorthy K. p16INK4A and familial melanoma. 2003.

[26] Rayess H, Wang MB, Srivatsan ES. Cellular senescence and tumor suppressor gene p16. Int J Cancer 2012 Apr 15;130(8):1715-25.

[27] Sharpless E. The INK4a/ARF locus and melanoma. 2003 May 19.

[28] Meyle KD. Genetic risk factors for melanoma. 2009 Oct.

[29] Hayward N. New developments in melanoma genetics. 2000 Jul.

[30] Dahl C, Guldberg P. The genome and epigenome of malignant melanoma. APMIS 2007 Oct;115(10):1161-76.

[31] Anichini A. APAF-1 signaling in human melanoma. 2006 Jul 18.

[32] Anichini A. APAF-1 signaling in human melanoma. 2006 Jul 18.

[33] Mustika R. Decreased expression of Apaf-1 with progression of melanoma. 2005 Feb.

[34] Gray-Schopfer V, Wellbrock C, Marais R. Melanoma biology and new targeted therapy. Nature 2007 Feb 22;445(7130):851-7.

[35] Hussein MR, Haemel AK, Wood GS. Apoptosis and melanoma: molecular mechanisms. J Pathol 2003 Mar;199(3):275-88.

[36] Pustisek N, Situm M. UV-radiation, apoptosis and skin. Coll Antropol 2011 Sep;35 Suppl 2:339-41.

[37] Nakano K. PUMA, a novel proapoptotic gene, is induced by p53. 2001 Mar.

[38] Zinkel S, Gross A, Yang E. BCL2 family in DNA damage and cell cycle control. Cell Death Differ 2006 Aug;13(8):1351-9.

[39] Yang G, Zhang G, Pittelkow MR, Ramoni M, Tsao H. Expression profiling of UVB response in melanocytes identifies a set of p53-target genes. J Invest Dermatol 2006 Nov;126(11):2490-506.

[40] Karst AM. PUMA expression is significantly reduced in human cutaneous melanomas. 2005 Feb 3.

[41] Bisso A. p73 as a pharmaceutical target for cancer therapy. 2011.

[42] Conforti F, Sayan AE, Sreekumar R, Sayan BS. Regulation of p73 activity by post-translational modifications. Cell Death Dis 2012;3:e285.

[43] Johnson J, Lagowski J, Sundberg A, Kulesz-Martin M. P53 family activities in development and cancer: relationship to melanocyte and keratinocyte carcinogenesis. J Invest Dermatol 2005 Nov;125(5):857-64.

[44] Chen F, Wang W, El-Deiry WS. Current strategies to target p53 in cancer. Biochem Pharmacol 2010 Sep 1;80(5):724-30.

[45] de LJ, Ly LV, Lodder K, Verlaan-de VM, Teunisse AF, Jager MJ, et al. Synergistic growth inhibition based on small-molecule p53 activation as treatment for intraocular melanoma. Oncogene 2012 Mar 1;31(9):1105-16.

[46] Sauter ER, Takemoto R, Litwin S, Herlyn M. p53 alone or in combination with antisense cyclin D1 induces apoptosis and reduces tumor size in human melanoma. Cancer Gene Ther 2002 Oct;9(10):807-12.

[47] Bedikian AY, Millward M, Pehamberger H, Conry R, Gore M, Trefzer U, et al. Bcl-2 antisense (oblimersen sodium) plus dacarbazine in patients with advanced melanoma: the Oblimersen Melanoma Study Group. J Clin Oncol 2006 Oct 10;24(29):4738-45.

Chapter 3

Interaction Between the Immune System and Melanoma

Norma E. Herrera-Gonzalez

Additional information is available at the end of the chapter

http://dx.doi.org/10.5772/54939

1. Introduction

No scientist can escape being fascinated by the complexity of the interplay between innate and adaptive immunity in order to monitor tissue homeostasis, to protect against infectious pathogens and to eliminate damaged cells. One of the most important tasks of the Immune System is to distinguish between "self" and "foreign". Cancer is formed of cells that suffer several mutations but form still part of the individual body. All types of cancer are caused by the progressive growth of the progeny of a single transformed cell. Curing this disease requires that all the malignant cells have to be removed or destroyed without damaging the patient. To achieve this task the own body has to distinguish between the cells of "the tumor" and their "other cellular" counterparts.

The initial thought that the immune system has indeed a protective role in tumor development has changed enormously in the past years. In the last few years, it has been experimentally shown that the Immune system itself can facilitate tumor development and progression and functions to promote or select tumor variants with reduced immunogenicity.

Decades of intensive investigation have made it increasingly clear that the interplay between immunity and cancer is complex. Next, there is some information about how the immunosurveillance hypothesis has been confronted through all these years since the early 70's [1].

2. Immunosurveillance hypothesis confrontation

The first approach to the interplay between cancer and the Immune system, was done by Stutman. He used nude mice and methylcolantreno (MCA) to produce tumors in both, nude and their wild type counterparts [2]. The conclusion was that nude mice did not form more chemically induced tumors compared with the controls, nor did they show a shortened tumor latency period after carcinogen injection. The similarity between immune-competent and nude mice was consistent in subsequent experiments that employed mice of different ages, different doses of carcinogen, etc. These findings were also supported by Rygaard who showed no differences in tumor formation in a study of 10 800 nude mice over a period of 5-7 months [3]. It is now clear that nude mice are not completely immunocompromised since they have detectable populations of functional $\alpha\beta$ T cell receptor bearing lymphocytes [4]. Furthermore, these studies were done before the discovery of NK cells, which are thymus independent and $\partial\gamma$ T cells, a subset of lymphocytes which may develop extrathymically. Later on, experiments based also on models of MCA–induced tumor formation showed that mice lacking either the IFN¥ receptor or STAT1, the transcription factor essential for the signalling of IFN¥ receptor, were found to be 10-20 times more sensitive than wild-type mice to the MCA tumor formation [5]. In studies of mice lacking the TCRβ chain or the TCRγ chain, MCA treatment of either mice increased the incidence of fibrosarcomas as compared with controls, showing that both T cells subsets are critical for protecting in this particular model of tumor development.

Shankaran in 2001 used targeted mice that lack RAG-1 or RAG 2 (recombination activating gene). These enzymes are essential for the repair of double stranded DNA breaks and they are solely in the lymphoid compartment. All this means that RAG deficient mice fail to rearrange lymphocyte antigen receptors and lack of NKT, T and B cells. When these mice were injected with MCA, 26 of 26 RAG deficient mice developed sarcomas. In contrast, 5 of 20 wild type mice developed spontaneous neoplásia [6].

The previous experiments show clearly the participation of some components of the Immune System in order to avoid the formation of tumors. However, these results are specifically for the MCA model, where its carcinogenesis mechanism is different from all the other types of cancer. Even more, these findings were obtained in murine models. However, if cancer immunosurvellience exists in mice, does exists in humans?

3. Is this immune protection similar in humans?

Scientist turned back to look if immunodeficient or immunosuppressed patients and individuals with primary immunodeficiencies had greater incidences of cancer. Early studies of transplanted patients who were subjected to immunosuppressive agents actually showed higher relative risk for cancer development. The answer was affirmative but, most of this higher risk was due to the development of tumors that were of viral origin. For example, non-Hodgking's lymphoma, Kaposi's sarcoma and carcinomas of the genitourinary and anogenital areas where all of these are linked to infection with Epstein-Barr virus, human herpesvirus 8 and HPV. A review of data from thirty years of Transplant Tumor Registry found that transplanted patients showed two times more relative risk to develop melanoma over the general population [7].

It has also been reported that there is evidence showing a positive correlation between the presence of lymphocytes in a tumor (TILs) and an increase in the patient's survival. Sorting more than 500 patients with primary melanoma who had more than 7 years of follow up, showed that patients in the brisk tumor infiltrating lymphocytes response survived two times longer than patients absent of TILs in their tumors. Later on, researchers reported the same prognostic correlation when studied the presence of TIL's in melanomas that had metastasized to lymph nodes [8]. The previous studies show that the presence of lymphocytes in the tumor may increase life survival. However, these patients after some time still die due to the progression and migration of melanoma to other vital organs, therefore, the Immune system do not resolve the tumor.

4. Cancer occur in immunocompetent individuals

The protective role of the Immune System is not completely effective to eliminate tumors. In order to explain this failure, it has been proposed that three stages exist in humans during this process: a) Elimination, where the Immune system is capable of destroying neoplastic cells by the innate immunity effectors; b) Equilibrium, specific effectors that eliminate the tumor are induced but, at the same time, selective pressure is generated on tumor cells, as a result mutated neoplastic variants occur; c) Escape, the tumor variants that survive become more resistant to identification and/or elimination by the Immune System and consequently the tumor grows. This process has been called "Cancer immunoediting" to describe more accurately the dual host-protecting and tumor sculpting actions of the Immune System shaping a neoplastic disease.

This hypothesis explains the observation that tumors often become clinically evident years after their molecular origin. At the end of this equilibrium between the immune system and tumor growth, the immune response allows for the outgrowth of a subpopulation of tumor cells. Factors contributing early neoplastic cells to survive, grow and invade are released by the immune system itself.

The major tumor type that occurs with increased frequency in immunodeficient individuals are virus-associated tumors, so immune surveillance is critical for control of this type of tumors, while the immune system does not normally respond to the neoantigens derived from the multiple genetic alterations in spontaneously arising tumors. Studies in mice have also revealed that when these are induced for immunodeficiency, show a high susceptibility to virally induced tumors and a greater tendency to develop spontaneous lymphomas compared with immunocompetent mice [8].

5. Does the immune system control each type of cancer?

All types of cancer share several characteristics, some of the most studied are uncontrolled growth, resistance to apoptosis, motility, proteolytic capacity and adhesion. However, each type of cancer also may have completely different etiologies (physical, chemical and/or biological), cell type of origin, mechanism of transformation, anatomical localization, histolo-pathological features, mortality rate, tumor markers, etc.

6. Melanoma: Its origins and incidence

Melanoma, an aggressive malignancy arising from melanocytes, is one of the most lethal of all skin cancers due to its great capacity to produce metastasis and its high chemoresistance [9]. It causes approximately 80% of skin cancer related deaths worldwide and is considered to be the most common mainly fatal malignancy of young adults mainly in Europe, Australia, New Zealand and United States of America where many people is red-haired with blue or green eyes. This disease is predominantly of populations with lighter skin color (Fitzpatrick I, II III) and the incidence is around tenfold lower in populations with darker skin color (Fitzpatrick IV, V and IV). The list of risk factors in developing melanoma is long but the main risk factors are: blond or red hair, numerous freckles and tendency to burn and tan poorly.

Over the past 55 years, the incidence of melanoma in most developed countries has risen faster than any other cancer type. Incidence rose dramatically between 1950 and 2000 (approximately 10% every year) particularly in some countries where caucasian population are. Melanoma provides one of the best examples of how genetics and environment interact in the pathogenesis of cancer. Incidence is strongly related to race and geographic location [10].

Primary melanoma progresses generally through two phases: a) the radial growth phase, is the horizontal spreading of transformed melanocytic cells inside the epidermis and small groups of invasive cells limited to the upper part of the dermis, and b) the vertical growth phase, is the invasion of melanoma cells into the deeper dermis and subcutaneous tissues.

7. Primary melanoma development

Most melanomas (with the exception of acral melanomas) are caused by exposure to UVB. This radiation can damage melanocyte DNA, causing hundreds of mutations including in genes controlling cell cycle progression and signal transduction pathways. UVB radiation may induce pyrimidine dimers, primarily thymidine di-nucleotides. So, lesions not repaired by nucleotide excision repair can lead to GC---→AT transitions, leaving a mutagenic mark. The epidemiological evidence for a role of solar exposure in melanoma (especially in Caucasian populations) is very strong. Some studies have suggested that total accumulated exposure to sun is a very important factor whereas long-term occupational exposure may be protective. UV irradiation induces also morphological and functional alterations in epidermal Langerhans' cell. The involvement of TNFα in the emigration of Langerhans' cells from UV-exposed skin into the regional lymph nodes has been reported. However, it may exist other non-mutagenic mechanisms involved such as immune suppression, UV induction of melanocyte growth factors by damaged keratinocytes, or UV production of mutagenic oxidative radicals during inflammation. UVB, can also weaken both the innate and adaptive immune systems by promoting the release of IL-10 by Langerhans cells [11] and by favoring the infiltration of IFNγ-producing macrophages. These cytokines possess activities as immunosuppressive and pro-angiogenic respectively [12].

It is important to mention that there are different molecular subtypes of melanomat, which may show a totally different antigenic profile depending on the number and quality of genetic alterations. These subtypes are superficial spreading, lentigo maligna, nodular and acral melanoma. The phenotype of malignancy is a reflexion of genetic events altering the RNA and protein expression patterns of normal cells. It has been observed that in general all metastatic melanoma generally displays resistance to treatment with antineoplastic drugs. Additionally, these therapies are severely toxic to the patients and their side effects include fatigue, malaise and a higher risk for non-melanoma cancers [13]. Superficial spreading melanoma is the most common melanoma in the first world countries and can occur at any site and at any age. About 80% of superficial spreading melanoma occur *de novo*. The classic lesions show variation in pigmentation and pagetoid spread of melanoma cell in epidermis [14]. Superficial spreading melanomas usually occur in younger patients than nodular or lentigo malign melanomas. They typically involve intermittently sun-exposed anatomical sites such as the trunk, back and extremities.

8. From melanocyte to melanoma

The epidermis contains keratinocytes and two types of dendritic cells, a) Langerhans' cells which are professional presenting cells playing an essential role in cellular response mainly to microorganisms but apparently also to tumor antigens; and b) melanocytes. Langerhans' cells are located in the suprabasal layer of the epidermis, whereas melanocytes are located amongst the basal layer of the epidermis, hair bulb, eyes, ears and meninges. Melanin pigment is produced by melanocytes in their specific cytoplasmic organelles called melanosomes. Melanin pigment synthesis by each melanocyte is transferred to an average of 36 keratinocytes. The transferred melanin forms a cap at the top of nucleous of mitotically active basal cells and prevent the UV damaging effects on nucleus.

Melanoma arises through a complex process of cellular mutations and a loss of keratinocyte control over growth and differentiation [15]. As malignant melanoma progresses, it develops through interaction between dysfunctional melanocytes and the tumor microenvironment. This progression is accompanied with changes in both keratinocytes and local adhesion molecules allowing for the formation of nevocyte nests at the dermal-epidermal junction [16].

As mentioned earlier, the progression from healthy melanocyte to melanoma occurs through both mutations within the tumor and through alterations of the cellular environment around the melanoma. In the skin, tissue homeostasis is critical in cellular regulation as well as immune control, and melanoma disrupts this regulation through multiple processes. Differentially expressed genes that are mutated during this multistep process conduct towards the transformation of melanocytes to melanoma. A great number of genes and proteins have been reported to play an essential role in this transformation. Some of these are listed: BRAF, cKIT, PTEN, p16,p53, cyclin1, ARF, K-RAS. Differentially expressed genes between melanocytes and melanoma cells impact in the expression of somehow "different" surface membrane expression of certain proteins (TAAs) that may play an important role for immune recognition and their elimination. In addition to mutation-derived tumor associate antigens (TAAs), melanoma is known to express normal, melanocytic lineage-related antigens (gp100, MART-1) that are not recognized by the immune system owing to some form of tolerance to self antigens [17].

9. The immune system in health

The immune system is highly elaborated, with a diversity of stop and go mechanisms essential to accomplish different tasks. It is composed of many cell types and mediators that interact with non-immune cells in a complex and dynamic way to ensure protection against foreign pathogens but at the same time maintaining tolerance to self-antigens (such as tumor cells in a way). The immune system has two completely different compartments –adaptive and innate, differing these on antigen specificity, timing of activation and cellular composition. These cells have communication networks that allow rapid responses to tissue injury. Innate immune cells, such as dendritic cells (DC) natural killer (NK) cells, macrophages, neutrophils, basophils, eosinophils and mast cells are the first line of defense against foreign antigens and damaged cells.

10. The innate immune system and inflammation

When tissue homeostasis is broken, sentinel macrophages, DC and mast cells release cytokines, chemokines, matrix remodeling proteases (MMP) and reactive oxygen species (ROS), inducing migration and infiltration of more leukocytes into damaged tissue, this process is called inflammation. Although inflammation is important in tissue repair and erradication of harmful pathogens, unresolved, chronic inflammation that happens when the offending agent is not removed, can be detrimental to the host. Immune cells infiltration in the absence of pathogens is also characteristic of cancer, and these cells can definitely influence the growth and progression of this disease. The destructive cycles that are initiated inside the tissues by failure to commit either arm of the immune system, can result in excessive tissue remodeling, loss of tissue architecture due to tissue destruction and finally DNA and protein alterations due to oxidative stress.

So, one might question, why does inflammation potentiate cancer development rather than protect against it. Neoplastic microenvironments enhance chronic pro-tumorigenic inflammatory state [18]. The inflammatory microenvironment of neoplastic tissues is characterized by the presence of host leukocytes both in the supporting stroma and among the tumor cells, with macrophages, dendritic cells, mast cells, and T cells being differentially distributed [19].

Macrophages represent up to 50% of the tumor mass and are key cells in chronic inflammation. These cells constitute an extremely heterogeneous population, which differentiate into distinct macrophages types, identified as M1 (or classically activated) and M2 (or alternatively activated) [20]. These cells respond to microenvironment signals with polarized functional programs [21]. M1 type macrophages produce Th1 cytokines and predominate in earlier stages of the disease. In contrast, M2 type macrophages secrete factors which favor immunosuppression and tumor development, so they prevail in more advanced disease. Initially, these cytokines have regulatory roles in the tumor microenvironment through growth inhibition, but these functions are lost as tumors slowly progress to a state of immunosuppression. This is the case for IL-6 when is released during initial tumor formation by keratinocytes and macrophages inhibits tumor proliferation. However, in late stages of melanoma progression undergoes transition to stimulator [22].

Mutations and genetic polymorphisms in crucial genes that regulate cytokine function, metabolism and leukocyte survival have also been implicated as aetiological factors in chronic inflammation [23]. Population based studies reveal that individuals who are prone to chronic inflammatory diseases have an increased risk of cancer development [24].

11. The adaptive immune system and melanoma

Melanoma usually remains refractory to immunologic control even when these cells are relatively immunogenic compared to other cancer types. Being melanoma a disease generated by autologous cells, should be possible to instruct the organism to fight against it?

The adaptive immune system is composed of the antigen presenting cells (APC) that include dendritic cells (DC), the most effective APCs and CD4+ and CD8+ T cells. CD4+ T cells include both T helper and regulatory T cell (Treg) populations. In order to initiate an adaptive immune response, APC can activate T cells by efficiently processing exogenous as well as endogenous antigens and present them to T cells through the major histocompatibility complex (MHC). T cells recognize their targets by detecting peptide fragments derived from these foreign or damaged proteins. There are two types of MHC, class I and II. One of the most important features of both molecules is an outer extracellular domain that forms a long pocket in which peptide fragments are located. The most important differences between the two classes of MHC molecules are in the source of the peptides they contain and carry to the cell surface. CD8+ and CD4+ T cells interact with melanoma through contact with MHC class I and II on their cell surface, respectively.

12. Defects in antigen processing and presentation

Presentation of tumor-associated antigens (TAA) on MHC class I by APCs is a crucial step for the differentiation and expansion of CD8+ T cells against TAAs and the eventual destruction of tumor cells.

Melanoma cells have been observed to downregulate MHC class I expression, so preventing any T cell activation and tumor elimination [25]. This tumor has strategies to avoid CD8+ detection and activation. There is clinical evidence that support this statement, since patients with metastatic melanoma show detectable CD8+ T cells specific for melanoma antigens, however, the tumor is not eliminated [26]. Other mechanisms that have been described in this context in melanoma include downregulation of MHC class II antigens [27]. One example is the low expression of HLA-DM, a nonclassical Class II MHC responsible for peptide loading into MHC class II and the removal of the invariant chain li peptide (CLIP) [28]. Melanoma cells also differentially express acidic cathepsins which process endogenous and exogenous antigens in endolysosomal compartments. Their limited activity results in poor Ag processing and the generation of useless antigenic determinants, which are unable of stimulating T cells [29]. Melanoma also has been found to lack the IFNϑ-inducible lysosomal thiol reductase (GILT), essential enzyme for the functional reduction of cysteinylated or oxidized proteins and peptides. The presence of GILT in endolysosomal compartments enhances the acidic cathepsin processing of TAAs and MHC class II components, and the functional processing of cystein-sylated or oxidized peptides for an excellent CD4+ T cell activation. All these defects result in the presentation of a range of nonfunctional peptides which fail to stimulate interacting CD4+ cells, limiting the effects of CD8+ cytotoxic responses.

13. Failure in costimulatory signals

After the Ag processing and the loading of tumor derived peptides into the MHC class II groove, this complex is translocated to the cell surface for presentation to T cells. CD4+ T cells recognize functional class II complexes with antigenic peptides and tight junction binding occurs between the TCR and the class II/Ag complex. CD4+ molecules on T cells then bind to a different site on the MHC class II molecule and T cells receive their first stimulation signal [30]. A second signal is required for activation of the T cell. If the T cells receive a stimulatory signal from the tumor in the form of CD80/CD86 (B7-1, B7-2) binding to T cell expressed CD28, then T cells become activated and may give an anti-tumor response. The most studied immune checkpoint molecule in activated T cell is CTLA-4. It is a high affinity receptor for the ligand B7 expressed by APCs. Ligation is thought to deliver an inhibitory signal, in contrast to CD28. CTLA-4 blockade is thought to act primarily by increasing effector T-cell function.

Coestimulatory molecules are often modified on melanoma cells inhibiting T cell activation, since it has been shown to express high levels of CTLA-4 [31]. Tumors exploit this process, functionally silencing CD4+ T cell activation and shifting the environment to a T regs setting.

Coinhibitory signaling pathway mediated by PD-1 ligand is expressed by activated T cells. It is considered a marker of T cell exhaustion, as engagements by its ligands PDL-1 (B7-H1] and PDL-2 results in T cell inhibition and apoptosis. Of particular interest is the finding that tumor-infiltrating or peri-tumoral lymphocytes in melanoma patients express PD-1 and have impaired effector function [32]. Study shows that melanoma expresses high levels of the ligand for PD-1, PD-1L which during TCR-MHC interaction sends a death signal to both CD4+ and CD8+ T cells causing them to undergo apoptosis [33]. A number of different subtypes of cancer, as well as lymphocytes and APCs in the tumor environment have also been shown to express ligands for PD-1 which may act to suppress PD-1 expressing T cells [34].

14. Immunosupressive tumor microenvironment and cytokines

An upregulation of immunossupressive cytokines such as IL-6, IL-10, TNFα, TGFβ and VEGF is promoted by melanoma microenvironment. The release of these cytokines attracts immunossupressive cells: myelo-derived suppressive cells, tumor associated macrophages, or tolerogenic DCs in the tumor microenvironment.

Polak reported that melanoma cells, melanoma recruited myeloid suppressor cells and Tregs actively secrete IL-10 to induce tolerized T cells and DC. [35] They showed tolerogenic DCs and Tregs present in all stages of disease progression. However, the expression of IL-10 and IDO increased with melanoma progression with the highest production in positive lymph nodes. Their work also suggests that TGFβ2 renders DCs tolerogenic, although for the case of lymph nodes, IDO and TGFβ1 have a higher impact. This mechanism of tumor-associated immunosuppression probably inhibits the immune response to the tumor and may explain the discrepancy between the induction of systemic immunity by anti-melanoma vaccines and their poor impact in the clinic.

It has also been reported that PGE2 is produced by melanoma associated fibroblasts and immature myeloid cells. Luft found that immature monocytes-derived DC that encountered pro-inflammatory cytokines in the presence of PGE2 acquired migratory capacity, but secreted low levels of cytokines. This suggest that not all mature stages of DCs are destined to migrate to lymphoid organs and the sequence in which stimuli are encountered significantly affects which functions are expressed [36]. Additionally, PGE2 inhibits NK T cells activity, once more resulting in changes in the tumor microenvironment towards immunossupression [37]. COX-2 is a multifunctional enzyme that is involved in prostaglandin biosynthesis, and it is upregulated in neoplastic tissues [38]. In several human epithelial cancers, expression of COX-2 correlates with poor prognosis. The crucial molecules that mediate these effects are not yet known, though they might include the PGE2 receptor EP2 subtype (PTGER2) [39].

15. Upregulation of regulatory T cells

Regulatory Tregs comprise 5% to 10% of the total peripheral CD4+T cell population. The main role of Tregs is to inhibit cytotoxic T cell response against self-antigens and maintain systemic tolerance to self-antigens. Tregs constitutively express CD25 (IL-2 receptor α chain) on their cell surface and suppresses CD4+ and CD8+ effector T cells through the release of immunosuppressive molecules, consumption of IL-2 and direct cell to cell contact [40]. The shift to tumor progression results in part, from the alteration in the type and characteristics of TILs within the tumor. These changes include the enhancement of CD4+CD25+FoxP3+Tregs, since in melanoma, particularly in advanced disease states, Tregs are the primary infiltrating lymphocyte where they inhibit all antitumor activity through direct contact inhibition, and the release of high levels of IL-10 [41]. Once activated these cells, are anergic and are able to block the proliferation of effector cells. A study suggests that high serum concentrations of Tregs are associated with poor prognosis, poor treatment responses and an increased risk of recurrence [42]. Human studies depleting Tregs prior to adoptive cell transfer (ACT) improved the effectiveness of treatment. Patients challenged with melanoma antigen peptides, MelanA/MART-1 and gp-100, developed significant induction of peptide specific CD8+ T cells in 90% of them. This study shows that depletion of Tregs in vivo, results in enhanced immune functions and substantial development of antigen-specific CD8+ T cells in vaccinated individuals [43]. Tregs may be harmful for individuals fighting tumors, since under these circumstances the immune system needs maximal activation, but as common tumor antigens are largely self-antigens, suppression of potentially self-reactive T cells by Tregs may be counterproductive in this specific process.

16. Melanoma, an abberrant HLA-G expression

It was previously mentioned that loss or down-regulated of classical MHC class I on melanoma cells is one of the most important mechanisms enabling tumor cells to escape from immune anti-tumor responses. Very similar to tumor cells, fetal cells do not express classical MHC class I molecules, instead these cells express the non-classical HLA-G molecules. The multiple immune suppressive properties of this molecule strongly imply that HLA-G is part of a tolerogenic system. HLA-G exerts exclusively immunossupressive functions, which impair both the innate as well as the acquired immunity by multiple mechanisms. Firstly, the immune effector functions of cytotoxic T lymphocytes and NK cells are inhibited in the case of target cells expressing HLA-G [44]. Secondly, APC expressing HLA-G, inhibit the proliferation of CD4+ T cells, induce CD4+ T cell anergy and cause the differentiation of CD4+ T cells into regulatory cells (Tregs), which as we mentioned previously these cells possess the competence to inhibit the effector function of other T cells. Thirdly, the binding of HLA-G to DC results in disruption of DC maturation, in inhibition of antigen presentation, and in induction of immunosuppressive T cells. Soluble HLA-G molecules fulfill the same tasks as membrane-bound ones. Beyond it sHLA-G molecules are able to inhibit cell cycle progression in T lymphocytes and to mediate the induction of apoptosis on activated T and NK cells [45].

HLA-G is unique in its heterogeneous and unusual molecular structure. Contrary to classical MHC class I molecules HLA-G displays with 23 different alleles a limited polymorphism, in which all amino acid exchanges are located outside the peptide binding groove. Therefore, the diversity of peptides bound by HLA-G is very restricted relatively to classical class I molecules [46]. Thus, it is very unlikely, that this molecule represents a target molecule for the T cell receptor inducing the anti-tumor response. The lymphocyte differentiation marker CD8+ is a classical receptor for MHC class I and as a co-receptor with the TCR during the recognition of peptides being presented by MHC class I. Both, HLA-G and classical HLA class I molecules bind with the same affinity to CD8+. The engagement of sHLA-G molecules with CD8+ results in the induction of apoptosis via the Fas/FasL pathway.

17. Immunotherapy in melanoma: Disappointing results

Recent progress toward an understanding of the interactions between the host's immune system and melanoma has led to the realization that tumor cells have devised many strategies to evade the immune attack. Evasion mechanisms can either be pre-existing, arise through outgrowth of escape mutants or take place during tumor-sculpting actions by the immune system as was proposed in the "Cancer Immunoediting" hypothesis [47]. One of these strategies of tumor-immune escape is represented by the acquistion of FasL expression that may enable cancer cells to deliver death signals to activate Fas-positive T lymphocytes [48]. However, despite all the data accumulated in the support of the FasL counterattack hypothesis, there are many studies in contradiction showing that FasL can also have proinflammatory effects in some contexts [49]. To explain these conflicting findings, it is proposed that the maintenance of immune privileged in tumors depend not only on FasL itsel but also on the production of massive immunosuppressive factors (previously mentioned). The final outcome of an effective antitumor response is determined by a delicate interplay among activating and inhibitory regulatory pathways and the removal of inhibitory signals may be very useful in addition to other therapeutic approaches.

Depending on the subtype of melanoma, patients with metastatic melanoma have a median survival of 8 months and 1 year survival rates of 10 to 15%. The two FDA approved treatments for melanoma are dacarbazine-based chemotherapy and IL-2 with objective response rates below 18% [50]. Several clinical trials in stages IIB-IV of cutaneous melanoma utilizing vaccination with multiple peptides derived from MART-1, gp-100, tyrosinase and MAGE had very limited success in those patients [51].

Nonspecific therapies including the use of monoclonal antibodies against CTLA-4 have leaded to some considerable responses, but this agent has low response rates (12% to 15%) in patients with advanced melanoma.

Active therapeutic immunization has been pursued in clinical trials using a host of tumor vaccines, but these have shown disappointing response rates [52]. The development of therapeutic cancer vaccines is very complex, and it has been learned that stimulation and suppression are the two sides to the coin of manipulation of the immune system and the latter might be increased with the multiple use of a specific vaccine.

Cancer/testis (CT) antigens represent promising targets for immunotherapy because they are expressed in a wide variety of epithelial cancers but are restricted in their expression in normal adult tissues to cells in the testis which lack expression of MHC class I and are not susceptible to damage by T cells that recognize these products. Other members of the CT family of antigens include NY-ESO-1, LAGE-!, SSX1-5, CTp11, CT7, etc. Melanoma cells produce the CT antigens at different frequencies, so more studies are needed to solve if some of these marker proteins might be useful in further clinical studies. The NY-ESO antigen is expressed in 15 to 40% of highly prevalent tumors such as breast, lung, prostate and melanomas. To test the effectiveness of adoptive immunotherapy with genetically engineered cells that target the NY-ESO-1 antigen, phase I clinical trials of cancer vaccines were tried using peptides [53], recombinant vaccinia and fowlpox viruses encoding full-length NY-ESO-1 [54], or recombinant NY-ESO-1 protein [55], but have failed to demonstrate a clinical benefit in patients with advanced disease.

Adoptive cell therapy (ACT) using tumor reactive TILs following host lymphodepletion can lead to objective responsive rates of around 40% and durable responses in patients with refractory melanoma. This ACT used tumor antigen-specific lymphocytes that were initiated in vitro from single-cell enzymatic digests or small fragments of resected tumor specimens and expanded to large numbers before infusion [56]. However, this therapy requires sophisticated cell processing and *in vitro* lymphocyte culturing for long periods. These requirements have technical, regulatory, and logistic challenges that have limited the use of antigen specific TILs as a biological therapy.

Recently, Rosenberg and his group, reported responses of around 45% in patients with melanoma. In their adoptive immunotherapy trial to treat melanoma they used genetic engineering of T cells to express a CT antigen-specific TCR. They reported great variation in levels of T cell persistence between the patients and did not seem to be associated with clinical response to therapy. These findings indicate that treatments using TCRs directed against NY-ESO-1 are effective at mediating tumor regression in some patients (two of eleven patients demonstrated complete regression that persisted after one year) [57]. Given the small number of patients treated in their trial, it is difficult to evaluate the significance of these results.

18. Conclusion

The accumulated data indicate that the outcome of an immune response toward a tumor is largely determined by the type of immune response elicited. A tumor-directed immune response involving CD8+ T cells, CD4+ Th1 cells and NK appears to protect against tumor development and progression.

The future looks promising for melanoma immunotherapy, even with the disadvantages that researchers in the area and clinicians still face nowadays. Most vaccine trials have failed to show an important response rate or an impact on survival. The overall situation, is problematic and it has become clear that large tumors display a setting in which vaccination has a limited role; the most amenable clinical context to assay antitumor vaccination, would be patients in which the existence of micrometastasis, is highly probable. In this case, the immune system has fewer obstacles to surmount. Melanoma patients with satges II and III of the disease could benefit from such therapy.

Of note is the report by Robbins and coworkers in 2011, where they used an adoptive transfer of autologous T cells transduced with a TCR directed against NY-ESO-1, a cancer/testis antigen expressed in 40% of metastatic melanomas, but not in any normal adult tissues except the testis.

They reported two of 11 patients with complete regressions that persisted after one year. Potential strategies that may enhance responses including immunization with recombinant vaccines encoding the NY-ESO-1 antigen, elimination of host Tregs and cotransduction of TCR constructs with genes that encode cytokines such as IL-12 should be taken into account in the future.

Author details

Norma E. Herrera-Gonzalez

Molecular Oncology Laboratory, Posgraduate Section, Superior School of Medicine, IPN, Prol Salvador Diaz Miron y Carpio, Col Sto. Tomas, Mexico

References

[1] Kenneth MurphyPaul Travers, and Mark Walport, Inmunobiología de Janewey, 7th Ed. In: Capítulo 15: Manipulación de la respuesta inmunitaria. Garland Science, New York, NY, pp., 978-0-81534-123-9, 2008-672.

[2] Stutman, O. Tumor development after 3-methylcholanthrene in immunologically deficient athymicnude mice. Science (1974). , 1974, 183-534.

[3] Rygaard, J, & Povlsen, C. O. The mouse mutant nude does not develop spontaneous tumours. An argument against immunological surveillance. Acta Pathol. Microbiol. Scand. (B) Microbiol. Immunol. (1974). , 1974, 82-99.

[4] Maleckar, J. R, & Sherman, L. A. The composition of the T cell receptor repertoire in nude mice. J Immunol. (1987). Jun 1;, 138(11), 3873-6.

[5] Kaplan, D. H, Shankaran, V, Dighe, A. S, Stockert, E, Aguet, M, Old, L. J, & Schreiber, R. D. Demonstration of an interferon γ-dependent tumor surveillance system in immunocompetent mice. Proc. Natl. Acad. Sci. USA (1998). , 1998, 95-7556.

[6] Shankaran, V, Ikeda, H, Bruce, A. T, White, J. M, Swanson, P. E, Old, L. J, & Schreiber, R. D. IFN_ and lymphocytes prevent primary tumour development and shape tumour immunogenicity. Nature (2001). , 2001, 410-1107.

[7] Penn, I. Malignant melanoma in organ allograft recipients. Transplantation (1996). , 1996, 61-274.

[8] Mihm, M. C. Jr. Clemente, C.G. & Cascinalli, N. Tumor infiltrating lymphocytes in lymph node melanoma metastses: a histopathologic prognostic indicator and an expression of local immune response. Lab. Invest. (1996). , 1996, 74-43.

[9] Herrera- González, N. E. Aco Flores A.Y. El melanoma en México. Revista de Especialidades Médico-Quirúrgicas (2010). , 15(3), 161-164.

[10] Balch, C. M, Houghton, A. N, Sober, A. J, Soong, S-J, Atkins, M. B, & Thompson, J. F. Cutaneous Melanoma. 5th ed. St. Louis, MO: Quality Medical Publishing, (2009). 101576262766

[11] Beissert, S, & Schwarz, T. Ultraviolet-Induced Immunosuppression: Implications for Photocarcinogenesis. Cancer Treatment and Research, (2009). Part II, 109-121., 146

[12] Zaidi, M. R, Davis, S, Noonan, F. P, Graff-cherry, C, Hawley, T. S, Walker, R. L, Feigenbaum, L, Fuchs, E, Lyakh, L, Young, H. A, Hornyak, T. J, Arnheiter, H, Trinchieri, G, Meltzer, P. S, De Fabo, E. C, & Merlino, G. Interferon-γ links ultraviolet radiation to melanomagenesis in mice. Nature. (2011). Jan 27;, 469(7331), 548-53.

[13] Kamposioras, K, Pentheroudakis, G, Pectasides, D, & Pavlidis, N. Malignant melanoma of unknown primary site. To make the long story short. A systematic review of the literature. Crit Rev Oncol Hematol. (2010). May;, 78(2), 112-26.

[14] Bandarchi, B, Ma, L, Navab, R, Seth, A, & Rasty, G. From melanocyte to metastatic malignant melanoma. Dermatol. Res. Pract. (2010).

[15] Shirakata, Y. Regulation of epidermal keratinocytes by growth factors. J Dermatol Sci. (2010). Aug; , 59(2), 73-80.

[16] Hsu, M. Y, & Meier, F. Herlyn M: Melanoma development and progression: a conspiracy between tumor and host. Differentiation (2002). , 70, 522-536.

[17] Mortarini, R, Piris, A, Maurichi, A, Molla, A, Bersani, I, et al. Lack of terminally differentiated tumor-specific CD8+ T cells at tumor site in spite of antitumor immunity to self-antigens in human metastatic melanoma. Cancer Res (2003). , 2003, 63-2535.

[18] Zou, W. Immunosuppressive networks in the tumour environment and their therapeutic relevance. Nature Rev. Cancer (2005). , 5, 263-274.

[19] Nakayama, T, Yao, L, & Tosato, G. Mast cell-derived angiopoietin- 1 plays a critical role in the growth of plasma cell tumors. J. Clin. Invest. (2004). , 114, 1317-1325.

[20] Martinez, F. O, Helming, L, & Gordon, S. Alternative activation of macrophages: An immunologic functional perspective. Annu. Rev. Immunol. (2009). , 27, 451-483.

[21] Gordon, S. Alternative activation of macrophages. Nat. Rev. Immunol. (2003). , 3, 23-35.

[22] Lu, C. and Kerbel RS: Interleukin-6 undergoes transition from paracrine growth inhibitor to autocrine stimulator during human melanoma progression. J Cell Biol (1993).

[23] Parsonnet, J. Molecular mechanisms for inflammation- promoted pathogenesis of cancer. The Sixteenth International Symposium of the Sapporo Cancer Seminar. Cancer Res.(1997). , 57, 3620-4.

[24] Balkwill, F, Charles, K. A, & Mantovani, A. Smoldering and polarized inflammation in the initiation and promotion of malignant disease. Cancer Cell (2005). , 7, 211-217.

[25] Cabrera, C. M. The double role of the endoplasmic reticulum chaperone tapasin in peptide optimization of HLA class I molecules. Scand. J. Immunol. (2007). , 65, 487-93.

[26] Harlin, H, Kuna, T. V, Peterson, A. C, Meng, Y, & Gajewski, T. F. Tumor progression despite massive influx of activated CD8 (+) T cells in a patient with malignant melanoma ascites. Cancer Immunol. Immunother. (2006). , 55, 1185-1197.

[27] Goldstein, O. G, Hajiaghamohseni, L. M, Amria, S, Sundaram, K, Reddy, S. V, & Haque, A. Gamma-IFN-inducible-lysosomal thiol reductase modulates acidic proteases and HLA class II antigen processing in melanoma. Cancer Immunol Immunother. (2008). Oct;, 57(10), 1461-70.

[28] Norton, D. L, & Haque, A. Insights into the Role of GILT in HLA Class II Antigen Processing and Presentation by Melanoma. J Oncol (2009).

[29] Goldstein, O. G, Hajiaghamohseni, L. M, Amria, S, Sundaram, K, Reddy, S. V, & Haque, A. Gamma-IFN-inducible-lysosomal thiol reductase modulates acidic proteases and HLA class II antigen processing in melanoma. Cancer Immunol Immunother. (2008). Oct; , 57(10), 1461-70.

[30] Chambers, C. A. The expanding world of co-stimulation: the two-signal model revisited. Trends Immunol. (2001). , 22, 217-223.

[31] Weber J: Overcoming immunologic tolerance to melanoma: targeting CTLA-4 with ipilimumab (MDX-010). (2008). *Oncologist*.

[32] Ahmadzadeh, M, Johnson, L. A, Heemskerk, B, Wunderlich, J. R, Dudley, M. E, White, D. E, & Rosenberg, S. A. Tumour antigen-specific CD8 T cells infiltrating the tumour express high levels of PD-1 and are functionally impaired. Blood (2009). , 114, 1537-1544.

[33] Pilon-thomas, S, Mackay, A, Vohra, N, & Mule, J. J. (2010). Blockade of programmed death ligand 1 enhances the therapeutic efficacy of combination immunotherapy against melanoma. J Immunol 2010; , 184(7), 3442-9.

[34] Thompson, R. H, Gillett, M. D, Cheville, J. C, Lohse, C. M, Dong, H, Webster, W. S, Krejci, K. G, Lobo, J. R, Sengupta, S, Chen, L, Zincke, H, Blute, M. L, Strome, S. E, Leibovich, B. C, Kwon, E. D, & Costimulatory, B. H1 in renal cell carcinoma patients: Indicator of tumor aggressiveness and potential therapeutic target. Proc Natl Acad Sci USA (2004). , 101, 17174-17179.

[35] Polak, M. E, Borthwick, N. J, Gabriel, F. G, Johnson, P, Higgins, B, Hurren, J, Mccormick, D, Jager, M. J, & Cree, I. A. Mechanisms of local immunosuppression in cutaneous melanoma. Br J Cancer (2007). , 96(12), 1879-87.

[36] Luft, T, Jefford, M, Luetjens, P, Toy, T, Hochrein, H, Masterman, K. A, Maliszewski, C, Shortman, K, Cebon, J, & Maraskovsky, E. Functionally distinct dendritic cell (DC) populations induced by physiologic stimuli: prostaglandin E2 regulates the migratory capacity of specific DC subsets. Blood (2002). , 100(4), 1362-72.

[37] Balsamo, M, Scordamaglia, F, Pietra, G, Manzini, C, Cantoni, C, Boitano, M, Queirolo, P, Vermi, W, Facchetti, F, Moretta, A, Moretta, L, Mingari, M. C, & Vitale, M. Melanoma-associated fibroblasts modulate NK cell phenotype and antitumor cytotoxicity. Proc Natl Acad Sci U S A (2009). , 106(49), 20847-52.

[38] Dannenberg AJ & Subbaramaiah KTargeting cyclooxygenase-2 in human neoplasia: rationale and promise. Cancer Cell (2003). , 4-431.

[39] Chang, S. H, Ai, Y, Breyer, R. M, Lane, T. F, & Hla, T. The prostaglandin E2 receptor EP2 is required for cyclooxygenase 2- mediated mammary hyperplasia. Cancer Res. (2005). , 65, 4496-4499.

[40] Camisaschi, C, Casati, C, Rini, F, Perego, M, De Filippo, A, Triebel, F. d. r, Parmiani, G, Belli, F, Rivoltini, L, & Castelli, C. LAG-3 Expression Defines a Subset of CD4+CD25highFoxp3+ Regulatory T Cells That Are Expanded at Tumor Sites. The Journal of Immunology (2010).

[41] Baumgartner, J, Wilson, C, Palmer, B, Richter, D, Banerjee, A, & Mccarter, M. Melanoma induces immunosuppression by up-regulating FOXP3 (+) regulatory T cells. J Surg Res (2007). , 141(1), 72-7.

[42] Vence, L, Palucka, A. K, Fay, J. W, Ito, T, Liu, Y. J, Banchereau, J, & Ueno, H. Circulating tumor antigen-specific regulatory T cells in patients with metastatic melanoma. Proc Natl Acad Sci U S A (2007). , 104(52), 20884-9.

[43] Mahnke, K, Schonfeld, K, Fondel, S, Ring, S, Karakhanova, S, Wiedemeyer, K, Bedke, T, Johnson, T. S, Storn, V, Schallenberg, S, & Enk, A. H. Depletion of CD4+CD25+ human regulatory T cells in vivo: kinetics of Treg depletion and alterations in immune functions in vivo and in vitro. Int J Cancer (2007). , 120(12), 2723-33.

[44] Le Gal FARiteau B, Sedlik C, Khalil-Daher I, Menier C, Dausset J, et al. HLA-G-mediated inhibition of antigen-specific cytotoxic T lymphocytes. Int Immunol. (1999). , 11, 1351-6.

[45] Contini, P, Ghio, M, Poggi, A, Filaci, G, Indiver, F, et al. Soluble HLA-A,-B,-C and-G molecules induce apoptosis in T and NK CD8+ cells and inhibit cytotoxic T cell activity through CD8 ligation. Eur J Immunol (2003). , 33(1), 125-34.

[46] Paul, P, Cabestre, F. A, Ibrahim, E. C, Lefebvre, S, Khalil-daher, I, et al. Identification of HLA-G7 as a new splice variant of the HLA-G mRNA and expression of soluble

HLA-G5,-G6, and-G7 transcripts in human transfec ted cells. Hum Immunol (2000). , 61(11), 1138-49.

[47] Dunn, G. P, Bruce, A. T, Ikeda, H, Old, L. J, & Schreiber, R. D. Cancer immunoediting: from immunosurveillance to tumor escape. Nat. Immunol. (2002). , 3, 991-998.

[48] Whiteside, T. L. Tumor-induced death of immune cells: its mechanisms and consequences. Semin Cancer Biol (2002). , 12, 43-50.

[49] Simon, A. K, Gallimore, A, Jones, E, Sawitzki, B, Cerundolo, V, & Screaton, G. R. Fas ligand breaks tolerance to selfantigens and induces tumor immunity mediated by antibodies. Cancer Cell (2002). , 2, 315-322.

[50] Tsao, H, Atkins, M. B, & Sober, A. J. Management of cutaneous melanoma. N Engl J Med (2004). , 351, 998-1012.

[51] Slingluff CL JrPetroni GR, Olson W, Czarkowski A, Grosh WW, et al. Helper T-cell responses and clinical activity of a melanoma vaccine with multiple peptides from MAGE and melanocytic differentiation antigens. J Clin Oncol (2008). , 26, 4973-4980.

[52] Rosenberg, S. A, & Yang, J. C. Restifo NP: Cancer immunotherapy: Moving beyond current vaccines. Nat Med (2004). , 10, 909-915.

[53] Bender, A, Karbach, J, Neumann, A, Jager, D, Al-batran, S. E, et al. LUD 00-009: phase 1 study of intensive course immunization with NY-ESO-1 peptides in HLA-A2 positive patients with NY-ESO-expressing cancer. Cancer Immun (2007). , 1.

[54] Jager, E, Karbach, J, Gnjatic, S, et al. Recombinant vaccinia/fowlpox NY-ESO-1 vaccines induce both humoral and cellular NY-ESO-specific immune responses in cancer patients. Proc Natl Acad Sci U S A 103:14453-14458, (2006). , 1.

[55] Nicholaou, T, Ebert, L. M, Davis, I. D, Mcarthur, G. A, Jackson, H, Dimopoulos, N, Tan, B, Maraskovsky, E, Miloradovic, L, Hopkins, W, Pan, L, Venhaus, R, Hoffman, E. W, Chen, W, & Cebon, J. Regulatory T-cell-mediated attenuation of T-cell responses to the NY-ESO-1 ISCOMATRIX vaccine in patients with advanced malignant melanoma. Clinical cancer research: an official journal of the American Association for Cancer Research. (2009). , 2166-2173.

[56] Dudley, M. E, Yang, J. C, Sherry, R, Hughes, M. S, Royal, R, Kammula, U, Robbins, P. F, Huang, J, Citrin, D. E, Leitman, S. F, et al. Adoptive cell therapy for patients with metastatic melanoma: evaluation of intensive myeloablative chemoradiation preparative regimens. J Clin Oncol (2008). , 26, 5233-5239.

[57] Robbins, P. F, et al. Tumor regression in patients with metastatic synovial cell sarcoma and melanoma using genetically engineered lymphocytes reactive with NY-ESO-1. J. Clin. Oncol. 29, 917-924 ((2011).

Chapter 4

MITF: A Critical Transcription Factor in Melanoma Transcriptional Regulatory Network

Jiri Vachtenheim and Lubica Ondrušová

Additional information is available at the end of the chapter

http://dx.doi.org/10.5772/55191

1. Introduction

Melanocytes are specialized cells found predominantly in the skin and eyes that form the pigment melanin, a polymer composed of several types of subunits formed from L-3,4-dihydroxyphenylalanine. Melanin is deposited in subcellular particles called melanosomes. Cutaneous melanocytes originate from neural-crest progenitors that migrate to the skin during embryonic development. In the skin, melanocytes reside in the basal layer of the epidermis and are present also in hair follicles. Skin melanocytes form an epidermal unit composed of one melanocyte having long cellular processes and about 30 keratinocytes.

Melanocytes are found also in a benign nevus, a common lesion observed in the skin which is a precursor of malignant melanoma. In the nevus, the melanocytes (called nevocytes) are morphologically different and although nevi are benign and the melanocytes in them are senescent, they may develop, though rarely, into melanoma, a highly malignant tumor whose incidence is rising steadily in western countries. Smaller part of melanoma tumors (approximately 10-15%) occurs in families with hereditary predisposition (Hansson, 2010). Most familial melanomas harbour germline mutations in the CDKN2A gene encoding the p16INK4 protein, a cdk inhibitor. Much smaller number of hereditary cases has germline mutations resulting in amino acid substitutions in the p14ARF or CDK4 proteins. Sporadic cases of melanoma predominate and can be grouped into four clinical subtypes: acral lentiginous melanoma, nodular melanoma, lentigo maligna and superficial spreading melanoma (SSM), which is by far the most common form of melanoma and develop into vertical-growth phase (VGP) melanoma. Lentigo maligna and SSM are most frequently associated with intermittent UV exposure (Gray-Schopfer et al., 2007).

About 60-70% of melanomas harbour mutations of the B-RAF gene (Davies et al., 2002) (in the vast majority the mutation is V600E), while mutations of N-RAS are present in about 10–25%

of all tumors. Activating N-RAS and B-RAF mutations demonstrate mutual exclusivity in melanomas. B-RAF mutations are present already in nevus cells, conferring senescence to these cells by a mechanism known as oncogene-induced senescence, possibly explaining the low rate of malignant transformation of nevi. Activation of these two oncogenes triggers the MEK-ERK kinase cascade that is almost invariantly activated in melanomas; however, other signaling pathways can probably activate the cascade. Therefore, small molecule inhibitors of kinases in the pathway are considered as a promising tool for melanoma treatment (Solit et al., 2006; Bogenrieder and Herlyn, 2011). Although B-RAF inhibitors seem to be rational antimelanoma drugs, resistance occurs in a large proportion of patients, because other stimuli may also activate MAPKs (Alcala and Flaherty, 2012). Many other genes are deregulated during melanoma progression, mainly antiapoptotic genes and genes which are involved in the invasiveness, migration, and metastasis of melanoma, many of which are regulated by MITF-M (microphthalmia-associated transcription factor), a pivotal transcription factor of the melanocyte lineage (Figure 1).

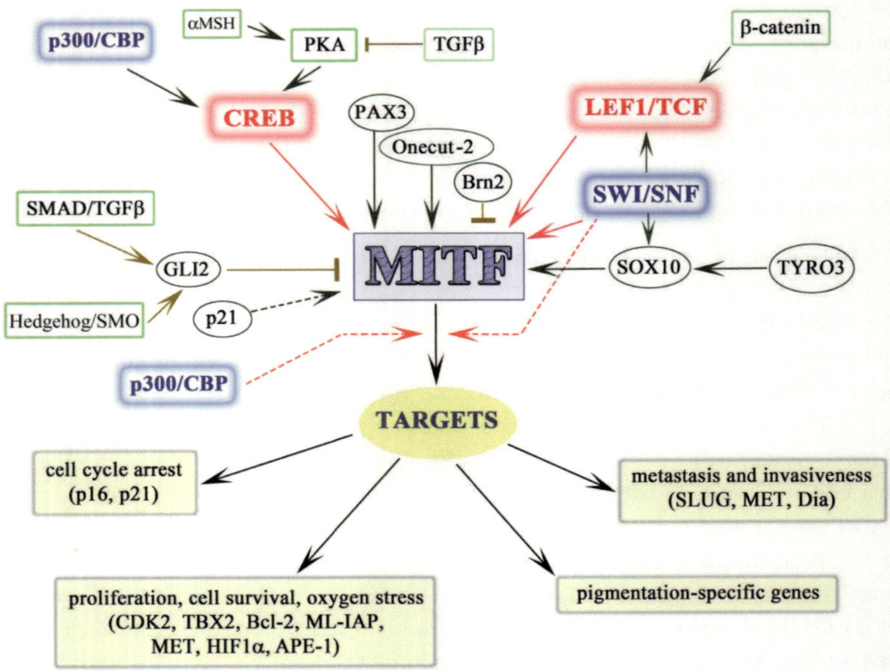

Figure 1. Transcriptional network of MITF-M in melanoma. The picture shows upstream MITF-M activators and main downstream transcription targets. The blue boxes indicate transcriptional coactivators and red boxes denote two transcription factors probably having more important role for the MITF-M expression in melanoma. Broken lines indicate that not all MITF-M targets may be coactivated by indicated epigenetic coactivators.

http://dx.doi.org/10.5772/55191

2. Regulation of MITF expresion

MITF gene locus encodes a transcription factor of the basic-helix-loop-helix-leucine zipper (bHLH-LZ) type, belonging to a large family of bHLH factors comprising also for example the myc oncogenes. Together with TFE3, TFEB, and TFEC, MITF-M constitutes a small bHLH subfamily sharing high sequence similarity. MITF gene was identified twenty years ago and cloned from a microphthalmic and hypopigmented mutant mouse having transgene-insertion at the MITF locus (Hodgkinson et al., 1993). The MITF locus has at least nine promoters producing corresponding MITF isoforms which differ in the first exon and share exons 2-9 (reviewed by Steingrimsson et al., 2004; Levy et al., 2006). Only the MITF-M isoform is melanocyte-specific and expressed exclusively in melanocytes and melanoma cells, whereas some other tissues (osteoclasts, mast cells, heart muscle) express other isoforms of MITF. MITF-M determines the specification of the melanocyte lineage during the embryonic development and stands centrally in the transcriptional network of pigment cells, regulating a number of genes involved not only in melanocyte differentiation and pigment formation (Vachtenheim and Borovansky, 2010; Yajima et al., 2011), but also in the survival, migration, proliferation, invasion and metastasis of melanoma cells (Figure 1).

Regulation of MITF-M transcription is complex and several positive regulators activate the expression (Figure 1), having the corresponding binding motifs in the melanocyte-specific MITF-M promoter. Transcription factor LEF-1/TCF, one of the effectors of the β-catenin pathway, activates MITF-M promoter (Yasumoto et al., 2002). This pathway has been demonstrated to be highly activated in melanoma cells with MITF-M being the necessary mediator of the final pro-survival cellular effects (Widlund et al., 2002; Sinnberg et al., 2011). Transcription factors Sox10 and Pax3 also upregulate MITF-M transcription (Watanabe et al., 1998; Potterf et al., 2000). Sox10 is also stimulated by protein kinase TYRO3, another positive MITF-M regulator in melanoma (Zhu et al., 2009).

CREB is an another transcription factor activating MITF-M expression. The αMSH hormone increases cAMP level, therefore activates PKA (protein kinase A) and the consequence is an increased MITF-M expression and pigmentation. Recently, it has been described that TGF-β represses protein kinase A activity and therefore reduces the CREB-dependent transcription of the MITF-M promoter (Pierrat et al., 2012). CREB requires the coactivators p300/CBP. These proteins, which are histone acetyltransferases, interact with MITF-M and are believed to coactivate at least some MITF-M target genes (Sato et al., 1997; Price et al., 1998). Furthermore, the phosphorylation of serine 73 is required for MITF-M-p300 interaction, at least after the Kit signaling (Hemesath et al., 1998). Controversially, however, it has been observed that MITF-M with mutation of this serine and the N-terminus truncated (including the S73) MITF-M construct were fully capable of activating promoter-reporter and the endogenous target tyrosinase (Vachtenheim et al., 2007).

Whereas the role of p300/CBP in coactivating endogenous targets might be disputable, another prominent epigenetic mechanism has been found to be crucial for MITF-M expression. The chromatin remodeling complex SWI/SNF has been found to be essential for the MITF-M expression in melanoma cells (Vachtenheim et al., 2010). The chromatin remodeling complex

SWI/SNF is composed of about 10-12 proteins and exists in the cells as several subcomplexes capable of changing the local structure of chromatin at the promoter sites. It has important functions in expression of various lineage specific genes and plays an essential function in basic cell processes that include mainly regulation of transcription, DNA replication and repair, and homologous recombination. The SWI/SNF is strongly implicated in human cancer, as several SWI/SNF subunits has been reported missing or strongly downregulated in tumors, and numerous experimental findings suggest that this complex functions as a tumor suppressor (reviewed by Reisman et al., 2009; Wilson and Roberts, 2011). The complex requires at least one ATPase subunit (Brg1 or Brm) and the presence of ATPase Brg1 and Brm is mutually exclusive in the subcomplexes. The components of SWI/SNF are generally highly expressed in melanoma cell lines and at least one ATPase of the complex, Brg1 or Brm, is always present in melanoma cell lines (Vachtenheim et al., 2010; Keenen et al., 2010). The positive effect of SWI/SNF on MITF-M transcription is direct, since both Brg1 and Brm were recruited to the MITF-M promoter in vivo, as revealed by chromatin immunoprecipitation assays (Vachtenheim et al., 2010). In addition, it is possible that SWI/SNF augment the MITF-M expression through LEF-1/TCF because Brg1 interacted with β-catenin and the SWI/SNF complex enhanced transcription of LEF-1/TCF downstream genes (Barker et al., 2001). Recently, we have found (Ondrušová et al., submitted) that Brg1 knockdown in melanoma cells downregulates also Sox10, an upstream MITF-M regulator, so this mechanism might also contribute to the MITF-M regulation. It is intriguing that for most cancers, SWI/SNF complex is a clear tumor suppressor, whereas a small number of cancer types has been recognized (prostate cancer, gastric and colorectal cancer, and melanoma) for which the SWI/SNF seems to function as a tumor promoter, probably by upregulating genes required for proliferation, antiapoptotic activity, invasivity or other characteristics of cancer cells.

It should be noted that the cut-homeodomain transcription factor Onecut-2 (OC-2) also stimulates MITF-M promoter activity. It binds to its promoter (although no OC-2 binding sites were found in the promoter region) and overexpression of ectopic OC-2 in transfected cells stimulates MITF-M promoter activity. Moreover, OC-2 is expressed in melanocytes (Jacquemin et al., 2001). We observed that even cdk inhibitor p21, which itself is a target of MITF-M, is its transcriptional activator (Sestakova et al., 2010). It probably stimulates the CREB pathway and is widely expressed in melanoma cell lines and tumors, and presumably protects malignant cells against apoptotic stimuli.

The POU domain containing transcription factor Brn-2 (N-Oct-3) has been recognized as a repressor of MITF-M expression in melanoma cells (Goodall et al., 2008). Brn-2 bound to MITF-M promoter both in gel-shift assays and in chromatin immunoprecipitation, indicating a direct repression. An inverse correlation between Brn-2 and MITF-M expression was found in melanomas and transfection assays showed that expression of exogenous Brn-2 substantially repressed the MITF-M promoter-reporter. Brn-2 also marked the subpopulation of low MITF-M cells in melanomas (which are heterogenous in MITF-M expression) and these cells displayed low proliferation but high invasiveness (also see below).

One of the effectors of the Hedgehog signaling, transcription factor GLI2, which also mediates the effect of the TGF-β/SMAD pathway, is another repressor of MITF-M expression (Javelaud et al., 2011). GLI2 expression inversely correlates with MITF-M expression in melanoma cell lines, and GLI2 and M-MITF represses each other's expression (Javelaud et al., 2011). The GLI2 expressing cells with low MITF-M level resemble in biological properties the Brn-2 positive tumor cells (see above), having more invasive and migratory behavior. The Hedgehog pathway is derailed in melanoma (Stecca et al., 2007) acting mainly via GLI1 but does not have inhibitory activity on MITF-M expression. Obviously more investigation is required to elucidate the function of the Hedgehog and TGF-β/SMAD pathways and GLI effectors in melanoma.

3. Downstream targets of MITF

A large number of genes is transcriptionally regulated by MITF-M. Which genes are activated also depends on how high is the level of MITF-M and whether the regulation occurs in normal or malignant melanocytes (Goodall et al., 2008; Carreira et al., 2006; Javelaud et al., 2011). Intriguingly, besides many pro-proliferative and pro-survival genes that are regulated by MITF-M, cell cycle inhibitors p21 and p16 are also its targets (Carreira et al., 2005; Loercher et al., 2005), presumably mainly in normal melanocytes or at higher levels of MITF-M, which favor differentiation (Figure 1). MITF-M interacts with the Rb protein (Yavuzer et al., 1995) which cooperates with MITF-M to induce p21 (Carreira et al., 2005). Importantly, MITF-M regulates almost all genes the products of which are involved in specific melanocyte differentiation, i.e. the formation of the pigment melanin and its deposition into melanosomes. The enzymes involved in melanin formation are tyrosinase and tyrosinase-related proteins 1 and 2 (TRP-1 and TRP-2, also known as dopachrome tautomerase, Dct). Even many genes encoding structural melanosomal proteins and factors involved in the melanosome motility are regulated by MITF-M (reviewed in Vachtenheim and Borovansky, 2010). Interestingly, exceptional melanoma cell lines which are transcriptionally silent for MITF-M and do not express the downstream genes tyrosinase, TRP-1, and TRP-2, do not express these markers even after the exogenous transfer of MITF-M, so these cell lines are MITF-M nonresponsive (Vachtenheim et al., 2001). It is therefore likely that the loss of all melanoma markers did occur in these cell lines concomitantly with their absolute dedifferentiation during the loss of MITF-M expression, after which they in fact do not biochemically resemble melanomas.

MITF-M transcriptionally activates a number of genes that act prosurvivally in melanomas. The cyclin dependent kinase 2, which proved crucial in melanoma proliferation (Du et al., 2004) is an important target of MITF-M. MITF-M further regulates HIF1α, a hypoxia response factor (Busca et al., 2005) and APE-1/Ref-1, through which MITF regulates cellular response to ROS (Liu et al., 2009). The c-Met, a receptor kinase for the hepatocyte growth factor, has proinvasive features and promotes metastatic process in several tumors including melanoma. c-Met has been shown to be a target of MITF-M. Gel shift assays with melanoma cell nuclear extracts demonstrated binding by endogenous MITF-M protein to the c-Met promoter at the consensus MITF-M binding site and exogenous MITF-M activated the c-Met expression (McGill et al., 2006). Additionally, MITF-M is a transcriptional activator of Tbx2 gene (Carreira et al., 2000). T-box family of transcription factors are crucial in embryonic development. Tbx2 has been implicated in morphogenesis of a wide range of organs including limbs, kidneys, lung, mammary gland, and heart. Tbx2 is expressed in melanoma cell lines in positive correlation with MITF-M. Tbx2 promoter contains a consensus MITF-M recognition element to which MITF-M is recruited and activates Tbx2 expression (Carreira et al., 2000). As Tbx2 is overexpressed in several cancers including melanoma and plays a role in suppressing senescence, MITF-M modulates the survival of melanoma cells also via this factor.

MITF-M also upregulates the expression of clearly antiapoptotic genes. First, it activates the general antiapoptotic protein Bcl-2 (McGill et al., 2002), which is important for the survival of both melanoma and melanocyte lineage. Second, melanoma inhibitor of apoptosis (ML-IAP, livin) is a potent inhibitor of apoptosis in melanoma and is directly regulated by MITF-M (Dynek et al., 2008). It was shown that MITF-M was recruited to the ML-IAP promoter by chromatin immunoprecipitation and gel shift assays, activated ML-IAP promoter-reporter, and downregulation of MITF-M abrogated ML-IAP expression. The SLUG protein was reported to be a crucial determinant of melanoma metastasis, and its gene is also upregulated by MITF-M (Gupta et al., 2005). Another important gene regulated by MITF-M is Dia (DIAPH1, encoding the diaphanous-related formin Dia1). Increased MITF-M level favors expression of Dia and higher proliferation of melanoma cells. On the contrary, lower MITF-M downregulates Dia but the cdk inhibitor p27 is stabilized resulting in slower proliferation but higher invasive potential. Thus, a "rheostat" model is proposed where MITF-M levels determine the proliferation, differentiation, and invasiveness of melanoma cells (Carreira et al., 2006). Noteworthy, many other genes were identified as potential MITF-M targets, by the microarray analysis (Hoek et al., 2008). The SWI/SNF complex has been shown to be an important coactivator for many target genes, especially those involved in pigment formation, in human melanoma cell lines (Keenen et al., 2010). Of the two ATPases of the complex, Brg1 seems to be more important than Brm since its knockdown downregulates the MITF-M target genes more efficiently than Brm knockdown (Vachtenheim et al., 2010).

MITF-M is considered to be a melanoma oncogene because mutations and amplifications were found in patients′ samples (Garraway and Sellers, 2006; Levy et al., 2006; Cronin et al., 2009). Copy gains at the MITF locus were found in about 10% melanoma samples and mutations of the MITF-M pathway were also described, even in the Sox10 gene (Cronin et al., 2009). Recently, novel MITF-M mutation, E318K, has been identified. This mutation is a germline allele variant (Yokoyama et al., 2011). E318K MITF-M encodes a protein with impaired sumoylation of MITF-M and differential regulation of several MITF-M targets. For example, the mutant enhances MITF-M protein binding to the HIF1α promoter, a MITF-M known target, and increases its transcriptional activity (Bertolotto et al., 2011; Yokoyama et al., 2011). The presence of this allele constitutes more than fivefold risk factor for melanoma and renal cell carcinoma. Further, the mutant protein enhanced melanocytic and renal cell carcinoma clonogenicity, migration and invasion, further implicating this MITF-M variant as a risk factor for these two cancers (Bertolotto et al., 2011). Together, as MITF-M is strictly required for the embryonic development of melanocytes, maintains the survival of melanoma, and gene amplifications and mutations in the protein coding region have been found, it is considered as a lineage addiction oncogene.

http://dx.doi.org/10.5772/55191

Acknowledgements

This work was supported by a grant NT/11229-3 (to J.V.) from the Ministry of Health (IGA, MH) and the institutional research project PRVOUK-P25/LF1/2. L.O. participates in the PhD program at Charles University in Prague, Third Faculty of Medicine, Czech Rep.

Author details

Jiri Vachtenheim* and Lubica Ondrušová

*Address all correspondence to: jiri.vachtenheim@lf1.cuni.cz

Laboratory of transcription and cell signaling, Institute of Medical Biochemistry and Laboratory Diagnostics, Charles University, Prague, First Faculty of Medicine, Czech Republic

Conflict of interest The authors state no conflict of interest.

References

[1] Alcala, A. M. Flaherty KT: BRAF inhibitors for the treatment of metastatic melanoma: clinical trials and mechanisms of resistance. Clin.Cancer Res. 18:33-39, (2012).

[2] Barker, N, Hurlstone, A, Musisi, H, et al. The chromatin remodelling factor Brg-1 interacts with beta-catenin to promote target gene activation. EMBO J. 20:4935-4943, (2001).

[3] Bertolotto, C, Lesueur, F, Giuliano, S, et al. A SUMOylation-defective MITF germline mutation predisposes to melanoma and renal carcinoma. Nature 480:94-98, (2011).

[4] Bogenrieder, T. Herlyn M: The molecular pathology of cutaneous melanoma. Cancer Biomark. 9:267-286, (2011).

[5] Busca, R, Berra, E, Gaggioli, C, et al. Hypoxia-inducible factor 1{alpha} is a new target of microphthalmia-associated transcription factor (MITF) in melanoma cells. J.Cell Biol. 170:49-59, (2005).

[6] Carreira, S, Goodall, J, Aksan, I, et al. Mitf cooperates with Rb1 and activates expression to regulate cell cycle progression. Nature 433:764-769, (2005). , 21Cip1.

[7] Carreira, S, Goodall, J, Denat, L, et al. Mitf regulation of Dia1 controls melanoma proliferation and invasiveness. Genes Dev. 20:3426-3439, (2006).

[8] Carreira, S, & Liu, B. Goding CR: The gene encoding the T-box factor Tbx2 is a target for the microphthalmia-associated transcription factor in melanocytes. J.Biol.Chem. 275:21920-21927, (2000).

[9] Cronin, J. C, Wunderlich, J, Loftus, S. K, et al. Frequent mutations in the MITF pathway in melanoma. Pigment Cell Melanoma Res. 22:435-444, (2009).

[10] Davies, H, Bignell, G. R, Cox, C, et al. Mutations of the BRAF gene in human cancer. Nature 417:949-954, (2002).

[11] Du, J, Widlund, H. R, Horstmann, M. A, et al. Critical role of CDK2 for melanoma growth linked to its melanocyte-specific transcriptional regulation by MITF. Cancer Cell 6:565-576, (2004).

[12] Dynek, J. N, Chan, S. M, Liu, J, et al. Microphthalmia-associated transcription factor is a critical transcriptional regulator of melanoma inhibitor of apoptosis in melanomas. Cancer Res. 68:3124-3132, (2008).

[13] Garraway, L. A. Sellers WR: Lineage dependency and lineage-survival oncogenes in human cancer. Nat.Rev.Cancer 6:593-602, (2006).

[14] Goodall, J, Carreira, S, Denat, L, et al. Brn-2 represses microphthalmia-associated transcription factor expression and marks a distinct subpopulation of microphthalmia-associated transcription factor-negative melanoma cells. Cancer Res. 68:7788-7794, (2008).

[15] Gray-schopfer, V, & Wellbrock, C. Marais R: Melanoma biology and new targeted therapy. Nature 445:851-857, (2007).

[16] Gupta, P. B, Kuperwasser, C, Brunet, J. P, et al. The melanocyte differentiation program predisposes to metastasis after neoplastic transformation. Nat.Genet. 37:1047-1054, (2005).

[17] Hansson J: Familial cutaneous melanomaAdv.Exp.Med.Biol. 685:134-145, (2010).

[18] Hemesath, T. J, Price, E. R, Takemoto, C, et al. MAP kinase links the transcription factor Microphthalmia to c-Kit signalling in melanocytes. Nature 391:298-301, (1998).

[19] Hodgkinson, C. A, Moore, K. J, Nakayama, A, et al. Mutations at the mouse microphthalmia locus are associated with defects in a gene encoding a novel basic-helix-loop-helix-zipper protein. Cell 74:395-404, (1993).

[20] Hoek, K. S, Schlegel, N. C, Eichhoff, O. M, et al. Novel MITF targets identified using a two-step DNA microarray strategy. Pigment Cell Melanoma Res. 21:665-676, (2008).

[21] Jacquemin, P, Lannoy, V. J, & Sullivan, O. J, et al: The transcription factor onecut-2 controls the microphthalmia-associated transcription factor gene. Biochem.Biophys.Res.Commun. 285:1200-1205, (2001).

[22] Javelaud, D, Alexaki, V. I, Pierrat, M. J, et al. GLI2 and M-MITF transcription factors control exclusive gene expression programs and inversely regulate invasion in human melanoma cells. Pigment Cell Melanoma Res. 24:932-943, (2011).

[23] Keenen, B, Qi, H, Saladi, S. V, et al. Heterogeneous SWI/SNF chromatin remodeling complexes promote expression of microphthalmia-associated transcription factor target genes in melanoma. Oncogene 29:81-92, (2010).

[24] Levy, C, & Khaled, M. Fisher DE: MITF: master regulator of melanocyte development and melanoma oncogene. Trends Mol.Med. 12:406-414, (2006).

[25] Liu, F, Fu, Y, & Meyskens, F. L. Jr.: MiTF regulates cellular response to reactive oxygen species through transcriptional regulation of APE-1/Ref-1. J.Invest Dermatol. 129:422-431, (2009).

[26] Loercher, A. E, Tank, E. M, Delston, R. B, et al. MITF links differentiation with cell cycle arrest in melanocytes by transcriptional activation of INK4A. J.Cell Biol. 168:35-40, (2005).

[27] Mcgill, G. G, Haq, R, Nishimura, E. K, et al. c-Met expression is regulated by Mitf in the melanocyte lineage. J.Biol.Chem. 281:10365-10373, (2006).

[28] Mcgill, G. G, Horstmann, M, Widlund, H. R, et al. Bcl2 regulation by the melanocyte master regulator Mitf modulates lineage survival and melanoma cell viability. Cell 109:707-718, (2002).

[29] Pierrat, M. J, Marsaud, V, Mauviel, A, et al. Expression of Microphtalmia-Associated Transcription Factor (MITF), which is Critical for Melanoma Progression, is Inhibited by both Transcription Factor GLI2 and Transforming Growth Factor-beta. J.Biol.Chem. (2012). Epub ahead of print]

[30] Potterf, S. B, Furumura, M, Dunn, K. J, et al. Transcription factor hierarchy in Waardenburg syndrome: regulation of MITF expression by SOX10 and PAX3. Hum.Genet. 107:1-6, (2000).

[31] Price, E. R, Ding, H. F, Badalian, T, et al. Lineage-specific signaling in melanocytes. C-kit stimulation recruits CBP to microphthalmia. J.Biol.Chem. 273:17983-17986, (1998). , 300.

[32] Reisman, D, & Glaros, S. Thompson EA: The SWI/SNF complex and cancer. Oncogene 28:1653-1668, (2009).

[33] Sato, S, Roberts, K, Gambino, G, et al. CBP/as a co-factor for the Microphthalmia transcription factor. Oncogene 14:3083-3092, (1997). , 300.

[34] Sestakova, B, & Ondrusova, L. Vachtenheim J: Cell cycle inhibitor WAF1/ CIP1 as a cofactor of MITF expression in melanoma cells. Pigment Cell Melanoma Res. 23:238-251, (2010). , 21.

[35] Sinnberg, T, Menzel, M, Ewerth, D, et al. beta-Catenin signaling increases during melanoma progression and promotes tumor cell survival and chemoresistance. PLoS.One. 6: e23429, (2011).

[36] Solit, D. B, Garraway, L. A, Pratilas, C. A, et al. BRAF mutation predicts sensitivity to MEK inhibition. Nature 439:358-362, (2006).

[37] Stecca, B, Mas, C, Clement, V, et al. Melanomas require HEDGEHOG-GLI signaling regulated by interactions between GLI1 and the RAS-MEK/AKT pathways. Proc.Natl.Acad.Sci.U.S.A 104:5895-5900, (2007).

[38] Steingrimsson, E, & Copeland, N. G. Jenkins NA: Melanocytes and the microphthalmia transcription factor network. Annu.Rev.Genet. 38:365-411, (2004).

[39] Vachtenheim, J. Borovansky J: "Transcription physiology" of pigment formation in melanocytes: central role of MITF. Exp.Dermatol. 19:617-627, (2010).

[40] Vachtenheim, J, & Novotna, H. Ghanem G: Transcriptional repression of the microphthalmia gene in melanoma cells correlates with the unresponsiveness of target genes to ectopic microphthalmia-associated transcription factor. J.Invest Dermatol. 117:1505-1511, (2001).

[41] Vachtenheim, J, & Ondrusova, L. Borovansky J: SWI/SNF chromatin remodeling complex is critical for the expression of microphthalmia-associated transcription factor in melanoma cells. Biochem.Biophys.Res.Commun. 392:454-459, (2010).

[42] Vachtenheim, J, & Sestakova, B. Tuhackova Z: Inhibition of MITF transcriptional activity independent of targeting CBP coactivators. Pigment Cell Res. 20:41-51, (2007). , 300.

[43] Watanabe, A, Takeda, K, Ploplis, B, et al. Epistatic relationship between Waardenburg syndrome genes MITF and PAX3. Nat.Genet. 18:283-286, (1998).

[44] Widlund, H. R, Horstmann, M. A, Price, E. R, et al. Beta-catenin-induced melanoma growth requires the downstream target Microphthalmia-associated transcription factor. J.Cell Biol. 158:1079-1087, (2002).

[45] Wilson, B. G. Roberts CW: SWI/SNF nucleosome remodellers and cancer. Nat.Rev.Cancer 11:481-492, (2011).

[46] Yajima, I, Kumasaka, M. Y, Thang, N. D, et al. Molecular Network Associated with MITF in Skin Melanoma Development and Progression. J.Skin Cancer (2011).

[47] Yasumoto, K, Takeda, K, Saito, H, et al. Microphthalmia-associated transcription factor interacts with LEF-1, a mediator of Wnt signaling. EMBO J. 21:2703-2714, (2002).

[48] Yavuzer, U, Keenan, E, Lowings, P, et al. The Microphthalmia gene product interacts with the retinoblastoma protein in vitro and is a target for deregulation of melanocyte- specific transcription. Oncogene 10:123-134, (1995).

[49] Yokoyama, S, Woods, S. L, Boyle, G. M, et al. A novel recurrent mutation in MITF predisposes to familial and sporadic melanoma. Nature 480:99-103, (2011).

[50] Zhu, S, Wurdak, H, Wang, Y, et al. A genomic screen identifies TYRO3 as a MITF regulator in melanoma. Proc.Natl.Acad.Sci.U.S.A 106:17025-17030, (2009).

Chapter 5

The Role of Oxidative Stress in Melanoma Development, Progression and Treatment

Fabiana Henriques Machado de Melo,
Fernanda Molognoni and
Miriam Galvonas Jasiulionis

Additional information is available at the end of the chapter

http://dx.doi.org/10.5772/54937

1. Introduction

1.1. Reactive oxygen species: An overview

Oxygen free radicals or, more generally, reactive oxygen species (ROS) are products of normal cellular metabolism. They are well recognized for playing a contradictory dual role in living systems, sometimes deleterious sometimes beneficial, depending on cell type, genetic background and levels and types of species involved. Beneficial effects of ROS occur at low/moderate concentrations and involve modulation of signaling pathways and gene expression regulation. The harmful effect of free radicals is termed oxidative stress and can result in damage to cellular lipids, proteins and DNA. The balance between benign and deleterious effects of ROS is a decisive factor of living organisms and is controlled by mechanisms called redox regulation. This process protects cells from oxidative stress and maintains the redox homeostasis by modulating the redox state *in vivo* [17].

ROS are a group of chemically reactive molecules derived from partial reduction of molecular oxygen, comprising a family of radical and non-radical species. A radical species is a free electron-containing species, including superoxide anion ($O_2^{\bullet-}$) and its conjugated acid hydroperoxyl radical ($HO_2^{\bullet-}$), hydroxyl ($\bullet OH$), carbonate ($CO_3^{\bullet-}$), peroxyl ($RO_2^{\bullet}$) and the alkoxyl radical ($RO\bullet$). Non-radical species, such as H_2O_2, hydrogen chloride (HOCl), fatty acid hydroperoxides (FaOOH), reactive aldehydes and singlet oxygen, can be readily reduced into free electron-containing species [18]. The reactivity of the different ROS with other compounds is variable and depends on their processing into more reactive ROS and the diffusion capability. It was shown that $O_2^{\bullet-}$ and H_2O_2 do not exhibit strong reactivity with other biomolecules, because they are more stable and can diffuse away from their sites of formation. Additionally, H_2O_2 can diffuse through membranes into the extracellular space. In the other hand, •OH radical is highly reactive and probably accounts for most of the oxidative damage attributed to ROS. It half-live time is very short, approximately 10^{-9}s, so •OH produced *in vivo* reacts close to its side of formation. Iron regulation ensures that there is no free intracellular iron, however, *in vivo*, under stress conditions, an excess of superoxide releases "free iron" form iron-containing molecules. The released Fe^{2+} can participate in the Fenton reaction, generating highly reactive hydroxyl radical [19].

These reactive species are generated partly as by-products of cellular metabolism mainly during mitochondrial electron transport. Evidences implicating mitochondria as the principal source of ROS were based on the fact that isolated mitochondria can produce $O_2^{\bullet-}$ through (1) auto-oxidation of the flavin component of complex I (NADH hydrogenase) and/or (2) auto-oxidation of the ubisemiquinone at complex III. During the process of cellular respiration, electron transfer occurs from NADH and FADH through complexes in the mitochondrial membrane, leading to a proton gradient, which is necessary for ATP production. Oxygen is involved as an electron acceptor at the end of the electron transfer in respiration chain. The electron transfer in respiratory chain is not completely efficient due electrons leakage from electron transport chain [20]. Approximately 1-3% of the total oxygen consumed in aerobic metabolism produces $O_2^{\bullet-}$ instead of contributing to the reduction of oxygen to water [18] Direct or indirect damage to mitochondria can lead to electrons leak from electron transport chain, including oxidative modification of mitochondrial membrane lipids (e. g. cardiolipin), resulting in mitochondrial outer membrane permeabilization. So $O_2^{\bullet-}$ is continuously generated mainly at complex I and complex III due to transfer of electrons to molecular oxygen. Superoxide radical that is produced by complex I is released into the mitochondrial matrix, whereas complex III forms $O_2^{\bullet}$- both in the matrix and the inner mitochondrial space [21].

Another major source of ROS is NADPH oxidases, a family of membrane-bound enzymes that catalyze controlled production of $O_2^{\bullet-}$ by coupling NADPH-derived electrons to oxygen. The NADPH oxidase complex consist of a membrane heterodimeric flavocytochrome (cytochrome B559) comprising two subunits, gp91phox and p22phox, and four cytosolic proteins, p47phox, p67phox, p40phox and the small guanosine triphosphate (GTP)-binding protein Rac (1 and 2) that form a functional complex at the membrane [22,23].

Superoxide can be also produced in the cell through one-electron transfer reactions catalyzed by a number of enzymes including monoamine oxidase, xantina oxidase, cyclooxygenases, lipoxygenases and components of the cytochrome P450 system. Peroxisomes are known to produce H_2O_2, but not $O_2^{\bullet-}$, under physiologic conditions [24]. Exposition to chemotherapeutic drugs and UV irradiation also increases the amount of ROS in intracellular milieu [25,26].

Redox homeostasis is determined by the balance between ROS production and detoxification rates by various antioxidants systems. To maintain intracellular free radicals from many sources under tight control, cells have developed a series of defense mechanisms against ROS-induced oxidative stress. The maintenance of intracellular redox state is essential for regulation of signal transduction because alterations in ROS levels can modify proteins conformation and consequently their functions. Enzymatic anti-oxidant defenses include superoxide dismutase

(SOD), glutathione peroxidase (GPx), glutathione reductase (GPx) and catalase (CAT). Non-enzymatic antioxidants systems are represented by ascorbic acid (Vitamin C), carotenoids, flavonoids, glutathione (GSH), α-tocopherol (Vitamin E), thioredoxin and other antioxidants. Superoxide dismutase converts $O_2^{\bullet -}$ in the lesser reactive species H_2O_2 [18,27]. There are three different SODs, which are involved in superoxide neutralization depending on the site of superoxide production or diffusion. Cu,Zn-SOD-1 is located in the cytoplasm, MnSOD-2 in mitochondria and Cu,Zn-SOD3 in the extracellular space [28]. When H_2O_2 is present in peroxisomes, it is decomposed to H_2O and O_2 by catalase. In the cytoplasm, glutathione peroxidase catalyzes the reduction of H_2O_2 into H_2O via oxidation of glutathione [29, 30, 31].

The tripeptide glutathione is the abundant low-molecular-weight thiol antioxidant, constituting with thioredoxin, the major redox buffer of the mammalian cells. Glutathione is present in reduced (GSH) and in oxidized (GSSH) forms and the reduced form of glutathione is 10- to 100-fold higher than the oxidized form. Glutathione couple (2GSH/GSSG couple) is the main responsible for the cellular redox homeostasis and therefore is a representative indicator of oxidative stress [17]. Because cellular glutathione concentration is ~500- to 1000-fold higher than the other redox regulating proteins, changes in the ratio of reduced to oxidized glutathione reflect directly intracellular redox alterations [29]. The GSH/GSSG ratio is normally tightly regulated. Increased ROS levels result in an elevation of GSSH content, which is reduced to GSH by the NADPH-dependent glutathione reductase as well as thioredoxin/glutaredoxin systems. So, even in the presence of oxidative stress, the redox homeostasis can be maintained by increasing glutathione reductase activity or via elimination of GSSG from cells. Glutathione decreases intracellular ROS levels by acting as cofactor of several detoxifying enzymes against oxidative stress, e.g, glutathione peroxidase and glutathione transferase; participating in amino acid transport through the plasma membrane; regenerating vitamin C and E back to their active forms [32]. Glutathione also modulates the activity of thiol-dependent enzymes that contain cysteine residues sensitive to redox changes [33].The enzyme γ-glutamylcysteine synthase (γ-GCS), involved in GSH synthesis, is regulated by ROS levels. Oxidizing conditions that result in GSH depletion promote a conformation change in γ-GCS, increasing its activity and GSH synthesis, while physiological GSH concentrations reduces GSH synthesis through feedback inhibition mechanisms [33].

Peroxiredoxins (Prxs) are also considered important cell redox state-regulating enzymes. Prxs are a family of peroxidases that also reduce H_2O_2 and alkyl hydroperoxides to the corresponding water or alcohol. At least six isoforms of human Prxs (Prx1-6) were located in different subcellular compartments, particularly in mitochondria (Prxs3 and 5). Prxs are maintained in the reduced form by the thioredoxin /thioredoxin reductase system that in conjunction with the GSH/GR system maintains the cellular thiol-disulfide redox status in the cell [34].

The thioredoxin system comprises thioredoxin (Trx), thioredoxin reductase (TrxR) and NADPH. Trxs are small redox active proteins (about 12kDa) with a disulfide active site (Trx-S2) that is reduced to a dithiol (Trx-$(SH)_2$) by thioredoxin reductase (TrxR) using NADPH as electron donor. Mammalian Trx and TrxR are expressed as isoforms either in the cytosol and in the nucleus (Trx1 and TrxR1) or in mitochondria (Trx2 and TrxR2); in addition, there are testis-specific Trx/TrxR system (Trx3 and TrxR3). Unlike Trx, which is reduced by its own reductase, glutaredoxins (Grxs) are coupled to GSH/GR. There are four Grx isoforms in humans, Grx1, Grx-3 and Grx5 primarily cytosolic and Grx2 displays different splice variants, which are located in mitochondria and nucleus [35].

There is a body of evidence showing the involvement of ROS in regulation of innumerous signaling pathways that control important biological processes, including migration, differentiation, proliferation, apoptosis, stress adaptation and gene expression. ROS can modulate multiple transduction signals by activation of growth factor receptors (e.g. the c-MET, EGF and PDGF receptor), activation of early growth-related genes such as c-fos and c-jun, alterations in the activities of protein kinases, oxidative inactivation of phosphatases and activation of transcription factors [36]. In the other hand, increased ROS levels in tumor cells is influenced by numerous factors such as disrupted signaling pathways, altered expression of transcription factors, deregulation of antioxidant enzymes, mitochondrial dysfunction, aberrant cancer cell metabolism, alteration in proliferation and the acquisition of the metastatic phenotype [9, 37].

Redox regulation of signaling pathways occurs through modifications of redox-reactive cysteine residues on proteins, which depend on redox status of the cell and the concentration of ROS. Oxidation of these residues forms reactive sulfenic acid (-SOH) that can form disulfide bonds with nearby cysteine (-S-S-) or undergo further oxidation to sulfinic (-SO_2H) or sulfonic (-SO_3H) acid. These alterations induced by ROS modify the structure and activity of proteins, regulating their functions. These redox modifications are reversible by antioxidants systems, including thioredoxin and peroxiredoxin, contributing to the modulation of signal transduction [8].

2. Reactive oxygen species in cancer development

Since ROS can act as signaling molecules it is reasonable to think that depending on cell context ROS could participate in development of innumerous pathologies including cancer. There is accumulating evidence supporting this view. Levels of ROS are increased in many tumors and murine and human tumor cells lines, contributing to neoplastic transformation and tumor progression [13, 38, 39, 40]. By regulating signal transduction pathways, ROS is involved in the acquisition of cancer hallmarks including self-sufficiency in growth signals, insensitivity to growth inhibitory (anti-growth) signals, evasion of programmed cell death (apoptosis), limitless replicative potential, sustained angiogenesis, tissue invasion and metastasis, altered metabolism and inflammation [40, 41]. The accumulation of ROS participates in the tumor development of many types of cancer including melanoma, leukemia, gastric, prostate, breast and colon cancer [39, 42, 43, 44, 45].

One of the signaling pathways regulated by ROS that is implicated in oncogenic transformation is the mitogen-activated protein kinase (MAPK) cascade that consists of four major MAPKs: the extracellular signal-related kinases (ERK 1/2), the c-Jun N-terminal kinases (JNK), the p38 kinase (p38) and the big MAP kinase 1 (BMK1/Erk5). The apoptosis signal-regulated kinase 1 (ASK1), which regulates the JNK and p38 MAPK pathways, is activated under stress conditions by dissociation of the redox protein thioredoxin. ASK1 is activated when ROS oxidize two cysteine residues in the redox center of thioredoxin, inducing formation of an intramolecular disulfide bond and triggering this dissociation from ASK1 [8]. Activated p38 negatively regulates the malignant transformation induced by oncogenic H-Ras by inhibition of ERK pathway, induction of premature senescence or by cell cycle arrest triggered by p53 [46]. In fact, it was shown that p38 specifically impairs the malignant transformation induced by oncogenes that increase ROS levels (including Ras) by triggering apoptosis and decreasing the accumulation of ROS [47]. MAPK pathways are also activated by the direct inhibition of MAPK phosphatases by ROS. Downregulation of mitogen-activated protein kinase phosphatase (MKP)-3, a negative regulator of ERK1/2, was associated with ubiquitination/proteosome degradation mediated by high intracellular ROS accumulation such as hydrogen peroxide. The aberrant ERK activation contributes to tumorigenicity and chemoresistance of human ovarian cancer cells [48].

Another signaling pathway that contributes to malignant phenotype acquisition, participating in cell survival and proliferation, is the phosphoinositide 3-kinase (PI3K) pathway. Activation of this signal transduction is regulated by the phosphatase and tensin homology (PTEN) phosphatase. It was found that PI3K pathway is reversible regulated by the redox status of the cell by inactivation of PTEN through oxidation of the cysteine located in its catalytic domain [8].

ROS have also been implicated at all stages of the carcinogenic process since are capable of modulating gene expression through oxidative DNA damage and epigenetic alterations [38, 50]. ROS-induced DNA damage includes single- or double-stranded DNA breaks, purine, pyrimidine or deoxyribose modifications and DNA cross-links. DNA damage can result in arrest or induction of transcription, induction of signal transduction pathways, replication errors and genomic instability, all of which are associated with tumorigenesis [19, 51]. The most extensively studied DNA lesion is 8-OH-G, a potential biomarker of carcinogenesis [50]. This oxidative DNA lesion was shown to interfere in the binding of methyl binding proteins to 5-methylcytosines [52], and 8-OH-G located adjacent to the target cytosine can affect the affinity of DNA for DNMT3A [53]. These data indicate that 8-OH-G may play a role in the formation of aberrant DNA methylation patterns during tumor formation. Increased Dnmt1 and global DNA methylation levels were observed in murine melanocytes submitted to sustained stress condition associated with malignant transformation [38]. Increased ROS levels can also induce the recruitment of DNMT1 to damaged chromatin where, together with DNMT3B and members of the Polycomb repressive complex 4, they form a silencing complex in GC-rich areas that might explain cancer-specific aberrant DNA methylation and transcriptional repression [54]. Oxidative stress associated with inflammation also triggers redox signaling through inactivation of HDACs. The reduction of HDAC activity is associated with posttranslational modifications, such as carbonylation [55]. Together, these data suggest a connection among oxidative stress, DNA damage, epigenetic alterations and malignant transformation.

Chronic stress conditions in tumor cells are triggered by an imbalance between ROS production and the ability of cells to scavenge these species. Many studies have shown the increase in Nox expression and activity in transformed cell lines [9, 56, 57]. It was shown that constitutively activated isoform of $p21^{Ras}$, H-Ras^{v12}, in NIH-3T3 fibroblasts improved increased superoxide anion production by Nox1, and was functionally required for oncogenic Ras transformation [58]. Mitochondria dysfunction can lead to oxidative stress, which could be also implicated in cancer development. Besides defects in mitochondrial electron transport chain and prolonged hypoxia and glucose deprivation, disrupted cell signal transduction can also increase mitochondrial-derived ROS in cancer cells. In turn, alteration in mitochondrial bioenergetics modulates signal transduction. It was demonstrated that increased ROS production derived from mitochondria is induced by oncogenic K-Ras and is required to maintain anchorage-independent cell grow and proliferation [59].

Increased ROS levels in malignant cells can arise also from the alteration or inactivation of the antioxidant defense system. Low activities of CuZn-SOD, Mn-SOD, CAT and GPxs have been reported in a variety of transformed and malignant cells compared with their normal counterparts [19]. Decreased activity and expression of Mn-SOD was reported in melanoma, colorectal, prostatic and pancreatic carcinomas [19].

However, it is important to note that only under a mild elevation in intracellular $O_2^{\bullet-}$ and H_2O_2 signaling pathways stimulate proliferation. In the other hand, if the concentration of ROS in the cells is so high these effects can be completely reversed resulting in oxidative stress and death. In this way, cancer cells must render the intracellular milieu pro-oxidant, where ROS has a pro-life role [60], which is supported by the fact that MnSOD acts like a tumor suppressor gene. Many authors have shown the suppression of malignant phenotype after MnSOD re-expression [61, 62, 63]. In addition, intracellular $O_2^{\bullet}$- has the ability to regulate apoptosis sensitivity to a variety of apoptotic stimulus [12,13]. The inhibitory effect of $O_2^{\bullet}$- on cell death signaling can be attributed to caspase proteases, mediators of apoptotic signaling, inactivation by oxidative modifications [60] and by the increased expression of Bcl-2, which is associated with a pro-oxidant milieu [64].

3. Melanoma and oxidative stress

Cutaneous melanoma is a highly malignant tumor derived from pigment-producing melanocytes in the epidermis of the skin. Melanocytes are responsible for the synthesis of melanin in melanosomes, which in turn, is transferred to neighboring keratinocytes where it can protect DNA from UV radiation damage. Melanocytic transformation is triggered by sequential accumulation of genetic and epigenetic alterations that driven modifications in several genes and signaling transduction pathways leading to abnormal proliferation of melanocytes.

Melanoma is one of the most aggressive tumors with a high frequency of metastasis. The incidence and mortality rates of malignant melanoma have increased in the past few decades particularly in Europe and the United States. Although, the etiology of melanoma is not completely known, several molecular and cellular mechanisms have been shown to contribute to melanoma genesis. Chronic stress exposures induced, for example, by solar UV and inflammation are among risk factors for melanoma development [65,66].

Many authors have shown increased ROS levels in melanoma cells through multiple mechanisms [9, 12, 57]. It was also demonstrated that the ability of melanocytes and melanoma cells to respond to oxidative stress is different. While melanocytes have the capability of suppressing increased ROS levels, melanoma cells are unable to do that [67]. This redox imbalance has a central role in melanoma genesis. One of the reasons is that melanoma cells show decreased antioxidant capability characterized by reduced catalase, glutathione-S-transferase and MnSOD enzymatic activity and low levels of glutathione [68, 69], characterizing an aberrant redox state. Moreover, melanoma cells have constitutive abnormalities in their melanosomes [70]. More importantly, it was found that melanoma cells have increased superoxide anion and decreased hydrogen peroxide levels leading to an establishment of a pro-oxidant intracellular milieu and the activation of redox-sensitive transcription factors that enhance the aggressiveness seen in melanoma cells characterized by high proliferative rate and drug resistance [60].

Besides genetic alterations found in melanoma caused by UV, the involvement of ROS in epigenetic alterations was also described in melanoma cells. Increased Dnmt1 and global DNA methylation levels was observed in murine melanocytes submitted to sustained stress condition associated with malignant transformation [38]. The treatment of cells with superoxide anion scavenger abrogated the increase of both Dnmt1 and global DNA methylation level (unpublished results).

4. UV radiation, its connection with oxidative stress and melanoma development

Circumstantial and direct evidences show ultraviolet radiation (UVR) as major environmental risk factor for melanoma formation. One of the evidences is the fact that melanoma incidence is higher in population with light skin types [71]. Skin types depend on melanin production and there are two types of melanin, eumelanin and pheomelanin. People with light skin have more pheomelanin than eumelanin and it has been shown that eumelanin confers more protection against malignant melanoma [72, 73]. Melanin is an important chromophore in the skin which is able to absorb UVR, visible light and scavenge molecular oxygen and hydroxyl radicals, protecting DNA from adducts formation and breaks [4]. In addition, melanoma from sun-exposed areas has different gene mutations than melanoma from unexposed skin areas, suggesting the existence of a particular pathway in melanoma genesis associated with UV radiation [65].

Ultraviolet radiation is subdivided into long wavelength UVA, shorter UVB and shortest UVC. UVC is normally absorbed by ozone at atmosphere and generally does not reach human skin. UVB is absorbed by cells located at outermost layer of epidermis and can be directly absorbed by keratinocytes DNA, causing its damage by producing photoproducts such as cyclobutane pyrimidine dimmers [74]. Additionally, UVB can affect DNA indirectly through oxidative stress generation [75]. In other way, UVA radiation can penetrate deeper into skin and, in addition to be absorbed by keratinocytes, is also absorbed by melanocytes, dermal fibroblasts and other cell types [76]. UVA comprises the majority of UV radiation that reaches earth's surface (95%) and is poorly directly absorbed by DNA, but can indirectly affect DNA by causing reactive oxygen species (ROS) increase and oxidative stress [77]. Oxidative stress can lead to single and double strand DNA breaks, DNA adducts formation, as well lipids and protein peroxidation.

The specific contribution of UVB and UVA radiation to melanocytes malignant transformation is questionable because the majority of *in vivo* and *in vitro* studies focus on UVB radiation. Several studies in mice that develop malignant melanoma show a role of UVB in melanoma genesis, in contrast to this, the role of UVA is less clear. It has been demonstrated that UVB can activate an important differentiation and proliferation signaling pathway, the MAPK pathway, leading to AP1 translocation to nucleus [2]. AP-1 results from heretodimerization of c-Fos and c-Jun proteins, and this complex is important for proper induction of many genes involved in cellular damage protection and repair against ROS damage. This transcriptional factor can operate as an oncogene and it has been related with tumor drug resistance [78, 79]. Additionally, Ming and co-workers [81] showed that UVB radiation induces PTEN down regulation through ERK and AKT pathway activation. The phosphatase and tensin homolog PTEN is an important tumor suppressor gene that negatively regulates PI3K/AKT pathway and its loss is related with many tumors, including melanoma [81, 82, 83]. In contrast with these studies, Kabuyama and colleagues showed in 2001 that while c-Jun is activated in cells irradiated with UVB, ERK activation occurs at same cells only after UVA irradiation [2]. Interestingly, treatment with antioxidants was able to reverse such activations.

When compared to UVB, there are fewer studies showing long-wave UVA radiation role in skin cancer, including melanoma. Recent study in mice did not show an induction of melanoma by a single UVA dose [84]. Nevertheless, there are circumstantial evidences suggesting UVA role in melanoma formation once it gets through clothes in greater quantities than UVB and it comprises the majority of UV radiation. Moreover, UVA, like mentioned before, can penetrate deeper into skin than UVB. It has been shown that high UVA dose causes loss of reduced glutathione and reduces plasma membrane stability in human melanocytes [85]. Glutathione is an important cell antioxidant and loss of its reduced state may reflect the oxidative pressure within this melanocytes as well the plasma membrane stability, once oxidative stress can cause lipid peroxidation. In opposite way to this effect of UVA on melanocytes, this has only been shown before in keratinocytes after UVB irradiation [85]. In addition, a recent work showed an alternative role of melanin in mitochondrial DNA damage only during UVA irradiation, not UVB, providing evidences for dual role of melanin as both protector and damage agent [86]. The accumulation of mitochondrial DNA (mtDNA) mutations, through oxidative stress mechanisms, has been proposed to contribute to carcinogenic and aging process in many tissues, including skin [76, 86].

Regarding the link between UV radiation and oxidative stress in melanoma, it is important to mention the fact that both UVA and UVB irradiation can induce nitric oxide synthases (NOS) expression at skin [87, 88, 89]. Warren and colleagues showed, for example, that an intradermal injection of L-NAME (NOS inhibitor) prevented erythema caused by UV radiation exposition in rats [87]. In addition, nitric oxide in combination with superoxide anion can form peroxynitrite, which leads to lipids and proteins peroxidation. Additionally, peroxynitrite might oxidize tetrahydrobiopterin (BH4) NO syntases' cofactor, what could cause NOS uncoupling. A critical aspect of NOS function is the requirement for the cofactor BH4, its absence destabilize NOS, which becomes "uncoupled". Uncoupled NOS produces superoxide anion instead of nitric oxide [12]. NOS-dependent superoxide formation has central role in the pathology of vascular diseases like diabetes, hypertension and atherosclerosis, but less is known about this phenomenon in cancer [90, 91]. Nevertheless, results from our group showed for the first time the involvement of the uncoupled eNOS in the generation of superoxide in melanoma genesis [12].

As showed, a potential causative role of ultraviolet radiation in oxidative stress and melanoma genesis has been investigated; however, more studies are necessary to fully understand this association.

5. UV-induced inflammation, immunosuppression and melanoma

The exposure of skin to UV irradiation results in increased blood flow, infiltration by macrophages and neutrophils, as well higher levels of nitric oxide and prostaglandins [87, 92]. This phenomenon is clinically observed as inflammation. Other UV-induced mediators such as tumor necrosis factor (TNF) and interleukin-1α (IL-1α) also contribute to inflammation. The recruited inflammatory cells produce ROS that, like mentioned before, drive damage to lipids, proteins and DNA. This damage could lead to genetic and epigenetic alterations and contribute to cancer development [38, 93, 94]. ROS and NO can be associated with all steps of tumor progression, causing oncogene activation, tumor suppressor inhibition through mutations or aberrant epigenetic modifications, angiogenesis, local invasion and metastasis [95].

Another feature of UV radiation is the fact that it can cause local and systemic immunosuppression on skin. The precise mechanism is not fully elucidated, but DNA damage is regarded as fundamental inciting event, which leads to depletion of Langerhans cells from epidermis, interfering with antigen recognition [96, 97]. It was observed that immunosuppression induced by UVA radiation diminishes immune surveillance and allows cutaneous melanoma development in transgenic mice [84]. Some additional evidences suggest that NO might be involved in passing a "migration signal" to the Langerhans cells that stimulates them to migrate and leave epidermis [98]. In this way, nitrosative stress could be involved both in inflammation and immunosuppression mechanisms linked with carcinogenesis.

6. The role of NADPH oxidase enzymatic complex in melanoma genesis

Melanoma cells spontaneously generate ROS and present alteration in NOX expression. NOX family, that comprises *NOX1*, *NOX2* (also called gp91), *NOX3*, *NOX4* and *NOX5*, consists of catalytic subunit of NADPH oxidase enzymatic complex, one of cells' superoxide anion sources, as mentioned before. The active form of this multi-protein complex is also normally composed by transmembrane $p22^{phox}$ and cytosolic proteins, $p40^{phox}$, $p46^{phox}$, $p67^{phox}$ and Rac. It has been observed that while melanoma cells present NOX2, $p22^{phox}$, $p67^{phox}$ and *NOX4* expression, epidermal melanocytes express only $p22^{phox}$ and *NOX4* [99]. Moreover, NOX4, that does not present Rac cytosolic subunit, was found up regulated in several melanoma cell lines and it seems to be important to regulation of G2-M cell cycle progression [57]. Interestingly, Govindarajan and co-workers [9] showed that AKT signaling is responsible by NOX4 overexpression in melanoma cell line WM35. These authors also observed that these events seem to be necessary to conversion of melanoma with radial growth to melanoma with vertical growth behavior. In addition to *NOX4* role in melanoma, recent research paper showed increased *NOX1* protein level and activity in melanoma cell lines compared to melanocytes. The same work showed that NOX1 overexpression increases melanoma cells invasion on matrigel and stable clones overexpressing Nox1 exhibited epithelial-mesenchymal transition [100].

There are few studies about NOX role in melanoma and more studies in this area may elucidate how NADPH oxidases might regulate specific signaling pathways during melanocyte malignant transformation and melanoma progression.

7. Mitochondria dysfunction as a ROS source in melanoma and therapeutic target

Recently, the role of mitochondrial functions, such as redox regulation and oxidative phosphorylation in melanoma progression has become to be elucidated. It was shown that dysfunctional mitochondria affect melanoma cell survival and death and drug resistance [101]. Tumor cells normally produce ATP via glucose metabolism with concomitantly decrease in ATP production by oxidative phosphorylation [102]. Unlike most tumor cells, melanoma cells rely more on oxidative phosphorylation than glycolysis to produce ATP. Compared with solid tumor xenografts, human melanoma xenografts have one of the highest rates of oxygen consumption, a surrogate marker of oxidative phosphorylation [101, 103]. Moreover, non-glycolytic metabolic sources, such as the Krebs cycle, occur more frequently in melanoma cells compared with melanocytes [104]. It was also shown that a particular group of patients with advanced melanoma utilize oxidative phosphorylation for energy production in addition to glycolysis [105]. Consequently, the mitochondria of melanoma cells generate high levels of ROS. These features make mitochondria a potential chemotherapy target in melanoma. In fact, it was shown that the drug Elesclomol, that alter redox balance and induce oxidative stress, lead to melanoma cells apoptosis by inhibiting oxidative phosphorylation through down regulation of proteins from electron respiratory chain. In addition, it was also demonstrated that melanoma cells with high levels of lactate dehydrogenase (LDH) (***--q), with characterizes ATP production mainly by glucose metabolism, are more resistant to Elesclomol [101]. Analysis of patients with normal lactate LDH versus patients with high serum LDH levels showed that the increase in LDH levels is a prognostic factor for metastatic melanoma [106].

8. Melanin: A pro-oxidant molecule contributing to melanoma genesis

In normal melanocytes, melanin is generated from the successive oxidation of tyrosine by tyrosinase in sub organelles called melanosomes to protect DNA, including mitochondrial

DNA, from UV radiation-induced damage [86]. Moreover, melanin neutralizes the inflammatory response to radiation and acts like an antioxidant, suppressing superoxide anion, singlet oxygen and hydrogen peroxide [107]. However, in melanoma cells, melanogenesis itself is a source of ROS and oxidative stress because of malformed melanosomes and melanin synthesis disruption [108]. Therefore, depending on the melanin type and redox intracellular state, melanin can play a dual role, both as a photoprotector and as a photosensitizer [86]. In melanoma cells, melanosomes are poorly compartmentalized, with malformed or twinned membranes, occlusions within the melanin and evident fragments outside of melanosome [109]. The structural differences between melanosomes from melanocyte and melanoma cells are significant, as melanosomal compartmentalization protects the cell from the highly reactive small-molecules catechols that are generated as by products during melanogenesis [108]. Ultrastructural studies of human melanosomes also indicate that melanocytes generally have fewer melanosomes than malignant melanoma [110]. Melanin deregulation renders it a pro-oxidant with ability to increase ROS levels and damage DNA [111]. In addition, melanin exposition to radiation also renders it pro-oxidant [107]. It is important to note that disturbed melanin synthesis and chronic oxidative stress are present in dysplastic nevi, indicating that the switch of melanin to a pro-oxidant state occurs early in melanoma development [112].

Melanins are naturally associated with a number of metal ions and have the capability to accumulate metals. However, oxidized melanin has high affinity for metal ions *in vivo* and the binding of metal ions alters dramatically chemical properties of melanin, increasing it susceptibility to further oxidation and the rate of melanin bleaching [113]. Therefore, it was suggested that metals ions are associated to melanin conversion from a normal reducing status to a pro-oxidant state. The binding of divalent zinc or cooper to melanin increases the capability of melanin to react with oxygen by redox cycling and induces the increase in superoxide and hydroxyl radicals [113]. There are several studies implicating heavy metal ions, including zinc, cooper and cadmium, in the pathogenesis of melanoma [112, 114]. In fact, melanoma tumors accumulate high concentrations of Cu and other metals in comparison with melanocytes, which induce oxidative stress [115]. Moreover, Cu is a critical cofactor for the enzyme tyrosinase and is found in abundance in melanosomes from melanocytes and melanoma cells [107]. It was shown that the pro-oxidant state of melanin can be a selective target in melanoma. The treatment of melanoma cells with Zn and Cu dithiocarbamate complexes, which are known to increase the uptake of metal ions into the cell, augmented the redox cycling of melanin and the oxidative stress, leading melanoma cells to apoptosis. Interestingly, the treatment was less toxic to melanocytes [113].

Melanin synthesis is regulated mainly by the alpha-melanocyte stimulating hormones (α-MSH), which bind to the melanocortin 1 receptor (MC-1R) and activate the cAMP pathway, which in turn, triggers its downstream effector molecules Protein Kinase A (PKA) and cAMP-Responsive Element Binding (CREB) transcription factors to up-regulate the expression of microphtalmia-associated transcription factor (MITF). MITF induces the transcription of tyrosinase, the rate-limiting enzyme in the synthesis of melanin [116]. Recently, it was shown that melanin synthesis is regulated by Nox4-induced ROS in a feedback mechanism regulated by MITF signaling pathway in melanoma cells [37]. The expression of Nox4 and ROS production was increased by α-MSH and was dependent of MITF signaling. Expression silencing of Nox4 gene increased melanin formation through MITF and tyrosinase activation upregulation, unraveling a novel negative regulatory mechanism of pigmentation in melanoma cells. This could be an adaptive mechanism of melanoma cells submitted to chronic stress condition to maintain redox homeostasis: decreasing oxidative stress by inhibiting the synthesis of pro-oxidant melanin.

9. Uncoupled endothelial nitric oxide synthase as a superoxide anion source: Its role in melanocyte transformation and melanoma progression

There is a lot of evidence showing the involvement of inducible nitric oxide synthase (iNOS) in melanoma development. Its strong association with poor patient survival seems to indicate that iNOS is a molecular marker of poor prognosis or a putative target for therapy. All these studies show the role of nitric oxide, a free radical produced by NOS, in proliferation and apoptosis [118, 119]. Recently, the role of NO derived from eNOS in melanoma induced by chronic stress was shown [117]. In fact, $eNOS^{-/-}$ mice are resistant to tumor development [120, 121]. However, NOS can be also a source of superoxide anion [10, 11].

It has been extensively demonstrated that uncoupled NOS can generate superoxide, which has a central role in the pathogenesis of vascular diseases, such as diabetes, hypertension and atherosclerosis. NOS are homodimeric oxidoreductases that catalyze NO production from L-arginine guanidine nitrogen using molecular oxygen. The NOS reductase domain generates electron that flow from NADPH through FAD and FMN flavins and are transferred to the oxidase domain of the other monomer in which L-arginine oxidation occurs at the heme group in the active site. A critical aspect of NOS function is the requirement of the cofactor tetrahydrobiopterin (BH4). In its absence, NOS dimerization is lost and NOS catalytic activity becomes uncoupled. In this state, NADPH oxidation and molecular oxygen reduction are uncoupled from L-arginine hydroxylation and nitric oxide (NO) formation. However, electron transfer from NADPH to molecular oxygen is not inhibited, resulting in superoxide production [10, 11].

An *in vitro* murine melanocyte malignant transformation model was developed in our laboratory after submitted a non-tumorigenic melanocyte lineage, melan-a, to a chronic stressful condition [122], which resulted in the establishment of pre-malignant and melanoma cell lines. It was demonstrated that along tumor progression increased superoxide and decreased NO levels were produced. The treatment with L-sepiapterin, a BH4 precursor, decreased superoxide and increased NO levels in melanoma cells [12]. The abrogation of superoxide anion levels rendered melanoma cells less *anoikis*-resistant. More importantly, L-NAME, a NOS inhibitor that decreases superoxide anion levels, impaired the acquisition of a malignant phenotype by melan-a that was subjected to a sustained stressful condition [12, 38]. Moreover, the expression of GTP cyclohydrolase I, the rate-limiting enzyme in the synthesis of BH4, is decreased in melanoma cells (unpublished results). Together, these data show that the superoxide production by eNOS uncoupling may be important for melanoma cells survival and melanocyte malignant transformation. The possible use of BH4 as a chemo-preventive agent for melanoma development is under investigation in our laboratory.

10. Redox signaling in melanoma

The appropriate proceeding of tumor cells exposed to ROS is associated with activation of different signaling pathways that in turn regulate transcriptional changes that allow cells to respond and adapt to oxidative stress for maintenance of homeostasis. These alterations are regulated by redox sensors such as apurinic/apyrimidinic endonuclease (APE-1/Ref-1). APE/Ref-1 is a point of convergence for various redox-sensitive signals as well as being important in DNA repair. Many studies demonstrated that many survival, proliferation and anti-apoptotic signaling pathways are activated by APE/Ref-1–mediated transcription factors, such as AP-1, NF-κB, HIF-1α and p53, whose regulation occurs in both a redox-dependent and a redox-independent manner [36]. Elevated APE/Ref-1 was associated with decreased intracellular ROS levels as well as reduced oxidative DNA-damage lesions. However, the prolonged activation of APE/Ref-1 induced by a sustained stress condition, switches the cellular signaling to proliferation and apoptosis resistance. It was shown that increased expression of APE/Ref-1 and increased ROS levels play a role in malignant transformation by increasing anchorage-independent growth and colony formation [123]. Moreover, knockdown of APE/Ref-1 was shown to efficiently induce apoptosis, sensitization, or both to chemical treatments [124]. It is also well documented that elevated APE/Ref-1 is associated with chemo- and radio-resistance in a number of cellular systems. Recently, this group also suggested that APE/Ref-1 is involved in the regulation of metastasis produced by melanoma cells [125]. These studies suggested that, as an adaptive response induced by APE/Ref-1, this transcription factor besides efficiently repairs oxidative DNA damage, also regulates redox-sensitive signaling such as AP-1 and NF-κB, which are involved in melanoma genesis. In fact, it was demonstrated the increased expression of APE/Ref-1 in melanoma specimens and cells, which is predominantly found in the nucleus and contributed to the binding and activation of AP-1 and NF-κB [123, 124]. Therefore, all these properties make APE/Ref-1 a promise target for melanoma therapy.

A signaling pathway disrupted in melanoma cells that is redox-sensitive is the Ras/BRAF/MEK/ERK [126]. We have observed that activation of Ras-ERK signal transduction in melan-a melanocytes during loss of integrin-mediated cell-matrix contact is regulated and regulates superoxide anion levels which is associated with global DNA hypermethylation (unpublished results). This aberrant signaling seems to have a significant impact in melanoma genesis since the malignant transformation was drastically compromised when melan-a melanocytes were pre-treated with superoxide scavenger.

Another pathway involved in melanoma progression that is responsive to alterations in redox homeostasis is p38 signal pathway. In melanocytes exposed to oxidative stress and UV-irradiation, p38 is activated and induces the expression of p16I^{NK4A}, which in turn decreases ROS levels [127]. It can be a mechanism by which the tumor suppressor gene p16^{INK4A} protects melanocytes against malignant transformation. According to this point, it was shown by many authors that induction of apoptosis in melanoma cells is dependent on p38 activation [128, 129].

11. Antioxidant therapy for melanoma

Many cancer types have some imbalance in physiologic antioxidant levels compared with the cell of origin like was mentioned before in this chapter [130]. Moreover, levels of anti-oxidant enzymes and non-enzymatic antioxidants such as catalase, MnSOD, glutathione (GSH), vitamins E, C and A are all typically decreased in tumors [131]. Although mutations in MnSOD gene have been demonstrated in some melanomas, the other antioxidant enzymes were found with high activity in this type of cancer cells [61, 131].

The redox imbalance found in melanoma cells is implicated in the malignant phenotype of these cells, characterized by abnormal proliferation, apoptosis resistance and metastasis capability through regulation of key signaling pathways. These observations support the notion that melanoma could be targeted using antioxidant therapy.

One of antioxidants, approved by Food and Drug Administration (FDA) and used to treat pulmonary fibrosis, is N-acetylcysteine (NAC) [132]. Studies in mouse showed that orally administrated NAC reduced UV-induced squamous carcinoma [133]. Moreover, Cotter and colleagues showed that NAC protects melanocytes from oxidative stress and delays UV-induced melanoma growth in mice [134]. In addition, other studies observed that topical NAC reduced UV-mediated GSH depletion and peroxide induction in normal human skin [135, 136]. The antioxidant vitamin E delays or reduces UV-induced skin carcinogenesis in mice, through reduction in DNA damage, immunosuppression or both [137]. Other epidemiologic studies showed that increased vitamins D and C intakes have some influence in melanoma prevention [14].

As mentioned above, the redox transcription factor sensor APE/Ref-1 has a potential as a target for the development of a new chemopreventive agent against cancer. Using docking-and-scoring technology and virtual screening, resveratrol was found to dock in one of the two drug-treatable pockets located in the redox domain of APE/Ref-1 [124]. The inhibitory effects of resveratrol on APE/Ref-1 occurred mostly through its redox-regulating functions and might be the principal role on its pharmacological activities, which are implicated in the reduced AP-1 and NF-κB activities in many human cancers [138]. In studies using human melanoma cells, resveratrol was shown to inhibit, in a dose-dependent manner, the APE1/Ref-1-mediated DNA-binding of AP-1. Resveratrol was also shown to inhibit APE1/Ref-1 endonuclease activity and render melanoma cells more sensitive to treatment with the alkylating agent dacarbazine [124]. More recently, a small molecule called E3330 was developed and showed strong inhibition of APE/Ref-1 *in vitro* [139]. The use of E3330 inhibited the interaction between retinoic acid receptor and its DNA response elements, which is redox-sensitive and mediated by APE/Ref-1, and increased the differentiation and apoptosis of myeloid leukemia cells induced by retinoic acid [140]. Therefore, these compounds may represent a novel class of anticancer agents and promising candidates for *in vivo* studies.

Although promising, treatment of melanoma with antioxidants has not yet achieved the desired results. One hypothesis is that antioxidants can be used as chemopreventive drugs, since the main role of ROS seems to be in the early progression of melanoma, when the tumor is fully installed.

12. Conclusion

Melanocytes are naturally exposed to oxidative stress due to UV, UV-associated inflammation and metal ions accumulation. However, melanocytes have a great capability to regulate their redox homeostasis due increased antioxidant activity and redox buffer characteristic of melanin. The disruption of redox regulation in melanocytes is not clear, but seems to be a consequence of many factors, including decreased of antioxidant enzymes expression and activity as MnSOD and glutathione levels, the switch of melanin to a pro-oxidant molecule and disturbance of signaling pathways that control melanocytes proliferation. Therefore, increased ROS levels found in melanoma cells are not a simple consequence of altered metabolism, but instead seem to have a central role in melanocyte malignant transformation and in abilities acquired during tumor progression as chemoresistance. The establishment of a pro-oxidant microenvironment also contributes to melanoma progression, implicating inflammatory cells as essential sources of ROS. Many mechanisms are associated with ROS accumulation in melanoma cells, including mitochondria dysfunction, increased NADPH oxidase activity and NOS uncoupling. ROS are implicated in regulating several biological processes by acting downstream important signaling pathways. Moreover, ROS regulate gene expression by genetic and epigenetic alterations. Although ROS are implicated in all stages of melanocyte malignant transformation, the uses of antioxidants as therapeutic strategies have not been successful. However, its use as a chemopreventive strategy has been shown to be efficient. Hence, efforts should be concentrated in the studies of the use of antioxidants as chemopreventive drugs for melanoma.

Acknowledgements

This work was supported by FAPESP (2011/12306-1 to MGJ and 2008/50366-3 to FM) and CAPES (2867/10 to FHMM).

Author details

Fabiana Henriques Machado de Melo[1,2], Fernanda Molognoni[2] and
Miriam Galvonas Jasiulionis[2*]

*Address all correspondence to: mjasiulionis@gmail.com

1 Microbiology, Immunology and Parasitology Department, Universidade Federal de São Paulo, São Paulo, Brazil

2 Pharmacology Department, Universidade Federal de São Paulo, São Paulo, Brazil

References

[1] Fruehauf, J. P. Meyskens FL Jr. Reactive oxygen species: a breath of life or death? Clin Cancer Res. (2007). , 13(3), 789-94.

[2] Kabuyama, Y, Homma, M. K, Sekimata, M, & Homma, Y. Wavelength-specific activation of MAP kinase family proteins by monochromatic UV irradiation. Photochem Photobiol (2001). , 73(2), 147-52.

[3] Brar, S. S, Kennedy, T. P, Whorton, A. R, Sturrock, A. B, Huecksteadt, T. P, Ghio, A. J, & Hoidal, J. R. Reactive oxygen species from NAD(P)H:quinone oxidoreductase constitutively activate NF-kappaB in malignant melanoma cells. Am J Physiol Cell Physiol (2001). C, 659-76.

[4] Hussein, M. R. Ultraviolet radiation and skin cancer: molecular mechanisms. J Cutan Pathol (2005). , 32(3), 191-205.

[5] Ueda, Y, & Richmond, A. NF-kappaB activation in melanoma. Pigment Cell Res (2006). , 19(2), 112-24.

[6] Xanthoudakis, S, Miao, G, Wang, F, Pan, Y. C, & Curran, T. Redox activation of Fos-Jun DNA binding activity is mediated by a DNA repair enzyme. EMBO J (1992). , 11(9), 3323-35.

[7] Smeal, T, Binetruy, B, Mercola, D. A, Birrer, M, & Karin, M. Oncogenic and transcriptional cooperation with Ha-Ras requires phosphorylation of c-Jun on serines 63 and 73. Nature (1991). , 354(6353), 494-6.

[8] Ray, P. D, Huang, B. W, & Tsuji, Y. Reactive oxygen species (ROS) homeostasis and redox regulation in cellular signaling. Cell Signal. (2012). May;, 24(5), 981-90.

[9] Govindarajan, B, Sligh, J. E, Vincent, B. J, Li, M, Canter, J. A, Nickoloff, B. J, Rodenburg, R. J, Smeitink, J. A, Oberley, L, Zhang, Y, Slingerland, J, Arnold, R. S, Lambeth, J. D, Cohen, C, Hilenski, L, Griendling, K, Martínez-diez, M, Cuezva, J. M, & Arbiser, J. L. Overexpression of Akt converts radial growth melanoma to vertical growth melanoma. J Clin Invest (2007). , 117(3), 719-29.

[10] Cardounel, A. J, Xia, Y, & Zweier, J. L. Endogenous methylarginines modulate superoxide as well as nitric oxide generation from neuronal nitric-oxide synthase: differences in the effects of monomethyl- and dimethylarginines in the presence and absence of tetrahydrobiopterin. J Biol Chem (2005). , 280(9), 7540-9.

[11] Rabelink, T. J, & Luscher, T. F. Endothelial nitric oxide synthase: host defense enzyme of the endothelium? Arterioscler Thromb Vasc Biol (2006). , 26(2), 267-71.

[12] Melo, F. H, Molognoni, F, Morais, A. S, Toricelli, M, Mouro, M. G, Higa, E. M, Lopes, J. D, & Jasiulionis, M. G. Endothelial nitric oxide synthase uncoupling as a key medi-

ator of melanocyte malignant transformation associated with sustained stress conditions. Free Radic Biol Med (2011). , 50(10), 1263-73.

[13] Pervaiz, S, Ramalingam, J. K, Hirpara, J. L, & Clément, M. V. Superoxide anion inhibits drug-induced tumor cell death. FEBS Lett. (1999). Oct 15;, 459(3), 343-8.

[14] Jensen, J. D, Wing, G. J, & Dellavalle, R. P. Nutrition and melanoma prevention. Clin Dermatol. (2010). Nov-Dec; , 28(6), 644-9.

[15] Jang, M, Cai, L, Udeani, G. O, Slowing, K. V, Thomas, C. F, Beecher, C. W, Fong, H. H, Farnsworth, N. R, Kinghorn, A. D, Mehta, R. G, Moon, R. C, & Pezzuto, J. M. Cancer chemopreventive activity of resveratrol, a natural product derived from grapes. Science (1997). , 275(5297), 218-20.

[16] Lao, C. D, Demierre, M. F, & Sondak, V. K. Targeting events in melanoma carcinogenesis for the prevention of melanoma. Expert Rev Anticancer Ther (2006). , 6(11), 1559-68.

[17] Dröge, W. Free radicals in the physiological control of cell function. Physiol Rev. (2002). Jan;, 82(1), 47-95.

[18] Valko, M, Leibfritz, D, Moncol, J, Cronin, M. T, Mazur, M, & Telser, J. Free radicals and antioxidants in normal physiological functions and human disease. Int J Biochem Cell Biol. (2007). , 9(1), 44-84.

[19] Valko, M, Rhodes, C. J, Moncol, J, Izakovic, M, & Mazur, M. Free radicals, metals and antioxidants in oxidative stress-induced cancer. Chem Biol Interact. (2006). Mar 10;, 160(1), 1-40.

[20] Kang, J, & Pervaiz, S. Mitochondria: redox metabolism and dysfunction. Biochem Res. Int. 2012;(2012).

[21] Muller, F. L, Liu, Y, & Van Remmen, H. Complex III releases superoxide to both sides of the inner mitochondrial membrane. J Biol Chem. (2004). Nov 19;, 9(47), 49064-73.

[22] Altenhöfer, S, Kleikers, P. W, Radermacher, K. A, & Scheurer, P. Rob Hermans JJ, Schiffers P, Ho H, Wingler K, Schmidt HH. The NOX toolbox: validating the role of NADPH oxidases in physiology and disease. Cell Mol Life Sci. (2012). Jul;, 69(14), 2327-43.

[23] Lassègue, B. San Martín A, Griendling KK. Biochemistry, physiology, and pathophysiology of NADPH oxidases in the cardiovascular system. Circ Res. (2012). May 11;, 110(10), 1364-90.

[24] Valko, M, Izakovic, M, Mazur, M, Rhodes, C. J, & Telser, J. Role of oxygen radicals in DNA damage and cancer incidence. Mol Cell Biochem. (2004). Nov;266(1-2):37-56.

[25] Sander, C. S, Chang, H, Hamm, F, Elsner, P, & Thiele, J. J. Role of oxidative stress and the antioxidant network in cutaneous carcinogenesis. Int J Dermatol. (2004). May;, 43(5), 326-35.

[26] Yen, H. C, Li, S. H, Majima, H. J, Huang, Y. H, Chen, C. P, Liu, C. C, Tu, Y. C, & Chen, C. W. Up-regulation of antioxidant enzymes and coenzyme Q(10) in a human oral cancer cell line with acquired bleomycin resistance. Free Radic Res. (2011). Jun;, 45(6), 707-16.

[27] Policastro, L. L, Ibañez, I. L, Notcovich, C, Durán, H. A, & Podhajcer, O. L. The tumor microenvironment: characterization, redox considerations and novel approaches for ROS-targeted gene therapy. Antioxid Redox Signal. (2012). Jul 15.

[28] Zelko, I. N, Mariani, T. J, & Folz, R. J. Superoxide dismutase multigene family: a comparison of the CuZn-SOD (SOD1), Mn-SOD (SOD2), and EC-SOD (SOD3) gene structures, evolution, and expression. Free Radic Biol Med. (2002). , 33(3), 337-49.

[29] Circu, M. L, & Aw, T. Y. Reactive oxygen species, cellular redox systems, and apoptosis. Free Radic Biol Med. (2010). Mar 15;, 48(6), 749-62.

[30] Kulak, M. V, Cyr, A. R, Woodfield, G. W, Bogachek, M, Spanheimer, P. M, Li, T, Price, D. H, Domann, F. E, & Weigel, R. J. Transcriptional regulation of the GPX1 gene by TFAP2C and aberrant CpG methylation in human breast cancer. Oncogene. (2012). Sep 10.

[31] Ansenberger-fricano, K. Silva Ganini DD, Mao M, Chatterjee S, Dallas S, Mason RP, Stadler K, Santos JH, Bonini MG. The peroxidase activity of mitochondrial superoxide dismutase. Free Radic Biol Med. (2012). Aug 28.

[32] Pastore, A, Federici, G, Bertini, E, & Piemonte, F. Analysis of glutathione: implication in redox and detoxification. Clin Chim Acta. (2003). Jul 1;, 333(1), 19-39.

[33] Lu, S. C. Regulation of glutathione synthesis. Mol Aspects Med. (2009). Feb-Apr; 30(1-2):42-59.

[34] Wood, Z. A, Poole, L. B, & Karplus, P. A. Peroxiredoxin evolution and the regulation of hydrogen peroxide signaling. Science. (2003). Apr 25;, 300(5619), 650-3.

[35] Meyer, Y, Buchanan, B. B, Vignols, F, & Reichheld, J. P. Thioredoxins and glutaredoxins:unifying elements in redox biology. Annu Rev Genet. (2009). , 43, 335-67.

[36] Liu, H, Colavitti, R, Rovira, I. I, & Finkel, T. Redox-dependent transcriptional regulation. Circ Res. (2005). Nov 11;, 97(10), 967-74.

[37] Liu, G. S, Peshavariya, H, Higuchi, M, Brewer, A. C, Chang, C. W, Chan, E. C, & Dusting, G. J. Microphthalmia-associated transcription factor modulates expression of NADPH oxidase type 4: a negative regulator of melanogenesis. Free Radic Biol Med. (2012). May 1;, 52(9), 1835-43.

[38] Campos, A. C, Molognoni, F, Melo, F. H, Galdieri, L. C, Carneiro, C. R, Almeida, D, Correa, V, & Jasiulionis, M. MG. Oxidative stress modulates DNA methylation dur-

ing melanocyte anchorage blockade associated with malignant transformation. Neoplasia (2007). , 9(12), 1111-21.

[39] Kumar, B, Koul, S, Khandrika, L, Meacham, R. B, & Koul, H. K. Oxidative stress is inherent in prostate cancer cells and is required for aggressive phenotype. Cancer Res. (2008). Mar 15;, 68(6), 1777-85.

[40] Pani, G, Galeotti, T, & Chiarugi, P. Metastasis: cancer cell's escape from oxidative stress. Cancer Metastasis Rev. (2010). Jun;, 29(2), 351-78.

[41] Hanahan, D, & Weinberg, R. A. Hallmarks of cancer: the next generation. Cell. (2011). Mar 4;, 144(5), 646-74.

[42] Meyskens FL JrMcNulty SE, Buckmeier JA, Tohidian NB, Spillane TJ, Kahlon RS, Gonzalez RI. Aberrant redox regulation in human metastatic melanoma cell compared to normal melanocytes. Free Radic Biol Med. (2001). Sep 15;, 31(6), 799-808.

[43] Handa, O, Naito, Y, & Yoshikawa, T. Helicobacter pylori: a ROS-inducing bacterial species in the stomach. Inflamm Res. (2010). Dec;, 59(12), 997-1003.

[44] Hole, P. S, Darley, R. L, & Tonks, A. Do reactive oxygen species play a role in myeloid leukemias? Blood. (2011). Jun 2;, 117(22), 5816-26.

[45] Saxena, A, Tammali, R, Ramana, K. V, & Srivastava, S. K. Aldose reductase inhibition prevents colon cancer growth by restoring PTEN through modulation of miR-21 and FOXO3a. Antioxid Redox Signal. (2012). Sep 16.

[46] Vurusaner, B, Poli, G, & Basaga, H. Tumor suppressor genes and ROS: complex networks of interactions. Free Radic Biol Med. (2012). Jan 1;, 52(1), 7-18.

[47] Dolado, I, Swat, A, Ajenjo, N, De Vita, G, Cuadrado, A, & Nebreda, A. R. p. alpha MAP kinase as a sensor of reactive oxygen species in tumorigenesis. Cancer Cell. (2007). Feb;PubMed PMID: 17292829., 11(2), 191-205.

[48] Chan, D. W, Liu, V. W, Tsao, G. S, Yao, K. M, Furukawa, T, Chan, K. K, & Ngan, H. Y. Loss of MKP3 mediated by oxidative stress enhances tumorigenicity and chemoresistance of ovarian cancer cells. Carcinogenesis. (2008). Sep;, 29(9), 1742-50.

[49] Ambrus, C. M, Lajos, T. Z, Stadler, I, Stadler, A, Alfano, J, & Tulumello, J. A. Ambrus Jr. Myocardial release of non-transferrin-bound iron during cardio-pulmonary bypass surgery. J Med. (1999). , 30(3), 4-157.

[50] Franco, R, Schoneveld, O, Georgakilas, A. G, & Panayiotidis, M. I. Oxidative stress, DNA methylation and carcinogenesis. Cancer Lett. (2008). Jul 18;, 266(1), 6-11.

[51] Marnett, L. J. Oxyradicals and DNA damage. Carcinogenesis. (2000). Mar;, 21(3), 361-70.

[52] Valinluck, V, Tsai, H. H, Rogstad, D. K, Burdzy, A, Bird, A, & Sowers, L. C. Oxidative damage to methyl-CpG sequences inhibits the binding of the methyl-CpG bind-

ing domain (MBD) of methyl-CpG binding protein 2 (MeCP2). Nucleic Acids Res (2004). , 32(14), 4100-8.

[53] Maltseva, D. V, Baykov, A. A, Jeltsch, A, & Gromova, E. S. Impact of 7,8-dihydro-8-oxoguanine on methylation of the CpG site by Dnmt3a. Biochemistry (2009). , 48(6), 1361-8.

[54] Hagan, O, Wang, H. M, Sen, W, Destefano, S, Shields, C, Lee, S. S, Zhang, Y. W, Clements, E. G, Cai, Y, Van Neste, L, Easwaran, H, Casero, R. A, & Sears, C. L. Baylin SB. Oxidative damage targets complexes containing DNA methyltransferases, SIRT1, and polycomb members to promoter CpG Islands. Cancer Cell. (2011). Nov 15;, 20(5), 606-19.

[55] Escobar, J, Pereda, J, López-rodas, G, & Sastre, J. Redox signaling and histone acetylation in acute pancreatitis. Free Radic Biol Med. (2012). Mar 1;, 52(5), 819-37.

[56] Irani, K, Xia, Y, Zweier, J. L, & Sollott, S. J. Der CJ, Fearon ER, Sundaresan M, Finkel T, Goldschmidt-Clermont PJ. Mitogenic signaling mediated by oxidants in Ras transformed fibroblasts. Science. (1997). Mar 14;, 275(5306), 1649-52.

[57] Yamaura, M, Mitsushita, J, Furuta, S, Kiniwa, Y, Ashida, A, Goto, Y, Shang, W. H, Kubodera, M, Kato, M, Takata, M, Saida, T, & Kamata, T. NADPH oxidase 4 contributes to transformation phenotype of melanoma cells by regulating G2-M cell cycle progression. Cancer Res (2009). , 69(6), 2647-54.

[58] Mitsushita, J, Lambeth, J. D, & Kamata, T. The superoxide-generating oxidase Nox1 I functionally required for Ras oncogene transformation. Cancer Res (2004). , 64, 3580-3585.

[59] Weinberg, F, Hamanaka, R, Wheaton, W. W, Weinberg, S, Joseph, J, Lopez, M, Kalyanaraman, B, Mutlu, G. M, Budinger, G. R, & Chandel, N. S. Mitochondrial metabolism and ROS generation are essential for Kras-mediated tumorigenicity. Proc Natl Acad Sci U S A. (2010). May 11;, 107(19), 8788-93.

[60] Pervaiz, S, & Clement, M. V. Superoxide anion: oncogenic reactive oxygen species? Int J Biochem Cell Biol. (2007).

[61] Church, S, Grant, J, Ridnour, L. A, Oberley, L. W, Swanson, P. E, Meltzer, P. S, & Trent, J. M. Increased manganese superoxide dismutase expression suppresses the malignant phenotype of human melanoma cells. Proc Natl Acad Sci U S A. (1993). Apr 1;, 90(7), 3113-7.

[62] Weydert, C, Roling, B, Liu, J, Hinkhouse, M. M, Ritchie, J. M, Oberley, L. W, & Cullen, J. J. Suppression of the malignant phenotype in human pancreatic cancer cells by the overexpression of manganese superoxide dismutase. Mol Cancer Ther. (2003). Apr;, 2(4), 361-9.

[63] Venkataraman, S, Jiang, X, Weydert, C, Zhang, Y, Zhang, H. J, Goswami, P. C, Ritchie, J. M, Oberley, L. W, & Buettner, G. R. Manganese superoxide dismutase overex-

pression inhibits the growth of androgen-independent prostate cancer cells. Oncogene. (2005). Jan 6;, 24(1), 77-89.

[64] Low, I. C, Kang, J, & Pervaiz, S. Bcl-2: a prime regulator of mitochondrial redox metabolism in cancer cells. Antioxid Redox Signal. (2011). Dec 15;, 15(12), 2975-87.

[65] Von Thaler, A. K, Kamenisch, Y, & Berneburg, M. The role of ultraviolet radiation in melanomagenesis. Exp Dermatol. (2010). , 19(2), 81-8.

[66] West, X. Z, Malinin, N. L, Merkulova, A. A, Tischenko, M, Kerr, B. A, Borden, E. C, Podrez, E. A, Salomon, R. G, & Byzova, T. V. Oxidative stress induces angiogenesis by activating TLR2 with novel endogenous ligands. Nature. (2010). Oct 21;, 467(7318), 972-6.

[67] Meyskens FL JrChau HV, Tohidian N, Buckmeier J. Luminol-enhanced chemiluminescent response of human melanocytes and melanoma cells to hydrogen peroxide stress. Pigment Cell Res. (1997). Jun;, 10(3), 184-9.

[68] Borrello, S, De Leo, M. E, & Galeotti, T. Defective gene expression of MnSOD in cancer cells. Mol Aspects Med. (1993). , 14(3), 253-8.

[69] Picardo, M, Maresca, V, Eibenschutz, L, De Bernardo, C, Rinaldi, R, & Grammatico, P. Correlation between antioxidants and phototypes in melanocytes cultures. A possible link of physiologic and pathologic relevance. J Invest Dermatol. (1999). Sep;, 113(3), 424-5.

[70] Gidanian, S, & Mentelle, M. Meyskens FL Jr, Farmer PJ. Melanosomal damage in normal human melanocytes induced by UVB and metal uptake--a basis for the pro-oxidant state of melanoma. Photochem Photobiol. (2008). May-Jun;, 84(3), 556-64.

[71] Armstrong, B. K, & Kricker, A. The epidemiology of UV induced skin cancer. JPhotochem Photobiol B (2001).

[72] Tadokoro, T, Kobayashi, N, Zmudzka, B. Z, Ito, S, Wakamatsu, K, Yamaguchi, Y, Korossy, K. S, Miller, S. A, Beer, J. Z, & Hearing, V. J. UV-induced DNA damage and melanin content in human skin differing in racial/ethnic origin. FASEB J (2003). , 17(9), 1177-9.

[73] Wood, S. R, Berwick, M, Ley, R. D, Walter, R. B, Setlow, R. B, & Timmins, G. S. UV causation of melanoma in Xiphophorus is dominated by melanin photosensitized oxidant production. Proc Natl Acad Sci U S A (2006). , 103(11), 4111-5.

[74] Mukhtar, H, Forbes, P. D, & Ananthaswamy, H. N. Photocarcinogenesis--models and mechanisms. Photodermatol Photoimmunol Photomed (1999).

[75] Horikawa-miura, M, Matsuda, N, Yoshida, M, Okumura, Y, Mori, T, & Watanabe, M. The greater lethality of UVB radiation to cultured human cells is associated with the specific activation of a DNA damage-independent signaling pathway. Radiat Res (2007). , 167(6), 655-62.

[76] Birch-machin, M. A, & Swalwell, H. How mitochondria record the effects of UV exposure and oxidative stress using human skin as a model tissue. Mutagenesis (2010). , 25(2), 101-7.

[77] Cotter, M. A, Thomas, J, Cassidy, P, Robinette, K, Jenkins, N, Florell, S. R, Leachman, S, & Samlowski, W. E. Grossman D. N-acetylcysteine protects melanocytes against oxidative stress/damage and delays onset of ultraviolet-induced melanoma in mice.Clin Cancer Res (2007). , 13(19), 5952-8.

[78] Bhushan, A, Abramson, R, Chiu, J. F, & Tritton, T. R. Expression of c-fos in human and murine multidrug-resistant cells. Mol Pharmacol (1992). , 42(1), 69-74.

[79] Mishra, M. V, Bisht, K. S, Sun, L, Muldoon-jacobs, K, Awwad, R, Kaushal, A, Nguyen, P, Huang, L, Pennington, J. D, Markovina, S, Bradbury, C. M, & Gius, D. DNMT1 as a molecular target in a multimodality-resistant phenotype in tumor cells. Mol Cancer Res (2008). , 6(2), 243-9.

[80] Ming, M, Han, W, Maddox, J, Soltani, K, Shea, C. R, Freeman, D. M, & He, Y. Y. UVB-induced ERK/AKT-dependent PTEN suppression promotes survival of epidermal keratinocytes. Oncogene (2010). , 29(4), 492-502.

[81] Birck, A, Ahrenkiel, V, Zeuthen, J, Hou-jensen, K, & Guldberg, P. Mutation and allelic loss of the PTEN/MMAC1 gene in primary and metastatic melanoma biopsies. J Invest Dermatol (2000). , 114(2), 277-80.

[82] Chudnovsky, Y, Adams, A. E, Robbins, P. B, Lin, Q, & Khavari, P. A. Use of human tissue to assess the oncogenic activity of melanoma-associated mutations. Nat Genet (2005). , 37(7), 745-9.

[83] Mirmohammadsadegh, A, Marini, A, Nambiar, S, Hassan, M, Tannapfel, A, Ruzicka, T, & Hengge, U. R. Epigenetic silencing of the PTEN gene in melanoma. Cancer Res (2006). , 66(13), 6546-52.

[84] Noonan, F. P, Dudek, J, Merlino, G, & De Fabo, E. C. Animal models of melanoma: an HGF/SF transgenic mouse model may facilitate experimental access to UV initiating events. Pigment Cell Res (2003). , 16(1), 16-25.

[85] Larsson, P, Andersson, E, Johansson, U, Ollinger, K, Rosdahl, I, & Ultraviolet, A. and B affect human melanocytes and keratinocytes differently. A study of oxidativealterations and apoptosis. Exp Dermatol (2005). , 14(2), 117-23.

[86] Swalwell, H, Latimer, J, Haywood, R. M, & Birch-machin, M. A. Investigating the role of melanin in UVA/UVB- and hydrogen peroxide-induced cellular and mitochondrial ROS production and mitochondrial DNA damage in human melanoma cells. Free Radic Biol Med (2012). , 52(3), 626-34.

[87] Warren, J. B, Loi, R. K, & Coughlan, M. L. Involvement of nitric oxide synthase in the delayed vasodilator response to ultraviolet light irradiation of rat skin in vivo. Br J Pharmacol. (1993). Jul;, 109(3), 802-6.

[88] Kuhn, A, Fehsel, K, Lehmann, P, Krutmann, J, Ruzicka, T, & Kolb-bachofen, V. Aberrant timing in epidermal expression of inducible nitric oxide synthase after UV irradiation in cutaneous lupus erythematosus. J Invest Dermatol (1998). , 111(1), 149-53.

[89] Suschek, C. V, Bruch-gerharz, D, Kleinert, H, Förstermann, U, Kolb-bachofen, V, & Ultraviolet, A. radiation induces nitric oxide synthase-2 expression in human skin endothelial cells in the absence of proinflammatory cytokines. J Invest Dermatol 2001;Channon KM. Tetrahydrobiopterin: regulator of endothelial nitric oxide synthase in vascular disease. Trends Cardiovasc Med (2004). , 117(5), 1200-5.

[90] Hink, U, Li, H, Mollnau, H, Oelze, M, Matheis, E, Hartmann, M, Skatchkov, M, Thaiss, F, Stahl, R. A, Warnholtz, A, Meinertz, T, Griendling, K, Harrison, D. G, Forstermann, U, & Munzel, T. Mechanisms underlying endothelial dysfunction in diabetes mellitus. Circ Res. (2001). E, 14-22.

[91] Roe, N. D, & Ren, J. Nitric oxide synthase uncoupling: A therapeutic target in cardiovascular diseases. Vascul Pharmacol (2012). Feb 16.

[92] Teixeira, M. M, Williams, T. J, & Hellewell, P. G. Role of prostaglandins and nitric oxide in acute inflammatory reactions in guinea-pig skin. Br J Pharmacol (1993). , 110(4), 1515-21.

[93] Creppy, E. E, Traoré, A, Baudrimont, I, Cascante, M, & Carratú, M. R. Recent advances in the study of epigenetic effects induced by the phycotoxin okadaic acid. Toxicology (2002).

[94] Hitchler, M. J, & Domann, F. E. An epigenetic perspective on the free radical theory of development. Free Radic Biol Med (2007). , 43(7), 1023-36.

[95] Lechner, M, Lirk, P, & Rieder, J. Inducible nitric oxide synthase (iNOS) in tumor biology: the two sides of the same coin. Semin Cancer Biol (2005). , 15(4), 277-89.

[96] Schwarz, T. Photoimmunosuppression. Photodermatol Photoimmunol Photomed (2002). , 18(3), 141-5.

[97] Kanavy, H. E, & Gerstenblith, M. R. Ultraviolet radiation and melanoma. Semin Cutan Med Surg (2011). , 30(4), 222-8.

[98] Yuen, K. S, Nearn, M. R, & Halliday, G. M. Nitric oxide-mediated depletion of Langerhans cells from the epidermis may be involved in UVA radiation-induced immunosuppression. Nitric Oxide (2002). , 6(3), 313-8.

[99] Brar, S. S, Kennedy, T. P, Sturrock, A. B, Huecksteadt, T. P, Quinn, M. T, Whorton, A. R, & Hoidal, J. R. An NAD(P)H oxidase regulates growth and transcription in melanoma cells. Am J Physiol Cell Physiol (2002). C, 1212-24.

[100] Liu, F. Gomez Garcia AM, Meyskens FL Jr. NADPH Oxidase 1 OverexpressionEnhances Invasion via Matrix Metalloproteinase-2 and Epithelial-MesenchymalTransition in Melanoma Cells. J Invest Dermatol (2012). , 132(8), 2033-41.

[101] Barbi de Moura MVincent G, Fayewicz SL, Bateman NW, Hood BL, Sun M, Suhan J, Duensing S, Yin Y, Sander C, Kirkwood JM, Becker D, Conrads TP, Van Houten B, Moschos SJ. Mitochondrial respiration- an important therapeutic target in melanoma. PLoS One. (2012). e40690.

[102] Warburg, O. On the origin of cancer cells. Science. (1956). Feb 24;, 123(3191), 309-14.

[103] Kallinowski, F, Schlenger, K. H, Runkel, S, Kloes, M, Stohrer, M, Okunieff, P, & Vaupel, P. Blood flow, metabolism, cellular microenvironment, and growth rate of human tumor xenografts. Cancer Res. (1989). Jul 15;, 49(14), 3759-64.

[104] Scott, D. A, Richardson, A. D, Filipp, F. V, Knutzen, C. A, Chiang, G. G, Ronai, Z. A, Osterman, A. L, & Smith, J. W. Comparative metabolic flux profiling of melanoma cell lines: beyond the Warburg effect. J Biol Chem. (2011). Dec 9;, 286(49), 42626-34.

[105] Hersey, P, Watts, R. N, Zhang, X. D, & Hackett, J. Metabolic approaches to treatment of melanoma. Clin Cancer Res. (2009). Nov 1;, 15(21), 6490-4.

[106] Manola, J, Atkins, M, Ibrahim, J, & Kirkwood, J. Prognostic factors in metastatic melanoma: a pooled analysis of Eastern Cooperative Oncology Group trials. J Clin Oncol. (2000). Nov 15;, 18(22), 3782-93.

[107] Gidanian, S, & Mentelle, M. Meyskens FL Jr, Farmer PJ. Melanosomal damage in normal human melanocytes induced by UVB and metal uptake--a basis for the pro-oxidant state of melanoma. Photochem Photobiol. (2008). May-Jun;, 84(3), 556-64.

[108] Sarangarajan, R, & Apte, S. P. The polymerization of melanin: a poorly understood phenomenon with egregious biological implications. Melanoma Res. (2006). Feb;, 16(1), 3-10.

[109] Hearing, V. J. Determination of melanin synthetic pathways. J Invest Dermatol. (2011). Nov 17;131(E1):EE11., 8.

[110] Rhodes, A. R, Seki, Y, Fitzpatrick, T. B, & Stern, R. S. Melanosomal alterations in dysplastic melanocytic nevi. A quantitative, ultrastructural investigation. Cancer. (1988). Jan 15;, 61(2), 358-69.

[111] Wittgen, H. G, & Van Kempen, L. C. Reactive oxygen species in melanoma and its therapeutic implications. Melanoma Res. (2007). Dec;, 17(6), 400-9.

[112] Pavel, S, Van Nieuwpoort, F, Van Der Meulen, H, Out, C, Pizinger, K, Cetkovská, P, Smit, N. P, & Koerten, H. K. Disturbed melanin synthesis and chronic oxidative stress in dysplastic naevi. Eur J Cancer. (2004). Jun;, 40(9), 1423-30.

[113] Farmer, P. J, Gidanian, S, & Shahandeh, B. Di Bilio AJ, Tohidian N, Meyskens FL Jr. Melanin as a target for melanoma chemotherapy: pro-oxidant effect of oxygen and metals on melanoma viability. Pigment Cell Res. (2003). Jun;, 16(3), 273-9.

[114] Meyskens FL JrFarmer PJ, Yang S, Anton-Culver H. New perspectives on melanoma pathogenesis and chemoprevention. Recent Results Cancer Res. (2007). , 174, 191-5.

[115] Leonard, S. S, Harris, G. K, & Shi, X. Metal-induced oxidative stress and signal transduction. Free Radic Biol Med. (2004). Dec 15;, 37(12), 1921-42.

[116] Bertolotto, C, Abbe, P, Hemesath, T. J, Bille, K, Fisher, D. E, Ortonne, J. P, & Ballotti, R. Microphthalmia gene product as a signal transducer in cAMP-induced differentiation of melanocytes. J Cell Biol. (1998). Aug 10;, 142(3), 827-35.

[117] Barbieri, A, Palma, G, Rosati, A, Giudice, A, Falco, A, Petrillo, A, Petrillo, M, & Bimonte, S. Di Benedetto M, Esposito G, Stiuso P, Abbruzzese A, Caraglia M, Arra C. Role of endothelial nitric oxide synthase (eNOS) in chronic stress-promoted tumour growth. J Cell Mol Med. (2012). Apr;, 16(4), 920-6.

[118] Salvucci, O, Carsana, M, Bersani, I, Tragni, G, & Anichini, A. Antiapoptotic role of endogenous nitric oxide in human melanoma cells. Cancer Res. (2001). Jan 1;, 61(1), 318-26.

[119] Ellerhorst, J. A, et al. Regulation of iNOS by the mitogen-activated protein kinase pathway in human melanoma. Oncogene. (2006). Jun 29; 25(28):3956-62., 44.

[120] Lim, K. H, Ancrile, B. B, Kashatus, D. F, & Counter, C. M. Tumour maintenance is mediated by eNOS. Nature. (2008). Apr 3;, 452(7187), 646-9.

[121] Lampson, B. L, Kendall, S. D, Ancrile, B. B, Morrison, M. M, Shealy, M. J, Barrientos, K. S, Crowe, M. S, Kashatus, D. F, White, R. R, Gurley, S. B, Cardona, D. M, & Counter, C. M. Targeting eNOS in pancreatic cancer. Cancer Res. (2012). Sep 1;, 72(17), 4472-82.

[122] Oba-shinjo, S. M, Correa, M, Ricca, T. I, Molognoni, F, Pinhal, M. A, Neves, I. A, Marie, S. K, Sampaio, L. O, Nader, H. B, Chammas, R, & Jasiulionis, M. G. Melanocyte transformation associated with substrate adhesion impediment. Neoplasia. (2006). Mar;, 8(3), 231-41.

[123] Yang, S, Misner, B. J, & Chiu, R. J. Meyskens FL Jr. Redox effector factor-1, combined with reactive oxygen species, plays an important role in the transformation of JB6 cells. Carcinogenesis. (2007). Nov;, 28(11), 2382-90.

[124] Yang, S, Irani, K, Heffron, S. E, & Jurnak, F. Meyskens FL Jr. Alterations in the expression of the apurinic/apyrimidinic endonuclease-1/redox factor-1 (APE/Ref-1) in human melanoma and identification of the therapeutic potential of resveratrol as an APE/Ref-1 inhibitor. Mol Cancer Ther. (2005). Dec;, 4(12), 1923-35.

[125] Yang, S, & Meyskens, F. L. Apurinic/apyrimidinic endonuclease/redox effector factor-1(APE/Ref-1): a unique target for the prevention and treatment of human melanoma. Antioxid Redox Signal. (2009). Mar;, 11(3), 639-50.

[126] Palmieri, G, Capone, M, Ascierto, M. L, Gentilcore, G, Stroncek, D. F, Casula, M, Sini, M. C, Palla, M, Mozzillo, N, & Ascierto, P. A. Main roads to melanoma. J Transl Med. (2009). Oct 14;7:86.

[127] Jenkins, N. C, Liu, T, Cassidy, P, Leachman, S. A, Boucher, K. M, Goodson, A. G, Samadashwily, G, Grossman, D, & The, p. INK4A) tumor suppressor regulates cellular oxidative stress. Oncogene. (2011). Jan 20;, 30(3), 265-74.

[128] Selimovic, D, Hassan, M, Haikel, Y, & Hengge, U. R. Taxol-induced mitochondrial stress in melanoma cells is mediated by activation of c-Jun N-terminal kinase (JNK) and pathways via uncoupling protein 2. Cell Signal. (2008). Feb;20(2):311-22., 38.

[129] Lee, S, Kim, Y. K, Shin, T. Y, & Kim, S. H. Neurotoxic Effects of Bisphenol AF on Calcium-Induced ROS and MAPKs. Neurotox Res. (2012). Sep 21.

[130] Oberlay, T. D, & Oberlay, L. W. Antioxidant enzyme levels in cancer. Histol Histopathol. (1997). , 12, 525-535.

[131] Yohn, J, Norris, D, Yrastorza, D, Bruno, I, Leff, J, Hake, S, & Repine, J. Disparate antioxidant enzyme activities in cultured cutaneous fibroblasts, keratinocytes and melanocytes. J Invest Dermatol. (1991). , 97, 405-410.

[132] Maxwell, S. R. Prospects for the use of antioxidant therapies. Drugs (1995). , 49, 345-61.

[133] Agostini, D, Balansky, F, Camoirano, R. M, & De Flora, A. S. Modulation of light-induced skin tumors by N-acetylcisteine and/or ascorbic acid in hairless mice. Carcinogenesis (2005). , 26, 657-64.

[134] Cotter, M. A, Thomas, J, Cassidy, P, Robinette, K, Jenkins, N, Florell, S. R, Leachman, S, & Samlowski, W. E. Grossman D. N-acetylcysteine protects melanocytes against oxidative stress/damage and delays onset of ultraviolet-induced melanoma in mice. Clin Cancer Res. (2007). Oct 1;, 13(19), 5952-8.

[135] Goodson, A. G, Cotter, M. A, Cassidy, P, Wade, M, Florell, S. R, Liu, T, Boucher, K. M, & Grossman, D. Use of oral N-acetylcysteine for protection of melanocytic nevi against UV-induced oxidative stress: towards a novel paradigm for melanoma chemoprevention. Clin Cancer Res. (2009). Dec 1;, 15(23), 7434-40.

[136] Kang, S, Chung, J. H, Lee, J. H, et al. Topical N-acetylcysteine and genistein prevent ultraviolet-light-induced signaling that leads to photoaging in human skin in vivo. J Invest Dermatol (2003). , 120, 835-41.

[137] Ichihashi, M, Ahmed, N. U, Budiyanto, A, Wu, A, Bito, T, Ueda, M, & Osawa, T. Preventive effect of antioxidant on ultraviolet-induced skin cancer in mice. J Dermatol Sci (2000). S, 45-50.

[138] Kundu, J. K, Chun, K. S, Kim, S. O, & Surh, Y. J. Resveratrol inhibits phorbol ester-induced cyclooxygenase-2 expression in mouse skin: MAPKs and AP-1 as potential molecular targets. Biofactors. (2004).

[139] Luo, M, Delaplane, S, Jiang, A, Reed, A, He, Y, Fishel, M, & Nyland, R. L. nd, Borch RF, Qiao X, Georgiadis MM, Kelley MR. Role of the multifunctional DNA repair and redox signaling protein Ape1/Ref-1 in cancer and endothelial cells: small-molecule

inhibition of the redox function of Ape1. Antioxid Redox Signal. (2008). Nov;, 10(11), 1853-67.

[140] Fishel, M. L, Colvin, E. S, Luo, M, Kelley, M. R, & Robertson, K. A. Inhibition of the redox function of APE1/Ref-1 in myeloid leukemia cell lines results in a hypersensitive response to retinoic acid-induced differentiation and apoptosis. Exp Hematol. (2010). Dec;, 38(12), 1178-88.

Chapter 6

Expression of Matrix Metalloproteinases and Theirs Tissue Inhibitors in Fibroblast Cultures and Colo-829 and SH-4 Melanoma Cultures After Photodynamic Therapy

Aleksandra Zielińska, Małgorzata Latocha,
Magdalena Jurzak and Dariusz Kuśmierz

Additional information is available at the end of the chapter

http://dx.doi.org/10.5772/54935

1. Introduction

Metalloproteinases (MMPs) are a numerous group of proteolytic enzymes whose activity depends on Zn^{2+} and Ca^{2+} ions [1-2]. They participate in various physiological and pathological processes. They are engaged in the processes of restructuring and degradation of the basement membrane and components of the extracellular matrix (ECM) [3]. So far, 25 enzymes from that group have been characterized (22 in humans), as well as 4 their inhibitors (tissue inhibitors of metalloproteinases - TIMPs) [4-5]. Gene expression of metalloproteinases occurs in almost all cells: in fibroblasts, keratinocytes, macrophages, endothelium cells, Langerhans dendritic cells, neurons, microglial cells, myocytes, as well as in inflammatory infiltration cells: in monocytes, T lymphocytes [5]. Increased activity of metalloproteinases can be observed in various pathological states, i.e. in neoplastic growths, arthritis, periodontal diseases, atherosclerosis, dilated cardiomyopathy, myocardial infarction and diseases of the skin [6]. In case of neoplasms, a possible dependence is often mentioned: quantity and activity level of these enzymes can influence advancement of the tumour. Results of many studies show importance of the expression profile of various MMPs and their inhibitors on the prognosis and course of the disease [7]. Generally, changes in proportion of particular MMPs in the whole MMP pool negatively influence the prognosis. However, in some cases, like e.g. in colorectal cancer, changes in the expression profile due to increased expression of MMP-12 and MMP-9 are connected with longer survivability of the patient and decreased ability of neoplastic cells to cause metastasis [8, 9]. Studies on the amount of inhibitors metalloproteinase matrices (TIMPs) have proven that there is a relation between a high level of TIMP-1 and -2, and an unfavourable prognosis for the patient. The cause of an increase in concentration of TIMPs is probably higher expression of MMPs and an attempt to maintain an equilibrium between MMP and TIMP expression in a neoplastic process [7]. TIMPs may also favour neoplastic progression through inhibition of apoptosis of neoplastic cells (TIMP-1 and -2), stimulation of their growth (TIMP-2 and -3) or participation in the beginning of angiogenesis in a tumour (stimulation of VEGF secretion – TIMP-1) [10]. Moreover, TIMPs show activity independent from MMPs, e.g. they cause increased levels of anti-apoptotic protien BCL-XL [11] and have an influence similar to the growth factor [12]. Tests performed on animals also proved that TIMP-2, despite its name, is an important activator of MMP-2 [13].

1.1. Participation and role of MMPs in the course of a neoplastic process

There are six basic changes in the physiology of a cell which underlie neoplastic development [14]:

- self-delivery of signals that stimulate growth,
- lack of sensitivity to signals that inhibit growth,
- escape from apoptosis,
- unlimited proliferation,
- stimulation of angiogenesis,
- invasiveness and ability to create metastasis.

The studies conducted in the last few years confirmed participation of metalloproteinases in several stages of neoplastic development.

1.1.1. MMPs and regulation of growth of tumour cells

Three ways in which MMPs contribute to proliferation of tumour cells are known. Firstly, MMPs release precursors of some growth factors, such as e.g. TGF-α [15] that are related to the cell membrane. Secondly, MMPs may participate in the process of activation of those factors, e.g. MMP-24 and MMP-25 activate IGF factors (insulin-like growth factors) through proteolysis of IGF-BPs (insulin-like growth factor binding proteines). Thirdly, metalloproteinases influence composition of ECM and thus can indirectly regulate proliferation signals through integrins [16]. MMPs can also influence, in a negative way, growth of neoplastic cells through TGF-β or through participation in production of proapoptotic factors such as Fas ligand (FasL) or TNF-α [7].

1.1.2. MMPs and regulation of apoptosis

MMPs demonstrate both apoptotic and anti-apoptotic activity. MMP-3, -7, -9 and MMP-11 are metalloproteinases with particular significance attributed to them. It was proved that overexpression of MMP-3 in epithelial cells of mammals induce apoptosis, which is probably a result of laminin degradation [17-19], while MMP-7 can release cell membrane-related FasL – transmembrane stimulator of the FasL death receptor. Released FasL can induce apoptosis of neigh-

http://dx.doi.org/10.5772/54935

bouring cells or cause inhibition of neoplastic cells [20-21]. MMP-7 may also inhibit apoptosis through digestion of pro-HB-EGF (inactive form of the heparin-binding epithelial growth factor) and secretion of mature HB-EGF which support cell survival [22]. Anti-apoptotic influence of MMP-11 is often described with an example of IGFs (insulin-like growth factors) release, which can be factors that increase survivability of cells [23-24]. During apoptosis of endothelium, metalloproteinases also participate in digestion of VE-cadherin (vascular endothelial cadherin) [25] and cell adhesion molecules such as: PECAM-1 (a cell adhesion molecule from the immunoglobulin superfamily) and E-cadherin (epithelial cadherin). Degradation of the aforementioned cell adhesion molecules may be a cause for typical rounding of apoptotic cells [26].

1.1.3. MMPs and regulation of angiogenesis

An important factor in the growth of a tumour is creation of new blood vessels within its region [14]. Metalloproteinases play an important role as positive regulators of that process. Tests conducted on animals have proven that both endogeneous and synthetic inhibitors of metalloproteinases cause decreased angiogenesis [27]. Huge significance is here attributed to the following metalloproteinases: MMP-2, -9, -14, which directly influence the course of the angiogenic process, and MMP-19, which is expressed in blood vessel cells [28]. In case of MMP-2 overexpression, a development of a mysterious feature of $\alpha v \beta$-integrin was described within type-IV collagen. Blocking that spot with antibodies inhibits migration of endothelial cells in the process of *in vitro* angiogenesis and limits growth of the tumour [29]. MMP-9 causes higher availability of pro-angiogenic VEGF factor, however the mechanism of its action has not yet been explained [30]. It is believed that also MMP-14 contributes to the angiogenesis of the tumour as antibodies aimed at the catalytic domain of MMP-14 inhibit migration of endothelial cells, as well as invasiveness and creation of capillary vessels *in vitro* [31]. MMP-14 can also degrade fibrillary matrix which surrounds newly created blood vessels, which may potentially disable endothelial cells to further penetrate the tumour tissue [32]. MMPs also contribute to creation of molecules which are inhibitors of angiogenesis. Digestion of plasminogen by MMP-2, -3, -7, -9 and -12 results in creation of angiostatin [33]. MMP-3, -9, -12, -13 and MMP-20 may also be engaged in creation of endostatin (C-terminal fragment derived from type XVIII collagen of basement membranes) [34]. Both angiostatin and endostatin reduce proliferation of endothelial cells [35]. Additionally, endostatin may inhibit invasiveness of endothelial cells, acting as MMP-14 and MMP-2 inhibitor [36]. MMP-12 may also inhibit angiogenesis of the tumour through digestion and cutting off the receptor related to the cell membrane, that is urokinase-type plasminogen activator (u-PA), which is necessary in the process of invasion of endothelial cells into a fibrin matrix [37].

1.1.4. MMPs and invasiveness and metastasis

During metastasis, neoplastic cells have to overcome several barriers put in their way by ECM. Firstly, they have to get through the basement membrane of the endothelium and infiltrate the surrounding stroma. Then they have to infiltrate the blood or lymphatic vessels (intravasation), migrate through vessel walls to the surrounding tissue (extravasation) and create new, proliferable metastatic foci [3].

Digestion of lamina-5 by MMP-2 and MMP-14 contributes to creation of a digestion product, which facilitates cell movements. Such phenomenon can be observed in experimental *in vivo* tumours, while in case of human neoplasms a common location for both MMP-14 and lamina-5 was found [7. However, MMP-14 may also participate in digestion of CD44 receptor (the main receptor for hyaluronic acid) which resides on the surface of neoplastic cells. That receptor has an ability to bond MMP-9 and, therefore, attributes to the location of the enzyme on the surface of the cell. Such location of MMP-9 is necessary to initiate invasion of the tumour cells and angiogenesis within its boundaries. Therefore, MMP-14 may contribute to a decrease in MMP-9 activity on the surface of the cell, which subsequently may inhibit invasive properties of the tumour cells and angiogenesis [38].

Progression of the tumour is also connected with disturbance of the functioning of the E-cadherin cell adhesion molecule, which is digested by MMP-3 and MMP-7. Secretion of an E-cadherin fragment due to a cut attributes to the invasion of neoplastic cells in the paracrine way [39]. Digestion of E-cadherin also contributes to transformation of the epithelial cells into the mesenchymal tissue [40].

During the invasion of tumour cells, placement of metalloproteinases on the cellular invadopodia is necessary for them to acquire the ability of invasiveness. MMP-2, -9 and -14 are metalloproteinases identified as those which appear within the invadopodia, however the placement mechanisms are different for each of them [41].

Metalloproteinases also participate in late stages of the metastatic process when neoplastic cells have to intrude blood and lymphatic vessels, survive in them and, finally, evacuate from them. At that stage, the experimental models describe overexpression of MMP-9 and MMP-14, which correlates with the growth in number of neoplastic cells which survive in experimental tests of metastasis [42- 43].

It is believed that there are tissue-specific differences in occurrence of proteinases which initiate metastasis. Moreover, activity of TIMPs in those tissues, which in some cases inhibit recurrence of neoplastic foci, also seems to be different [7].

1.1.5. MMPs and immunological response

One of the characteristics of a neoplastic disease is occurrence of inflammatory responses [44]. The immunological system is able to recognize and attack neoplastic cells. However, those cells have an ability to "escape" supervision and control of the immunological system. Those phenomena may, to some extend, depend on metalloproteinases [7].

Inflammatory infiltration within a tumour contains cytotoxic T lymphocytes, NK cells and macrophages which target neoplastic cells. Proliferation of T lymphocytes is regulated by cytokine signals, precisely by interleukin-2 receptor-α (IL-2Rα) [7].

Metalloproteinases, including MMP-9, can only digest IL-2R⟨and in that way inhibit proliferation of T lymphocytes [7]. Metalloproteinases are also an activator of TGF-β [45], an important T lymphocyte response inhibitor targeted against neoplastic cells [46]. The product of digestion of ⟨1-proteinase inhibitor created by MMP-11 causes decreased sensitivity of neoplastic cells

http://dx.doi.org/10.5772/54935

to an attack from NK cells. MMPs may also target the chemokines themselves, which results in a growth or reduction of infiltration and migration of leukocytes [ADD CITATION]. MMP-9 shows ability to digest neutrophil chemotactic factor CXCL8 (interleukin-8; IL-8), therefore making it ten times more active. Moreover, MMP-9 inactivates the CXCL7 precursor (a Type-III connective tissue activating peptide; CTAP-III), CXCL4 (platelet factor 4; PF4) and CXCL1 (growth-related oncogene-α; GROα) [47].

MMP-1, -3, -9, -13, -14 can participate in digestion and inactivation of CXCL12 (stromal cell-derived factor 1, SDF-1) [48], which is a ligand for the CXCR4 receptor (SDF-1 chemokine receptor) located on the leukocytes. It is interesting that breast cancer cells also show expression of CXCR4, while inhibition of binding CXCL12 to CXCR4 through blockage with use of antibodies significantly reduces *in vivo* metastasis to lungs and lymph nodes. Therefore, digestion of CXCL12 by MMPs may inhibit metastasis [49].

Although the immunological system reacts to cancer cells and probably delays progression of the neoplastic disease, existence of a chronic inflammatory state may also influence development of tumours of the skin, breasts, prostate, ovary, mucous membrane of the stomach, large intestine, liver and bladder. In progression of neoplastic disease of animal models, inflammatory cells such as mastocytes, neutrophil granulocyte and macrophages participate in the process [44]. Those cells synthesize several types of MMPs, including -9, -12 and -14, therefore release of those MMPs may stimulate neoplastic progression [7].

1.2. Participation of MMPs in progression of melanoma

Melanoma belongs to the group of highly invasive neoplasms with high ability of metastasis through both blood and lymphatic vessels. Some studies suggest that various arrangements of proteolytic enzymes play an important role in progression of melanoma. Those include the plasmin activator system and the extracellular matrix group of metalloproteinases. Melanoma cells have an ability to produce many kinds of ECM metalloproteinases, including MMP-1, -2, -9, -13, -14, as well as other inhibitors: TIMP-1, -2, and -3. It is currently believed that metalloproteinases MMP-2 and MMP-9 play the most important roles in development of melanoma. It was proved that expression and activation of those proteinases is in close relation to the invasive and metastatic melanoma phenotype [50]. Those metalloproteinases are constitutively expressed in the most aggressive forms of melanoma. Their level of expression is strongly related to the atypia of melanocytes and differentiation of cells within the melanocytic nevi [51].

It was found that in case of both human and mouse melanoma cell lines, increased MMP-2, MMP-9 and MMP-14 (MT1-MMP) expression is related to an invasive form of the neoplasm [52]. Increase of MMP-2 is highly related to blood vessel metastasis. Clark's and Breslow's classification shows relation between a high level of MMP-2 expression and low survivability index, which is particularly typical for male patients [50]. Studies carried out by Zucker and Cao [53] proved that MMP-2 is undetectable *in situ* in human melanoma, however high level of an active form of that enzyme is present in the matrix of the primary tumour in advanced stages of melanoma and its metastatic forms. Their results were confirmed by research conducted by Vaisanen et al. [54], who proved that intensified expression of MMP-2 is a typical feature of invasive forms of melanoma and is an unfavourable prognostic factor. Increased level of MMP-2 expression in mRNA and proteins was also observed in case of the most aggressive melanoma cell lines (MV3, BLM), as well as xenografts derived from them. The pro-MMP-2 activation mechanism has not been fully discovered yet. An active form of MMP-2 directly regulates adhesion of melanoma cells and their proliferation to the ECM, facilitating the processes of migration and invasion [55].

It was also found that increased expression of MMP-14 (MT1-MMP) causes activation of MMP-2 on the surface of melanoma cells. MMP-2 activity is also regulated by presence of TIMP-2. On the one hand, an inhibitor may slow down MMP-2 and in that way limit growth of a tumour and invasion. On the other hand, TIMP-2 may also be directly engaged in activation of MMP-2 through formation of a complex with MMP-14, which is a receptor for MMP-2 on the surface of cells. Therefore, co-ordinated expression of MMP-2, MMP-14 and TIMP-2 leads to activation of MMP-2, while increased concentration of the said metalloproteinases and their inhibitor is also characteristic for other human neoplasms [50, 55].

The hypothesis that there is a dependence between activation of MMP-2 and overexpression of MMP-14 was also proved in the research conducted by Kurschat et al. [56]. They found that in case of abnormal human melanocytes, an increase in expression of both MMP-2 and MMP-14 is related to progression of the neoplasm. An *in situ* zymographic analysis confirmed presence of an active form of MMP-2 in the boundary cells of the tumour and in the surrounding matrix. Moreover, it was proved that the neoplastic cells which produce simultaneously MMP-2 and MMP-14 are often situated on the boundary between the stroma and the front of the invasive tumour cells [56].

Tests conducted on mice deprived of MMP-2 gene confirmed that MMP-2 synthesis is necessary for occurrence of metastasis [50].

Iida et al. [57] found that MMP-14 facilitates invasion of melanoma cells through matrigel, increases their ability to migrate through lamina-1, facilitates growth of the tumour in *in vitro* cell cultures and supports forming of melanoma cell colonies in agarose gel. Moreover, such influence of MMP-14 which causes increase of invasive abilities of melanoma and supports growth of the tumour does not depend on the operation of MMP inhibitors [57].

Participation of MMP-9 in progression of melanoma remains unexplained. So far, contradictory data has only been obtained as to the influence of MMP-9 expression on progression of melanoma. Experiments conducted on melanoma lines derived from advanced stages of the neoplasm proved existence of MMP-9 expression. However, no such occurrence was found in case of cell lines derived from early stages of melanoma [3]. What is more, research carried out by van den Oord et al. [58] shows that, in case of humans, MMP-9 probably undergoes expression only in the phase of horizontal growth of the tumour when it does not exceed 1.6 mm in height. No expression of metalloproteinase-9 was found in metastatic material [58]. Nikkola et al. [59] proved that a high level of MMP-9 in blood serum is typical for patients with vast metastasis and generally shorter survivability time when compared to patients with lower level of MMP-9 in the serum.

In case of experimental models, in which neoplastic tissue was implanted into rodents, MMP-9 was identified within the occurring tumour only when its cells were derived from advanced melanoma stages [50, 52]. Moreover, in case of organisms that constitutively expressed MMP-9, increased colonization of the lungs and metastasis were observed, while mice without the MMP-9 gene virtually had no secondary neoplastic foci. Those studies suggest that MMP-9, which is produced by both neoplastic and stroma cells, plays an important role in the occurrence of metastasis. Moreover, it is thought that expression of MMP-9 is a feature of neoplastic cells which participate in spontaneous metastasis to the lymph nodes and lungs. Therefore it seems that the process of selection of the cells which create *in vivo* metastasis favours those subclone cells which express MMP-9. As that selection is independent from the microenvironment and is not observed during experimental metastasis, it seems that MMP-9 participates in early stages of metastatic occurrence than in the later states, such as e.g. extravasation [50, 52].

An important role in the development of melanoma is also attributed to MMP-1 and MMP-3. Durako et al. [51] proved that gradation of Type-I and Type-IV collagen, as well as invasion of melanoma cells through matrigel both depend on expression of MMP-1. Nikkola et al. [59] demonstrated correlation between a high level of MMP-1 and MMP-3 in the tissue and a shorter survivability time, as well as a relation between expression of MMP-13 and parenchymal metastases. Increased progression of the neoplastic disease was observed at the beginning of a therapy in case of patients with higher level of metalloproteinases, while in case of patients with melanoma, MMP-13 activity was detected [59].

Due to the properties of TIMPs, it seems that an equilibrium between the level of active MMPs and their inhibitors may be a turning point for neoplastic progression. For example, it was proved that overexpression of TIMP-1, TIMP-2 and TIMP-3 can cause inhibition of melanoma invasion. On the other hand, *in situ* tests show that induction of TIMP-1 and -3 occurs in a late stage of melanoma tumour progression, which is a result of a complex interaction of the MMP/TIMP system. Increased expression of TIMPs can also inhibit metastasis, while simultaneously giving unfavourable prognosis due to TIMPs acting as stimulants to the growth of human melanoma cells [50].

The studies of Wandel et al. [60] show that stroma cells also participate in induction of the proteolytic potential of tumour cells. Therefore, expression of MMPs may occur not only in neoplastic cells but also in the surrounding fibroblasts, which proves participation of those cells in the process of melanoma progression [50]. Wander et al. [60] proved that both fibroblasts located in the direct vicinity of the *in vivo* melanoma lesion, as well as those stimulated with a medium derived from the *in vitro* culture of melanoma cells (the medium contained solvable factors secreted by melanoma cells, such as cytokines and growth factors) showed increased MMP-1 expression of mRNA and proteins. Moreover, a relation between that phenomenon and invasiveness of the tumour was observed.

As the presented data shows, it seems that ECM metalloproteinases play an important role in the development of the neoplastic process, including the melanoma tumour. Anomalies in the expression profile of MMPs not only influence the *in situ* growth of the tumour itself but particularly affect location and the way of induction of the metastatic process. This can suggest that various MMPs may play individual roles in particular stages of melanoma metastasis [52].

2. Photodynamic therapy in treatment of melanoma

Photodynamic therapy (PDT) is used in treatment of chosen pre-neoplastic states and early neoplastic stages, as well as for aesthetic and plastic purposes [61]. The basis of PDT is the interaction of laser light (usually long-wave infrared) with photosensitive molecules selectively accumulated in pathologically changed tissue, in presence of oxygen. Such interaction turns those molecules into their cytotoxic forms that, eventually, cause death of the cells, therefore highly selectively destroying pathological lesion in the tissue [62].

A possibility to use photodynamic therapy in treatment of melanoma is currently a subject of research conducted on both cell and animal cultures. Photosensitizers and their derivatives, such as Photofrin, ALA, Porphyrin IX, Vertoporphyrin and others, are currently being assessed or even used in clinical practice in case of other diseases. Simultaneously, very intensive research on newly synthesized compounds is being conducted [63 – 66]. The most attention is drawn to those photosensitizers which have the maximal absorption pattern shifted to the infrared, which allows the light to penetrate the tissue deeper and avoids its absorption by melanin. Laboratory studies also include analyses of mutual influence between molecules of particular photosensitizer and melanin. In case of Chlorin e6 and Polyvinylpyrrolidone complex (FOTOLON) used in our study, research conducted by Parkhots et al. [67] proved that presence of DOPA-melanin (up to 0.1 mg/ml concentration) does not influence the properties of the photosensitizer and those systems do not interact with each other, do not form any bonds nor complexes. However, even quite low concentration of melanin (up to 0.02 mg/ml) in the sample, despite its lack of influence on the rate of singlet oxygen creation in the medium, significantly lowers effectiveness of that reactive form of oxygen. Other studies which assessed mutual interactions of the melanin – photosensitizer - light system described occurrence of so called 'side reactions' [68]. Presence of endogeneous chromophores, including melanin, in surface layers of the illuminated tissue can significantly limit access of the light (especially that of shorter wavelengths). It may also result in so called 'photobleaching', which was confirmed for established parameters of the therapy [68].

First clinical trials with use of PDT in patients with melanoma are currently being conducted. However, the number of reports with successful application of that kind of therapy is still small. Due to very limited knowledge of the molecular and long-term effects of such therapy, the most common but still casuistic reports are related to application of PDT in the palliative therapy of metastatic melanoma. One such case was described by Fasanell and McGrath [69]. Those researchers proved effectiveness of the PDT therapy in treatment of melanoma metastasis to the duodenal ampulla. The therapeutic effect was immediately observed and lasted for a long time (13 months). Unfortunately, further observation was impossible due to death of the patient caused probably by metastasis to the brain and complications in a form of the intracerebral hemorrhage. Other cases of PDT application in the available literature concern patients with melanoma of the sight apparatus, lesions in the nasal area and sensitive parts of the face. There are also reports of successfully concluded therapies of iris melanoma [70], as well as descriptions of 14 patients with metastatic melanoma (13 of them previously treated with other methods) in which cases a successful elimination of all neoplastic cells was achieved after one treatment with PDT-chlorin e6 (in 8 cases) or after a series of therapeutic procedures (in 6 cases) [71].

3. Metalloproteinases in photodynamic therapy of melanoma

Photodynamic therapy (PDT) allows for selective elimination of pathological cells with use of light. The light illuminates chosen, mostly pathological, cells of the tissue which gathers photosensitizing substances. The cause of death of those cells are molecular changes that occur during the therapy. However, a question arises: if use of sublethal conditions (that depend on susceptibility of cells, their type, concentration of the photosensitizer, presence of oxygen or dose of radiation) does not increase resistance of the pathological cells to those conditions, leading to occurrence of a malignant phenotype and, in that way, increasing the possibility of metastasis.

More and more studies describe a co-relation between the degree of invasiveness of neoplastic cells and changes in expression of metalloproteinases (MMPs) ECM and their inhibitors (TIMs) located in both neoplastic cells and cells of the stroma - connective tissue of the tumour. Due to that, an attempt to assess influence of photodynamic therapy on changes in expression of chosen meta metalloproteinases MMP-2, MMP-9, MMP-14 and their inhibitors TIMP-1 and TIMP-2 was made in two cultures of melanoma: Colo-829 (melanotic type – a line taken from cells isolated from skin) and SH-4 (melanotic metastatic type – a line taken from cells isolated from pleural effusion; initial occurrence - skin; metastatic occurrence – lungs). The influence of photodynamic therapy on expression of chosen metalloproteinases and their inhibitors was analysed in melanoma cell cultures and regular fibroblast cultures (HFF-1 line – normal fibroblasts isolated from skin), the latter were exposed to factors secreted by melanoma cells after photodynamic therapy.

Chlorin e6 – PVP (Fotolon OAO; producer: Biełmedpreparaty) was used as a photosensitizer with concentration of 0.01 mg/ml of the growth medium. The photosensitizer was added to the growth medium in which cultures of a given cell line were grown. After the growth medium and the photosensitizer were added and an incubation period of 1 hour, cell cultures were illuminated with use of PDT-662 laser (Kriomed) with a wavelength of 662 nm in 5J, 10J and 20 J/cm^2 doses.

The analysis of chosen genes was carried out at the transcription stage with use of quantitative determination and QRT-PCR method. Determination of mRNA transcripts of the examined genes in whole-cell RNA extracts was conducted with use of a DNA Engine OPTICON™ fluorescence detector (MJ Research). After each amplification cycle, the number of PCR amplicons was determined based on the intensity of SYBR Green I fluorescent dye which binds to double-stranded DNA, a product of RT-PCR reaction, which has an ability to emit fluorescent light. In order to prepare the reacting QRT-PCR mixture, a stock QuantiTect Sybr Green RT-PCR Reagent Kit (Qiagen) was used. Amplimer identification was based on electrophoretic separation in 8% solution of silver-stained polyacrylamide gel.

Specificity of RT-PCR reaction was confirmed for each analysed sample on the basis of a thermal denaturation profile of the amplification product. The denaturation curve was established for a range of temperature between 50°C and 95°C. Rapid decrease in intensity of fluorescence was observed during denaturation of samples at the melting temperature (Tm) of the amplimer which was contained in that gene. This is due to the release of SYBR Green I dye from the double-stranded product of the PCR reaction.

The results of our study, representing a quantitative feature, were checked for normality by the Shapiro–Wilk test for each trial. In all cases, there was no reason to reject the hypothesis of normality. Thus, to verify the research hypothesis, parametric tests were used and the data is expressed as mean values ± standard deviations. Average results of two samples (trials) were compared using Student's *t*-test when the assumption of variance homogeneity was met, or Student's *t*-test with separate estimation of variance in case of the opposite situation. The homogeneity of variance for two samples (trials) was checked using Snedecor's *F*-test or Levene's test. Comparison of the average of one distinguished group (control) with the remaining experimental averages was made using Dunnett's test, after previously determining (by means of the *F*-test in variance analysis) the statistical significance of differences between analysed averages. When comparing the averages of at least three samples (trials), analysis of variance (ANOVA) was performed. The results for $p < 0.05$ were considered statistically significant. Statistica PL version 8 software was used for the statistical analysis.

The results of the study showed expression of mRNA in *MMP-2, MMP-9* (on a very low level), as well as *MMP-14* and *TIMP-2* of SH-4 metastatic melanoma cells. Only MMP9 and TIMP-2 transcripts were detected in Colo-829 melanoma cells (Table 1).

Melanoma cell line	MMP-2 [mRNA copy number/1 µg of total RNA]	MMP-9 [mRNA copy number/1 µg of total RNA]	MMP-14 [mRNA copy number/1 µg of total RNA]	TIMP-1 [mRNA copy number/1 µg of total RNA]	TIMP-2 [mRNA copy number/1 µg of total RNA]	β-aktyna [mRNA copy number1/µg of total RNA]
Colo-829	-	527	-	-	47255	3922322
SH-4	860	57	558459	-	1855586	12604750

Table 1. The mRNA copy number of β-actin, MMP-2, MMP-9, MMP-14 and TIMP-1 and TIMP-2 in melanoma cultures estimated by QRT-PCT method.

However, the results that show limited expression of MMPs in *in vitro* melanoma cell cultures are not surprising. It was even suggested that neoplastic cells themselves do not produce all proteolytic enzymes necessary to initiate the invasion and metastasis [72-74]. Some of those enzymes are probably produced exclusively by stimulated stroma cells [60]. For example, Wandel et al. [60] proved lack of MMP-1 expression in *in vitro* melanoma cell culture lines derived from the primary tumour and the following lines: A365, SK-Mel-13 and MeWo. Whereas Roomi et al. [ADD CITATION] confirmed that some MMP-2 and -9 expression cannot be observed in some *in vitro* types of carcinoma cells. However, Hofmann et al. [55] examined changes in expression of mRNA, MMP-1, -2, -3, -9 metalloproteinases and TIMP-1 and -2 inhibitors in a human model of *in vitro* and *in vivo* melanoma xenograft. The xenograft comprised eight melanoma cell lines with various intensity of maliciousness. Those experiments proved that mRNA level expression of MMP1 occurred in all melanoma cell lines. However, protein-level expression analysed with Northern Blot method could not be confirmed

http://dx.doi.org/10.5772/54935

which may suggest that the amount of MMP-1 in those cells was very small [55]. Presence of mRNA and MMP-2 protein was confirmed in all cell lines, however the highest level of expression, both in latent and active MMP-2 form was identified in the cells with the most malicious phenotype, those which were able to create metastatic foci – MV3 and BLM [55]. Presence of *MMP3* transcripts was confirmed only in three lines: in both most malicious (MV3 and BLM) and in the cell line 530, which did not have metastatic features. However, presence of MMP-3 protein characterized only MV3 and BLM lines. None of studied melanoma cell lines showed MMP-9 expression, yet mRNA and TIMP-1 and -2 protiens were identified in all of them [55]. Therefore, it seems that only the most aggressive melanoma cell lines demonstrate *in vitro* expression of most metalloproteinases, which determine their invasive abilities.

Results of the research for *MMP-2, MMP-9* and *MMP-14* mRNA, as well as *TIMP-1* and *TIMP-2* in SH-4 melanoma cells are shown in Table 1. They can confirm high invasiveness of those cells.

Photodynamic reaction conducted in Colo-829 and SH-4 melanoma cell lines with use of Fotolon causes inhibition of expression on the mRNA level for those metalloproteinases identified above or at least significantly decreases its value. It makes further analysis of influence of therapeutic conditions on expression of chosen *MMPs* and *TIMPs* in examined *in vitro* melanoma cell lines impossible and focuses the researchers' attention on fibroblasts stimulated with a growth media derived from melanoma cell cultures treated with PDT. For it has been confirmed that the invasive and metastatic processes occurring in tumours are results of ECM destruction caused by MMPs, which are produced by both melanoma and stroma cells. Neoplastic cells, due to secretion of various factors, such as growth factors and cytokines, can stimulate neighbouring fibroblasts, which form the stroma tissue of the tumour, to produce and change the level of expression of metalloproteinases [73]. Moreover, results of various studies suggest even that neoplastic cells themselves do not produce all proteolytic enzymes necessary to initiate the invasion and metastasis [72-74]. Some of those enzymes are probably produced only by stimulated stroma cells [60]. Wandel et al. [60] proved that fibroblasts gathered around the melanoma cells have an increased level of *MMP1* expression in comparison to those fibroblasts which have no contact with neoplastic cells. Stimulation of the fibroblasts who did not have any contact with neoplastic cells with the growth medium gathered from melanoma cell cultures leads to over 20 times higher number of *MMP1* transcripts when compared to unstimulated fibroblasts. Those have only three times higher level of expression when compared to rhe SK-Mel-13 line melanoma cells. Increase of *MMP1* expression was also observed on the protein level. Wandel et al. [60] proved statistically significant amounts of proteins between the unstimulated fibroblast cultures and those cultures which were stimulated with the growth medium gathered from melanoma cell cultures. Moreover, Zhang et al. [74] proved that MMP-2 and MMP-14 (MT1-MMP) metalloproteinases produced by fibroblasts attribute to higher invasiveness of *in vitro* HNSCC tumour (Head and Neck Squamous Cell Carcinoma) and stimulate its *in vivo* growth.

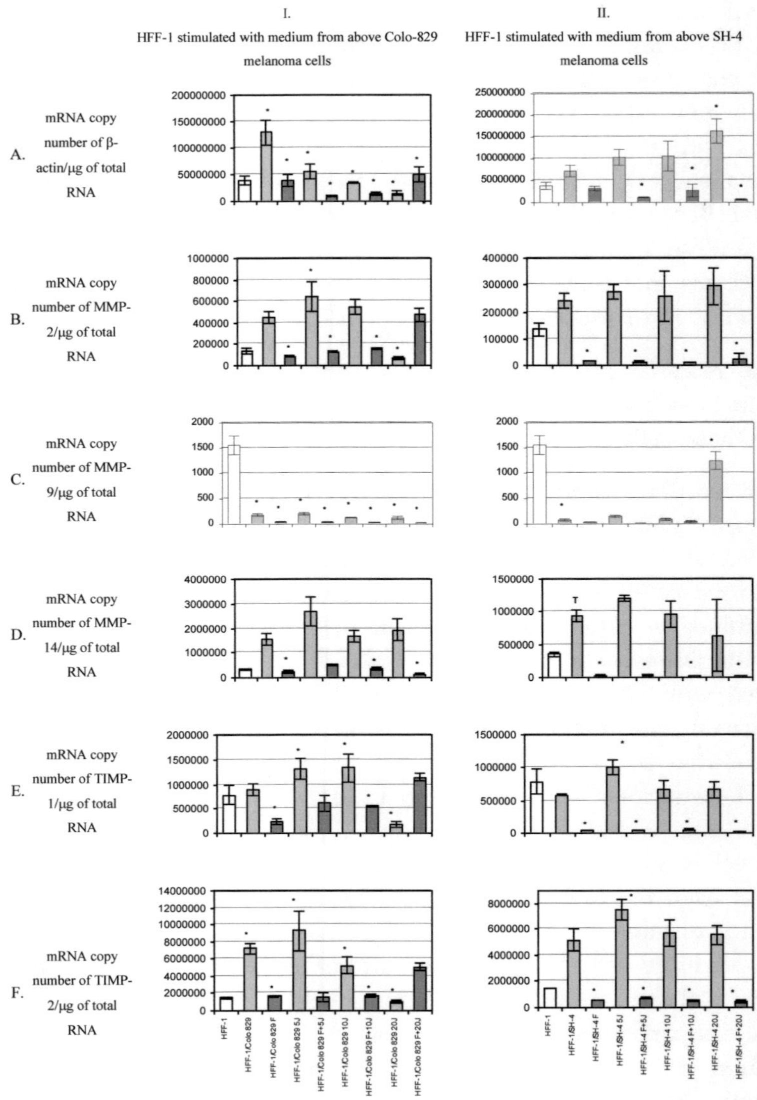

Figure 1. Comparison of (A) β-actin, (B) MMP-2, (C) MMP-9, (D) MMP-14, (E) TIMP-1, and (F) TIMP-2 gene expression at transcription level among fibroblast cultures HFF-1 stimulated with medium from above melanoma cultures from Colo-829 and SH-4 cell lines before and after PDT. The first and the second column (column I and II) show the changes of all chosen genes expression in the fibroblast cultures HFF-1 stimulated with medium from above melanoma cultures from appropriately Colo 829 and SH-2 cell lines. The statistically significant results are marked with the symbol „*" ($p<0,05$).

Results obtained for *MMP-2, MMP-9* and *MMP-14* metalloproteinases and their TIMP-1 and TIMP-9 inhibitors confirm processes observed in SK-Mel-13 melanoma line [60], including the

http://dx.doi.org/10.5772/54935

influence of factors secreted by melanoma cells on expression of metalloproteinases (at the mRNA level) and their inhibitors by fibroblast cells in *in vitro* conditions. The conducted research showed general growth of *MMP-2* and *MMP-14* metalloproteinase transcripts, as well as *TIMP-2* inhibitor, in fibroblast cells stimulated by the growth medium gathered from both Colo-829 and SH-4 melanoma cultures. However, statistical significance of the growth of expression on the mRNA level occurs only in the case of *TIMP-2* in fibroblast cultures stimulated by the growth medium gathered from Colo-829 (HFF-1/Colo-829) melanoma cultures ($p < 0.05$). In case of fibroblast cultures stimulated by the growth medium gathered from Colo-829 (HFF-1/Colo-829) and SH-4 (HFF-1/SH-4) cultures, a statistically significant decrease of the number of MMP-9 metalloproteinase transcripts was also observed ($p<0.05$). In most cases and independently from the applied radiation dose (5 J/cm^2, 10 J/cm^2 and 20 J/cm^2), stimulation of *in vitro* fibroblasts by the growth medium gathered from the melanoma cell cultures which were treated with PDT laser in presence of a photosensitizer causes a decrease of expression on the mRNA level in the examined *MMPs* and *TIMPs* in a statistically significant way ($p<0.05$) (Fig. 1).

Moreover, in case of normal fibroblast cultures stimulated with the growth medium gathered from Colo-829 melanoma cell cultures that were previously treated with PDT, an increase of the ratio between the number of *MMP2/TIMP2/MMP14* transcript copies can be observed when compared to HFF-1/Colo-829 cultures (Table 2, Fig.2).

Stimulated fibroblast cell cultures HFF-1	The proportion of mRNA copy number: MMP-2 : MMP-14 : TIMP-2			Interaction between the MMP-14:TIMP-2 proportion
HFF-1 (nonstimulated control cell culture)	**1 :**	**3 :**	**11**	-
HFF-1/Colo-829	**1 :**	**3 :**	**16**	**p = 0,0038**
HFF-1/Colo-829 F	1 :	3 :	19	
HFF-1/Colo-829 5J/cm^2	1 :	4 :	14	p = 0,6450
HFF-1/Colo-829 F+5J/cm^2 (PDT)	1 :	4 :	13	
HFF-1/Colo-829 10J/cm^2	1 :	3 :	10	p = 0,1832
HFF-1/Colo-829 F+10J/cm^2 (PDT)	1 :	2 :	10	
HFF-1/Colo-829 20J/cm^2	1 :	29 :	15	**p < 0,0001**
HFF-1/Colo-829 F+20J/cm^2 (PDT)	4 :	1 :	11	
HFF-1/SH-4	**1 :**	**4 :**	**21**	**p = 0,0086**
HFF-1/SH-4 F	1 :	1 :	34	
HFF-1/SH-4 5J/cm^2	1 :	4 :	27	**p < 0,0001**
HFF-1/SH-4 F+5J/cm^2 (PDT)	1 :	3 :	53	
HFF-1/SH-4 10J/cm^2	1 :	4 :	22	**p = 0,0060**
HFF-1/SH-4 F+10J/cm^2 (PDT)	1 :	2 :	42	
HFF-1/SH-4 20J/cm^2	1 :	2 :	19	p = 0,8270
HFF-1/SH-4 F+20J/cm^2 (PDT)	1 :	1 :	19	

Table 2. The comparition of the proportion of mRNA copy number of MMP-2, MMP-14 and TIMP-2 (MMP-2:MMP-14:TIMP-2) in the fibroblast cell cultures HFF-1 stimulated with media from above melanoma cultures from Colo 829 and SH-4 cell lines before and after PDT. The table shows also the interaction between the MMP-14:TIMP-2 proportion in case of pairs of the cell lines: with and without the Photolon (F) addition (the statistically significant results – interactions - are when p<0,05).

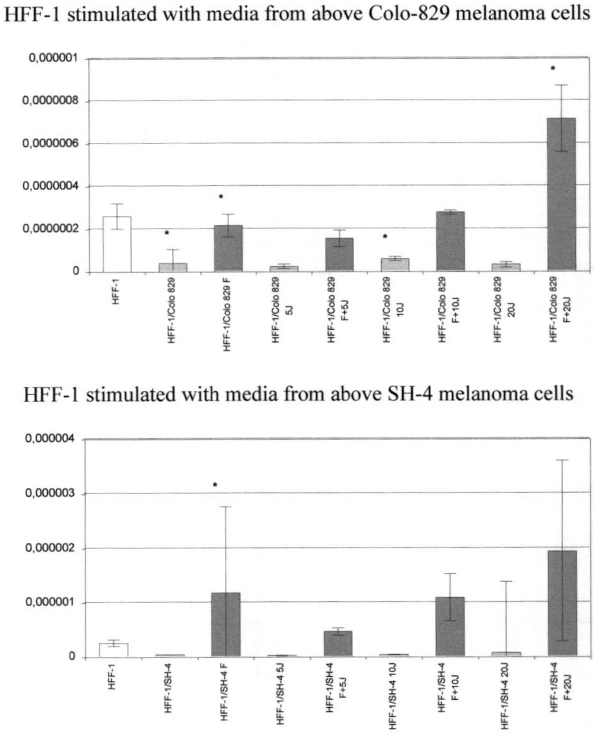

Figure 2. Comparison of the MMP-2/MMP-14/TIMP-2 mRNA copy number ratio among fibroblast cultures HFF-1 stimulated with media from above melanoma cultures from Colo 829 and SH-4 cell lines before and after PDT. The statistically significant results are marked with the symbol „*" (p<0,05).

Appropriate ratio of *MMP2/TIMP2/MMP14* gene transcripts guarantees correct course of MMP-2 activation. Increased MMP-14 expression causes activation of MMP-2 on the surface of melanoma cells. Activity of MMP-2 is also regulated by presence of TIMP-2. On the one hand, that inhibitor can influence MMP-2 and, in that way, limit growth of the tumour and invasiveness. On the other hand, TIMP-2 may be engaged in a direct way in activation of MMP-2 by forming a complex with MMP-14, which is a receptor for MMP-2 on the surface of cells. Therefore, only coordinated expression of MMP-2, MMP-14 and TIMP-2 causes activation of MMP-2 [50, 55].

It was also observed during gene tagging that a statistically significant decrease in the number of transcripts of examined genes ($p < 0.05$) in fibroblasts occurred due to stimulation with the growth medium gathered from those melanoma cell cultures which were not treated with PDT but had a photosensitizer added to them. Therefore, Fotolon alone probably causes so significant changes in synthesis and secretion of factors produced by neoplastic cells and later present in the growth medium that it also influences expression of *MMP* genes and fibroblast *TIMPs* (Fig. 1).

The research of expression of MMP-2, MMP-9 and MMP-14, as well as TIMP-1 and TIMP-2 in Colo-829 and SH-4 melanoma cells conducted and described in our study proves that *in vitro* photodynamic therapy of melanoma can cause changes in expression of *MMPs* and *TIMPs*. This may not happen in the melanoma cells themselves but certainly occurs in the connective stroma tissue of the tumour. Moreover, melanoma cells proved to be sensitive to both laser light and the photosensitizer alone.

The analysed ratio of MMP/TIMP copies is also significant, as it may influence later synthesis of proteins and effective activation of metalloproteinases. In most cases, the ratio decreases, which is particularly noticeable in case of cells stimulated with the growth medium from Colo-829. Due to the characteristics of TIMPs, it seems that the equilibrium between the level of active MMPs and their inhibitors may be a turning point in neoplastic progression. As noticed in the literature [50], overexpression of TIMP-1, TIMP-2 and TIMP-3 may be the cause of both inhibition of proteolysis and invasion of melanoma. However, *in situ* research proved that induction of TIMP-1 and -3, which occurs in a late stage of progression of melanocytic tumours, is mainly a result of a complex interaction within the MMP/TIMP system. Therefore, increased expression of TIMPs may inhibit the metastatic process, at the same time giving a bad prognosis [50, 59].

Demonstrated results of the study are related to the influence of PDT therapy on *in vitro* melanoma cultures. Unfortunately, this does not allow for a direct transfer of the observed processes into *in vivo* conditions. Therefore, those results cannot be the only premise to forecast changes of the phenotype in various types of melanoma cells treated with PDT in *in vivo* conditions, as the observed changes in parameters that describe the invasive potential of the tumour do not have to be related only to the speed of its growth and *in vivo* metastasis [74]. In order to understand better the influence that photodynamic therapy has on melanoma cells and the mechanisms triggered by the influence of laser light and a photosensitizer, it is necessary to conduct further, more detailed research. It is certain that changes of expression of *MMPs* and *TIMPs* on the protein level have to be examined in more detail. It is possible that other than mentioned in this study *MMPs* and *TIMPs* may influence the studied processes, depending on a type of melanoma in question. Moreover, the research needs to be conducted in both *in vitro* and *in vivo* conditions. Only after such extended amount of data is collected, a more detailed analysis and comparison of influence of PDT parameters can give a picture of effectiveness and safety of that kind of therapy on melanoma tumour cases.

4. Summary

Changes in transcriptional activity of *MMP2, MMP9, MMP14* genes, as well as *TIMP1* and *TIMP2,* in Colo-829 and SH-4 lines of cell cultures suggest that photodynamic therapy does not contribute to an increase of invasiveness of melanoma cells in relation to proteolytic enzymes of the extracellular matrix, even in sublethal conditions.

However, it should be noted that:

- presented results of *MMP2, MMP9, MMP14,* as well as *TIMP1 and TIMP2* expression are related only to the first stage of expression of examined genes (transcription), while the final effect (which is the amount of active form of enzyme proteins coded by those genes) also depends on a number of other factors,
- obtained data is valid for cells cultured in *in vitro* conditions, therefore, in order to formulate an explicit conclusion as to harmlessness of photodynamic therapy in relation to invasiveness of melanoma cells treated with PDT, this study should be treated as a starting point and similar research should be conducted in in vivo conditions.

Acknowledgements

This work was supported by a grant sponsored by Statutory Funds of the Medical University of Silesia (KNW-1-034/10) supported by the Polish Ministry of Science and Higher Education.

Author details

Aleksandra Zielińska, Małgorzata Latocha, Magdalena Jurzak and Dariusz Kuśmierz

Medical University of Silesia, Department of Cell Biology, Poland

References

[1] Curran S, Murray GI. Matrix metalloproteinases in tumor invasion and metastasis. Review article. Pathology 1999; 189: 300-308.

[2] Dziankowska-Bartkowiak B, Waszczykowska E, Żebrowska A. Udział metaloproteinaz i ich inhibitorów w patomechanizmie wybranych chorób skóry. Alerg Astma Immun 2004; 9: 71-79.

[3] Wideł MS, Wideł M. Mechanizmy przerzutowania i molekularne markery progresji nowotworów złośliwych. I. Rak jelita grubego. Post Hig Med Dośw 2006; 60: 453-470.

[4] Chaussain-Miller C, Fioretti F, Goldberg M, Menashi S. The role of matrix Metalloproteinases (MMPs) in human caries. J Dent Res 2006; 85: 22-32.

[5] Bogaczewicz J, Jasielski P, Mosiewicz A, Trojanowski T, Suchożebrska-Jesionek D, Stryjecka-Zimmer M. Rola metaloproteaz macierzy i tkankowych inhibitorów metaloproteaz w inwazji nowotworów pochodzenia neuroepitelialnego. Neurol Neurochir Pol 2006; 40: 404-412.

[6] Żebrowska A, Bogdańska M, Waszczykowska E. Metaloproteinazy i adamalizyny w patomechanizmie pemfigoidu. Post Dermatol Alergol 2005; 22: 283-287.

[7] Egeblad M, Werb Z. New functions for the matrix metalloproteinases in cancer progression. Nat Rev 2000; 2: 161-174.

[8] Yang W, Arii S, Gorrin-Rivas MJ, Mori A, Onodera H, Imamura M. Human macrophage metalloelastase gene expression in colorectal carcinoma and its clinicopathologic significance. Cancer 2201; 91: 1277-1283.

[9] Takeha, S, Fujiyama Y, Bamba T, Sorsa T, Nagura H, Ohtani H. Stromal expression of MMP-9 and urokinase receptor is inversely associated with liver metastasis and with infiltrating growth in human colorectal cancer: a novel approach from immune/ inflammatory aspect. Jpn J Cancer Res 1997; 88: 72-81.

[10] Jiang, Y, Wang M, Celiker MY, et al. Stimulation of mammary tumorigenesis by systemic tissue inhibitor of matrix metalloproteinase 4 gene delivery. Cancer Res 2001; 61: 2365-2370.

[11] Hayakawa T, Yamashita K, Ohuchi E, Shinagawa A. Cell growth-promoting activity of tissue inhibitor of metalloproteinases-2 (TIMP-2). J Cell Sci 1994; 107: 2373-2379.

[12] Yoshiji H, Harris SR, Raso E, et al. Mammary carcinoma cells over-expressing tissue inhibitor of metalloproteinases-1 show enhanced vascular endothelial growth factor expression. Int J Cancer 1998; 75: 81-87.

[13] Wang Z, Juttermann, R, Soloway PD. TIMP-2 is required for efficient activation of proMMP-2 *in vivo*. J Biol Chem 2000; 275: 26411-26415.

[14] Hanahan D, Folkman J. Patterns and emerging mechanisms of the angiogenic switch during tumorigenesis. Cell 1996; 86: 353-364.

[15] Peschon JJ, Slack JL, Reddy P, et al. An essential role for ectodomain shedding in mammalian development. Science 1998; 282: 1281-1284.

[16] Agrez M, Chen A, Cone RI, Pytela R, Sheppard D. The avb6 integrin promotes proliferation of colon carcinoma. The avb6 integrin promotes proliferation of colon carcinoma. J Cell Biol 1994; 127: 547-556.

[17] Alexander CM, Howard EW, Bissell MJ, Werb Z. Rescue of mammary epithelial cell apoptosis and entactin degradation by a tissue inhibitor of metalloproteinases-1 transgene. J Cell Biol 1996; 135: 1669-1677.

[18] Witty JP, Lempka T, Coffey R.J Jr, Matrisian LM. Decreased tumor formation in 7,12-dimethylbenzanthracene-treated stromelysin-1 transgenic mice is associated with alterations in mammary epithelial cell apoptosis. Cancer Res 1995; 55: 1401-1406.

[19] Sympson CJ. Talhouk RS, Alexander CM, et al. Targeted expression of stromelysin-1 in mammary gland provides evidence for a role of proteinases in branching morpho-

genesis and the requirement for an intact basement membrane for tissue – specific gene expression. J Cell Biol 1994; 125: 681-693.

[20] Powell WC, Fingleton B, Wilson CL, Boothby M, Matrisian LM. The metalloproteinase matrilysin proteolytically generates active soluble Fas ligand and potentiates epithelial cell apoptosis. Curr Biol 1999; 9: 1441-1447.

[21] Mitsiades N, Yu WH, Poulaki V, Tsokos M, Stamenkovic I. Matrix metalloproteinase-7-mediated cleavage of Fas ligand protects tumor cells from chemotherapeutic drug cytotoxicity. Cancer Res 2001; 61: 577–581.

[22] Yu WH, Woessner JF Jr, McNeish JD, Stamenkovic I. CD44 anchors the assembly of matrilysin/MMP-7 with heparin-binding epidermal growth factor precursor and ErbB4 and regulates female reproductive organ remodeling. Genes Dev 2002; 16: 307-323.

[23] Mañes S. Mira E, del Mar Barbacid M, et al. Identification of insulin-like growth factor – binding protein-1 as a potential physiological substrate for human stromelysin-3. J Biol Chem 1997; 272: 25706-25712.

[24] Baserga R. The contradictions of the insulin-like growth factor 1 receptor. Oncogene 2000; 19: 5574-5581.

[25] Herren B, Levkau B, Raines EW, Ross R. Cleavage of β-catenin and plakoglobin and shedding of VE-cadherin during endothelial apoptosis: evidence for a role for caspases and metalloproteinases. Mol Biol Cell 1998; 9: 1589-1601.

[26] Ilan N, Mohsenin A, Cheung L, Madri JA. PECAM-1 shedding during apoptosis generates a membrane – anchored truncated molecule with unique signaling characteristics. FASEB J 2001; 15: 362-372.

[27] Steinhusen U, Weiske J, Badock V, Tauber R, Bommert K, Huber O, et al. Cleavage and shedding of E-cadherin after induction of apoptosis. J Biol Chem 2001; 276: 4972-4980.

[28] Rodriguez-Manzaneque JC, Lane TF, Ortega MA, et al. Thrombospondin-1 suppresses spontaneous tumor growth and inhibits activation of matrix metalloproteinase-9 and mobilization of vascular endothelial growth factor. Proc Natl Acad Sci USA 2001; 98: 12485-12490.

[29] Netzer KO, Suzuki K, Itoh Y, Hudson BG, Khalifah RG. Comparative analysis of the noncollagenous NC1 domain of type IV collagen: identification of structural features important for assembly, function, and pathogenesis. Protein Sci 1998; 7: 1340-1351.

[30] Xu J, Rodriguez D, Petitclerc E, et al. Proteolytic exposure of a cryptic site within collagen type IV is required for angiogenesis and tumor growth *in vivo*. J Cell Biol 2001; 154: 1069-1080.

[31] Bergers G, Brekken R, McMahon G, et al. Matrix metalloproteinase-9 triggers the angiogenic switch during carcinogenesis. Nature Cell Biol 2000; 2: 737-744.

[32] Galvez BG, Matias-Roman S, Albar JP, Sanchez-Madrid F, Arroyo AG. Membrane type 1-matrix metalloproteinase is activated during migration of human endothelial cells and modulates endothelial motility and matrix remodeling. J Biol Chem 2001; 276: 37491-37500.

[33] Hiraoka N, Allen E, Apel IJ, Gyetko MR, Weiss SJ. Matrix metalloproteinases regulate neovascularization by acting as pericellular fibrinolysins. Cell 1998; 95: 365-377.

[34] Cornelius LA, Nehring LC, Harding E, et al. Matrix metalloproteinases generate angiostatin: effects on neovascularization. J Immunol 1998; 161: 6845-6852.

[35] Ferreras M, Felbor U, Lenhard T, Olsen BR, Delaisse J. Generation and degradation of human endostatin proteins by various proteinases. FEBS Lett 2000; 486: 247-251.

[36] O'Reilly MS, Boehm T, Shing Y, et al. Endostatin: an endogenous inhibitor of angiogenesis and tumor growth. Cell 1997; 88: 277-285.

[37] Kim YM. Jang JW, Lee OH, et al. Endostatin inhibits endothelial and tumor cellular invasion by blocking the activation and catalytic activity of matrix metalloproteinase. Cancer Res 2000; 60: 5410-5413.

[38] Koolwijk P, Sidenius N, Peters E, et al. Proteolysis of the urokinase-type plasminogen activator receptor by metalloproteinase-12: implication for angiogenesis in fibrin matrices. Blood 2001; 97: 3123-3131.

[39] Yu Q, Stamenkovic I. Localization of matrix metalloproteinase 9 to the cell surface provides a mechanism for CD44-mediated tumor invasion. Genes Dev 1999; 13: 35-48.

[40] Noe V, Fingleton B, Jacobs K, et al. Release of an invasion promoter E-cadherin fragment by matrilysin and stromelysin-1. J Cell Sci 2001; 114: 111-118.

[41] Birchmeier C, Birchmeier W, Brand-Saberi B. Epithelial – mesenchymal transitions in cancer progression. Acta Anat Basel 1996; 156, 217-226.

[42] Nakahara H, Howard L, Thompson EW, et al. Transmembrane/cytoplasmic domain-mediated membrane type 1-matrix metalloprotease docking to invadopodia is required for cell invasion. Proc Natl Acad Sci USA 1997; 94: 7959-7964.

[43] Kim J, Yu W, Kovalski K, Ossowski L. Requirement for specific proteases in cancer cell intravasation as revealed by a novel semiquantitative PCR-based assay. Cell 1998; 94: 353-362.

[44] Coussens LM, Werb Z. Inflammatory cells and cancer: think different! J Exp Med 2001; 193: F23-26.

[45] Yu Q, Stamenkovic I. Cell surface-localized matrix metalloproteinase-9 proteolytically activates TGF-band promotes tumor invasion and angiogenesis. Genes Dev 2000; 14: 163-176.

[46] Gorelik L, Flavell RA. Immune-mediated eradication of tumors through the blockade of transforming growth factor-b signaling in T cells. Nature Med 2001; 7: 1118-1122.

[47] Opdenakker G. Van den Steen PE, Van Damme J. Gelatinase B: a tuner and amplifier of immune functions. Trends Immunol 2001; 22: 571-579.

[48] McQuibban GA, Butler GS, Gong JH, et al. Matrix metalloproteinase activity inactivates the CXC chemokine stromal cell-derived factor-1. J Biol Chem 2001; 276: 43503-43508.

[49] Müller A, Homey B, Soto H, et al. Involvement of chemokine receptors in breast cancer metastasis. Nature 2001; 410: 50-56.

[50] Hofmann UB, Houben R, Bröcker EB, Becker JC. Role of matrix metalloproteinases in melanoma cell invasion. Biochimie 2005; 87: 307-314.

[51] Durko M, Navab R, Shibata HR, Brodt P. Suppression of basement membrane type IV collagen degradation and cell invasion in human melanoma cells expressing an antisense RNA for MMP-1. Biochim Biophys Acta 1997; 1356: 271-280.

[52] Hofmann UB, Eggert AAO, Blass K, Bröcker EB, Becker JC. Expression of matrix metalloproteinase in the microenvironment of spontaneous and experimental melanoma metastases reflects the requirements for tumor formation. Cancer Res 2003; 63: 8221-8225.

[53] Zucker S, Cao J. Measurement of matrix metalloproteinases in serum of patients with melanoma: snarled in technical pitfalls. Commentary on Nikkola et al., p. 5158. Clin Cancer Res 2005; 11: 5069-5070.

[54] Vaisanen A, Tuominen H, Kallioienen M, Turpeenniemi-Hujanen T. Matrix metaloproteinase-2 (72kD type IV collagenase) expression occurs in the early stage of human melanocytic tumor progression and may have prognostic value. J Pathol 1996; 180: 283-289.

[55] Ray JM, Stetler-Stevenson WG, Gelatinase A activity directly modulates melanoma cell adhesion and spreading. EMBO J 1995; 14: 908-917.

[56] Kurshat P, Wickenhauser C, Groth W, Kreig T, Mauch C. Identification of activated matrix metalloproteinase-2 (MMP-2) as the main gelatinolytic enzyme in malignant melanoma by in situ zymography. J Pathol 2002; 197: 179-187.

[57] Iida J, Wilhemson K L, Price M A et al. Membrane type-1 matrix metalloproteinase promotes human melanoma invasion and growth. J Invest Dermatol 2004; 122: 167-176.

[58] van den Oord J J, Paemen L, Opdenakker G, De Wolf-Peeters C. Expression of gelatinase B and the extracellular matrix metalloproteinase inducer EMMPRIN in benign

http://dx.doi.org/10.5772/54935

and malignant pigment cell lesions of the skin. Short Communication. Am J Pathol 1997; 151: 665-670.

[59] Nikkola J, Vihnen P, Vlaykova T, Hahka-Kemppinen M, Kahari VM, Pyrhonen S. High expression levels of collagenase-1 and stromelisin-1 correlate with shorter disease-free survival in human metastatic melanoma. Int J Cancer 2002; 97: 432-438.

[60] Wandel E, Raschke A, Hildebrandt G, et al. Fibroblasts enhance the invasive capacity of melanoma cells in vitro. Arch Dermatol Res 2002; 293: 601-608.

[61] Podbielska H, Sieroń A, Stręk W. Diagnostyka i terapia fotodynamiczna. Wrocław: Wydanie I, 2004.

[62] Castano AP, Demidova TN, Hamblin MR. Mechanisms in photodynamic therapy: Part one – Photosensitizers, photochemistry and cellular localization. Photodiagnosis and Photodyn Ther 2004; 1: 279-293.

[63] Kramer-Marek G, Serpa C, Szurko A, et al. Spectroscopic properties and photodynamic effects of new lipophilic porphyrin derivatives: Efficacy, localisation and cell death pathways. J Photochem Photobiol B 2006; 84, 1: 1-14.

[64] Tomečka M, Kolařova H, Džubak P, et al. Assessment of early apoptosis on tumour cell line G361 after photodynamic therapy. Scripta Med 2005; 78, 4: 205-210.

[65] Pasewicz A, Idziak D, Koloczek J, et al. Pair correlation function analysis of 5-(4-hexadecyloxyphenyl)-10,15,20-tri(4-pyridyl)porphyrin and 5-(4-methoxycarbonylphenyl)-10,15,20-tri(4-pyridyl)porphyrin. J Mol Struct 2008; 875, 1-3: 167-172.

[66] Grinholc M, Szramka B, Olender K, Graczyk A. Bactericidal effect of photodynamic therapy against methicillin-resistant Staphylococcus aureus strain with the use of various porphyrin photosensitizers. Acta Biochim Pol 2007; 54, 3: 665-670. on-line at: [www.actabp.pl].

[67] Wang HM, Jiang JQ, Xiao JH, Gao RL, Lin FY, Liu XY. Porphyrin with amino acid moieties: A tumor photosensitizer. Chem Biol Interact 2008; 127, 2: 154-158.

[68] Saji H, Song W, Furumoto K, Kato H, Engleman EG. Systemic Antitumor Effect of Intratumoral Injection of Dendritic Cells in Combination with Local Photodynamic Therapy. Clin Canc Res 2006; 12: 2568-2574.

[69] Usuda J, Hirata T, Ichinose Set al. Tailor-made approach to photodynamic therapy in the treatment of cancer based on Bcl-2 photodamage. Int J Oncol 2008; 33, 4: 689-696.

[70] Trichopoulos N, Damato B. Photodynamic therapy for recurrent hyphema after proton beam radiotherapy of iris melanoma. Graefes Arch Clin Exp Ophthalmol 2007; 245, 10: 1573-1575.

[71] Sheleg SV, Zhavrid EA, Khodina TV. Photodynamic therapy with chlorin e6 for skin metastases of melanoma. Photodermatol Photoimmunol Photomed 2004; 20: 21-26.

Chapter 7

MMP-2 and MMP-9 Expression in Canine Cutaneous Melanocytic Tumours: Evidence of a Relationship with Tumoural Malignancy

Isabel Pires, Joana Gomes, Justina Prada,
Dinora Pereira and Felisbina L. Queiroga

Additional information is available at the end of the chapter

http://dx.doi.org/10.5772/54878

1. Introduction

1.1. Melanocytic tumours

Melanocytic tumours derive from melanoblast and melanocyte transformation and occur both in humans and dogs [1-4]. These lesions are mainly found at skin, digits and oral cavity and eye [2,5,6]. Moreover, melanocytic tumours can be benign or malignant. Melanomas are aggressive tumours that can metastasize early in the course of the disease, both locally and in distant organs [3,7,8]. Whereas in mouth and eye, this type of tumour is generally malignant, at cutaneous level, and despite the difficulties of making a precise diagnosis, melanocytic tumours are usually benign. When malignant, they are very aggressive [3-5,8,9].

Generally, the tumour initially starts with a radial-growth phase, which can rapidly progress to a vertical-growth phase, a stage where melanoma cells have a high proliferation rate and a strong ability to metastasize [10]. Although early detection and improved surgical techniques had increase the patient survival, the prognosis of metastatic melanoma is still very poor due to the resistance to existing therapies [10,11]. Consequently, cutaneous melanoma, the most malignant tumour of the skin, still represents the leading cause of skin cancer deaths [10]; therefore, canine malignant melanoma is a life threatening disease, with up to 80% of affected dogs developing metastasis [12].

The similarities between human and canine melanoma, coupled with their similar environmental exposure, make spontaneous canine melanoma an excellent model in comparative pathology, for studying the correspondent disease in human counterpart [8,13-15]. These studies rely, primarily, on understanding the factors and mechanisms underlying tumour growth and dissemination, which, ultimately, allows the design and effective use of novel therapeutic strategies for cancer therapy [4,10,11,16].

The major hallmarks of cancer include migration, invasion, metastasis and angiogenesis [17]. An event intrinsically associated with the initial process of tumour invasion is similar to the epithelial-mesenchymal transition (EMT), a highly conserved and fundamental process of morphological transition that occurs during developmental processes; during this event, epithelial cells down-regulate cell–cell adhesion molecules and acquire a mesenchymal phenotype with reduced intercellular interactions and increased migratory capacity [17,18]. In addition, for cancer cells being able to continue growing and start migrating, new blood vessels have to be created by angiogenesis, being the new vessels easily penetrable by tumour cells due to their elevated permeability and reduced resistance [17-21].

Under normal circumstances, the extracellular matrix (ECM) constitutes one of the natural barriers against tumour spread [11,22-24]. Therefore, as cell dissemination from the primary tumour includes invasion of surrounding tissue and basement membranes, intravasation into the lymphatic or blood circulation, adhesion and extravasation into distant organs, degradation and remodeling of ECM by proteolytic enzymes are essential for tumour metastasis [5,17-19,25,26]. Thus, proteolytic enzymes have been considered important factors and potential molecular markers associated with tumour growth and invasion in several types of cancer, including melanoma [16,26,27], where prognostic markers are needed to predict the risk of progression, assess the clinical outcome and select optimal treatment strategies [4,10,16].

1.2. Matrix metalloproteinases

Proteolytic enzymes can be classified as exopeptidases or endopeptidases, based on their ability to cleave terminal or internal peptide bonds, respectively [28]. Proteases are proteolytic enzymes present in all organisms in different sizes, shapes and catalytic properties, but with the common ability to hydrolyze the internal bonds of various peptides [27,29].

Most proteases are classified as serine, cysteine, aspartic or matrix metalloproteinases (MMPs), according to their catalytic mechanism and inhibitor sensitivities [28,30]. The MMPs or matrixins were first described in 1962 by Gross and Lapiere [22,23] and are mostly known by their ability to degrade components of the ECM. This family of endoproteases has been considered essential in a number of normal physiologic processes as well as pathological events [24]; therefore, over the last years, the structure and function of MMPs and their roles in pathological processes, including cancer, have been intensively investigated in both human and veterinary medical research [19,27,29,31,32].

Currently, more than 25 different types of MMPs have been identified among vertebrates and the majority is expressed and has similar functions both in humans and dogs [16,27-29,33]. Nevertheless, MMPs have many similarities in their structure, sharing considerable homology within their major domains, including signal peptide, propeptide, catalytic and hemopexin-like domains [16,23,27,34]. Additionally, MMPs are zinc- and calcium-dependent for functional activity and, according to substrate specificities, domain organization and sequence similarities, they are classified into six groups: collagenases, stromelysins, matrilysins, membrane-type MMPs (MT-MMPs), gelatinases and other MMPs [16,23,27,35].

Collagenases are represented by MMP-1, MMP-8 and MMM-13 or collagenase -1, -2 and -3, respectively. Preferentially, they have affinity to collagen types I, II and III. Stromelysins are represented by MMP-3 and MMP-10 or stromelysin-1 and -2, respectively; they have specificity for laminin, fibronectin, elastin, gelatin and proteoglycans (MMP-11 is called stromelysin-3 but it is usually grouped with "other MMPs"). Matrilysins are represented by MMP-7 and MMP-26 or matrilysin-1 and -2, respectively; they have specificity for collagen IV, fibronectin, elastin and gelatin. The MT-MMPs are MT1, 2, 3, 4, 5 and 6 – MMP or MMP-14, -15, -16, -17, -24, and -25, respectively; they have specificity for collagen, gelatin, fibronectin and laminin [16,19,27,35,36]. Finally, the group of gelatinases includes MMP-2 and MMP-9 or gelatinases A and B, respectively. Gelatinases have a fibronectin domain into the catalytic site, which improves the degradation of denatured collagen (gelatin), type IV (basement membrane) collagen, type V collagen, fibronectin, plasminogen and elastin. The MMP-2, unlike MMP-9, digests type I, II, and III collagens [16,19,28,35].

There are a variety of cells expressing gelatinases. Typically, MMP-2 is produced by macrophages, T-cells, osteoblasts, endothelial and epithelial cells, fibroblasts, keratinocytes and chondrocytes. On the other hand, MMP-9 expression occurs in T-cells, neutrophils, leukocytes, endothelial and breast epithelial cells, osteoclasts, keratinocytes, monocytes, macrophages, and in connective tissue cells [19,23,30,37]. Furthermore, and despite their usual extracellular activity, several MMPs have been demonstrated as active proteases localized in nuclei of various human and animal cell types, including heart myocytes, brain neurons, breast and endothelial cells, fibroblasts and hepatocytes [26].

The degradation of ECM by MMPs essentially consists in the disruption and remodeling of structural barriers that enable the occurrence of extravascular tissue access and cellular invasion into the surrounding tissue stroma [22,23,38]. However, that process is more complex as it makes the ECM a major influence of cell behavior survival and communication, since it responds to signaling molecules and acts as ligand for cellular adhesion receptors [24,27,28]. Therefore, as MMPs alter and structurally organize ECM, thus altering matrix-derived signals, they are essential to sustain homeostasis, regulating several cellular processes that require ECM breakdown and modification, such as cell shape, movement, growth, differentiation, survival and apoptosis [16,19,28,34].

Generally, both MMP-2 and -9 participate in these processes, where MMP-2 has major roles reducing cell adhesion, stimulating cell migration and differentiation and acting as an anti-inflammatory factor; the MMP-9, on the other hand, may act as anti- or pro-inflammatory factor [35]. The gelatinases are also linked to the cell spreading and cytoskeletal changes during cell migration [19]. Moreover, MMPs substrates are not limited to ECM proteins; in fact they have the ability to cleave and activate one another, disrupt cell–cell contacts and cleave latent growth factors, proteinases and their inhibitors, blood clotting factors, cell surface receptors, adhesion molecules and intracellular substrates [19,24,28,34,39]. Therefore, MMPs, including gelatinases, are associated with many normal physiological events, such as embryonic development, reproduction, ovulation, wound healing, bone resorption, tissue morphogenesis, nerve growth and mammary gland development [16,23,30,34,38].

Usually, alternating cycles of proteolysis and its inhibition prevent an excessive proteolytic activity and tissue destruction [19]. Therefore, in most tissues, basal MMP production is normally very low [23,28,39]. The MMP-2, in particular, is widely distributed and is constitutively expressed by most cells with only modest up or downregulation under various conditions [19,29]; on the other hand, MMP-9 expression is normally induced and, while almost MMPs are constitutively secreted after their translation [29,30], MMP-9 can be packaged in neutrophils, being released during specific stimulation [19,23,26,30]. Nevertheless, endothelial cells can release both MMP-2 and -9 very quickly, indicating that they might originate from intracellular storage compartments [26].

At the transcription level, the expression of MMPs can be activated by cytokines and growth factors, including transforming growth factor-α and -β (TGF- α and β, respectively), tumour necrosis factor- α (TNF- α) interleukins (ILs), interferons, endothelial growth factor (EGF), basic fibroblast growth factor (bFGF), keratinocyte growth factor (KGF), nerve growth factor (NGF) and vascular endothelial growth factor (VEGF), among others [17,18,23,24,28]. In addition to soluble proteins, cell-matrix and cell-cell interactions, mediated by cell-adhesion molecules like epithelial (E)-cadherin and several integrins [21], can also stimulate the expression of MMPs [23]. At the post-transcriptional level, gene expression can be regulated through the stability of mRNA in the cytoplasm [30]. On the other hand, the expression of MMPs can be downregulated by targeting of extracellular components, intracellular growth factors, signal transduction pathways and suppressive factors, which include transforming growth factor-beta (TGF-β), retinoic acids and glucocorticoids [19,23,24,26].

Gelatinases are secreted into the ECM in an inactive or latent form, being called proenzymes or zymogens; the proenzyme secretion, activation and the inactivation of their activities by endogenous inhibitors represent additional regulation processes of these enzymes [18,19,23,30]. Initially, each MMP contains an amino-terminal (N-terminal) domain, called pre-domain, a signal sequence that guides the enzyme for synthesis and secretion in the extracellular environment in a zymogenic form; when that occurs, the pre-domain is lost and the latency of these enzymes is maintained by the cysteine in the pro-domain of the propeptide, which chelates the zinc ion bounded in the active site, formatting a bridge. This interaction can be further abolished by mechanical disruption or other processes (cysteine switch) leading to an intermediate activation, which is followed and completed by the activity of other extracellular proteases, including other MMPs, or even by autocatalytic cleavage; at the time of enzyme activation, the pro-domain is removed [16,23,35,38].

In both humans and dogs, pro-MMP-2 has 72 kDa and may be converted to the 62 or 66 kDa active forms by several enzymes, such as MMP-1,MMP -7, MMP-14, MMP-15, MMP-16, MMP-24, MMP-25, thrombin and plasmin; on the other hand, MMP-2 can activate MMP-1, MMP-13 and MMP-9. In addition to MMP-2, pro-MMP-9 (92 kDa) can be activated to the 82, 84 or 88 kDa active form by MMP-3, MMP-7, MMP-10, MMP-13, MMP-26 and plasmin [19,28,29,35]. In the particular case of MMP-9, the substrate binding to proenzime seems to be enough to trigger the cysteine switch. This may explain the fact that usually, the active MMP-9 is often absent in the tissues, despite the observation of its catalytic activity [19]. Furthermore, MMP-9 exists in plasma as a monomer, complexed as a dimer with a protein named lipocalin, present in activated neutrophils; the MMP-2, on the other hand, is strictly monomeric [19].

Moreover, except for matrilysin, all MMPs also have a hemopexin domain, which is a heme-binding peptide at the carboxyl-terminal (C-terminal) [16,23,27,29]. This additional domain is important in substrate recognition and in inhibitor binding [16,27]. The MMPs activity can be inhibited by zinc- and calcium-chelating agents and by specific naturally occurring tissue inhibitors of metalloproteinases (TIMPs), which augment cell adhesion and stabilize cell–cell contacts by inhibiting ECM degradation [16,19,23,26]. The TIMPs are secreted proteins, but may be found at the cell surface in most tissues and body fluids, in association with membrane-bound proteins; based on structure, four different types of TIMPs have been characterized: TIMP-1, -2, -3 and -4 [16,28,30,34].

Both TIMP-1 and TIMP-2 inhibits MMP-9, although TIMP-1 is more effective; on the other hand TIMP-2 inhibits proMMP-2 over 10-fold more effectively than TIMP-1. However, TIMP-2 has a bi-functional effect on MMP-2, inhibiting its activity in high concentrations, but regulating its activation when present in low levels, by associating to MT1-MMP and pro-MMP-2 at cell surface [28,30,34,38,39]. Like TIMP-1 and TIMP-2, TIMP-3 and TIMP-4 also may inhibit MMP-2 and -9; TIMP-4, particularly can also regulate MMP-2 by inhibiting its activator MT1-MMPs [30,34]. In addition, gelatinases, unlike other families, can be regulated by TIMPs before being activated, since these inhibitors can reversibly bind to MMP-2 and -9 zymogens [34,37]. Like MMPs, TIMPs also exhibit biological functions, including mitogenic activities on a number of cell types, which are independent of their MMP-inhibitory activities; therefore, TIMPs are also important regulators in cellular activities [34,38].

Another pos-translation regulation mechanism of MMPs activity is associated with their localization, where specific events concentrate proteinases in the pericellular microenvironment, within the vicinity of their targets [18,26,28,34]. These localization mechanisms also limit the access of TIMPs and the extent of proteolysis to discrete regions [19,26,28].

However, as a result of specific protein, genetic and/or epigenetic mutations [23,27-30], and reactive oxygen species influence [18], the functions of MMPs that are essential in normal conditions may develop into pathogenesis. When the regulatory mechanisms are compromised, MMPs production and activity may be abnormally diminished or increased, leading to an improperly ECM degradation [16,23,34,40,41]. Therefore, the occurrence of MMPs deregulation, particularly an increased gelatinase activity [16,19,34,39], is frequently associated with several human and canine pathological events, including: rheumatoid arthritis, inflammatory disorders of the gastrointestinal tract, cerebrovascular, cardiovascular, skin and lung diseases, and cancer [16,18,19,24,27,29,32].

1.3. Matrix metalloproteinases and cancer

The MMPs have been implicated in cancer for more than 40 years [18], being overexpressed in a wide range of malignant tumours in response to oncogenic cellular transformation [23,26], cytokines and several growth and angiogenic factors [16,19,23,26,42]. In addition, the complexity of the tumour microenvironment triggers a variety of regulatory cascades that determine the expression and function of several proteins; therefore, the tumour context is important, that is weather TIMPs and/or activating enzymes in the microenvironment are present or not [18].

Despite they are often produced by invasive cancer cells, most MMPs, under stimulation of ILs and growth factors, are produced by non-malignant stromal cells such as fibroblasts, endothelial cells and bone marrow-derived cells, including macrophages [5,17,19,21,43]. Furthermore, MMPs are typically required in the early stage of the tumour progression [19,20] due to their ability to degrade the ECM, basement membranes, growth-factor receptors, cytokines, chemokines, cell adhesion molecules, apoptotic ligands and angiogenic factors [17, 27,33], since that contributes to tumour proliferation, invasion, intravasation into circulation, extravasation, migration to metastatic sites and angiogenesis [16,19,21,26,27]. Therefore, several proteins, including MMPs, integrins, matrix proteins are gathered when the cells need to invade and migrate and come across a non-degraded ECM [19].

On the other hand, MMPs may deregulate the balance between growth and antigrowth signals in the tumour microenvironment [18,20,44]. Additionally, MMPs orchestrate inflammation, which is linked to cancer progression [18,19,43], and are also associated with mechanisms that cancer cells develop to avoid host immune response, mainly through the suppression of T-lymphocytes proliferation or by decreasing the tumour cells sensitivity to natural killer (NK) cells [19,23,25,26,31]. The MMP function is also involved with the ability of malignant cells to evade apoptosis, by cleaving ligands and receptors that transduce pro-apoptotic signals [18,23,24]. Furthermore, the overexpression of MMPs, gelatinases in particular, can also cause EMT and induce genomic instability [17,18]. Consequently, the presence of MMPs in malignant diseases, including gelatinases, is often correlated with highly aggressive tumours and low prognosis, both in humans and dogs [18,27,32,43,45].

However, the degradation of ECM components and other extracellular molecules, although under malignant stimulation, may generate fragments with new bioactivities that inhibit angiogenesis [18]. On the other hand, TIMPs expression in tumour tissue and stroma generally inhibits tumour cell growth, reduces the invasive and metastatic capacity of tumour cells and prevents angiogenesis [16,34,42,46,47]. Hence, it would be logical to assume that during cancer development, an high MMP:TIMP ratio would be present [44]. However, an excessive activity of MMPs may difficult tumour cell adhesion by destroying cell-matrix interactions or matrix signals required for cell migration, invasion and angiogenesis; therefore, even in cancer progression, a certain balance between MMPs and TIMPs is needed, in order to allow the remodeling of stromal tissues [19,20,26,44].

Among all MMPs, the gelatinases and respective proenzymes are two of the most important members in the development and invasion of tumour cells in several neoplasias. Both MMP-2 and MMP-9 are expressed in a variety of human [16,19,25,27,43,48] and canine [32,33,45,49-52] cancers, including lymphoma, glioma, ovarian, lung, bladder, pancreatic, prostate, renal, oral, gastric, and breast cancers, neuroblastoma, promyelotic leukemia, fibrosarcoma, osteosarcoma, cutaneous mast cell tumours and melanoma.

With respect to balance deregulation between growth and anti-growth signals, as MMPs substrates, latent growth factors can be activated by gelatinases [20]. For instance, they are able to release the active TGF-β, thus promoting angiogenesis and tumour metastasis [4,17-19,44]; on the other hand, TGF- β up-regulates the MMP-2, acting as a strong autocrine mediator of tumour cell invasion [4]. Moreover, neutrophil-derived pro-MMP-9 is not complexed with TIMP-1, being more readily activated to drive tumour angiogenesis by activating the basic fibroblast growth factor 2 (FGF-2) pathway [17,18]. Likewise, MMP-9 is implicated in vasculogenesis and regulates the bioavailability of bFGF and VEGF, the most potent inducer of tumour angiogenesis, which may also affect lymphangiogenesis [17-19,43,45]. The increased expression of MMP-2 is also associated with lymphatic invasion and lymph node metastases [18].

Additionally, not only the presence of MMPs, but also their cellular location plays a crucial role in cell invasion [53]; during invasion, the localization of MMPs to specialized cell surface structures is requisite for their ability to promote invasion [17]. Thus, the cell surface-bound gelatinases also play a role in cancer progress; in leukemic cells, for example, pro-MMP-9 interacts with intercellular adhesion molecule-1 (ICAM-1), enhancing tumour cell resistance to NK cell-mediated cytotoxicity [19,25,26]. Furthermore, the gelatinases cell surface activity has been found to be dependent of cell adhesion molecules, such as integrins, for tumour migration, invasion angiogenesis in many cancers [5,10,19,23,26,28].

In human melanoma cells, particularly, MMP-2 and -9 have been focus of attention in the last years, both in cutaneous [4,5,27,43,48,53-57], as well as in eye [11,58-62] and oral melanoma [6]. Although the role of MMPs in melanoma remains controversial [5,55], both gelatinases are often overexpressed in melanocytic tumours, frequently in advanced stages of melanoma, thus being associated to the most invasive and aggressive cases and to a low prognosis and patient outcome. The specific activation processes and the localization of MMPs during migration of melanoma cells is still poorly understood [5]; nevertheless, MMP-2 and -9 have been detected in a high number of vesicular organelles, which may be a way of achieving a rapid and directional proteolysis during cell migration, invasion and angiogenesis [26]. In veterinary medicine, as the best authors' knowledge only two studies concerning the gelatinases expression have been made in canine melanocytic tumours, one in cutaneous lesions [49] and the other in oral melanomas [51].

Conversely to the majority of the observations, there are several MMPs, including gelatinases, with the ability to negatively control some aspects of cancer progression. Particularly, MMP-2 and -9 are able to cleave plasminogen, which creates angiostatin, and MMP-9 can also cleave a basement membrane collagen type XVIII, creating a product named endostatin; both cleavage products can inhibit endothelial cell proliferation and angiogenesis [20,22,27,38,44]. Similarly a few studies indicate a positive correlation between increased TIMP levels and poor outcome in some human malignancies [40]. Although the significance of this event remains unclear, it seems that the role of each MMP and TIMP depends on the type of cell that produces the enzyme (tumour cell or stroma), the cancer stage, the tumour site (primary or metastasis), the substrate profile, the tissue of neovascularization and several microenvironmental factors [17-20]; however, the significance of this event remains unclear [20,27,44].

In the context of cancer therapy, several clinical trials have been developed in both humans and dogs, in order to inhibit MMP activity [18,32,52], particularly the activity of gelatinases, in several malignant diseases, including melanoma [27,42]. The majority of these studies are based on the use of TIMPs or synthetic inhibitors [20,26,27,42] and knockout experiments [19, 42], where MMP-2 and MMP-9 are absent. In addition, similar studies are based on the degradation of particular cell receptors that bind to gelatinases [19]. Although some these inhibition studies remain controversial, promising results have been observed, including the reduction of the growth and invasion of the more aggressive cases [19-21,26,27]. The presence of anti-tumour MMPs may be the underlying cause of lack of success of some of these clinical trials [27]; therefore, the dual role of MMPs in angiogenesis highlights the need to develop selective MMP inhibitors [20].

On the bases of what was previously described, MMPs are undeniably important factors influencing tumour behavior; however, there is still not enough knowledge about the function of individual MMPs in cancer [19,27]. As the dog has been considered a good model for studies of spontaneous melanoma [8,13-15] and since the role of MMPs in canine melanocytic tumours is still poorly explored and understood, the aims of the present work are to study the immunoexpression of MMP-2 and MMP-9 in canine cutaneous melanocytic tumours and the association between them and several pathological characteristics.

2. Material and methods

2.1. Tissue processing and tumour classification

From the archive of the Histopathology Laboratory of the University of Trás-os-Montes and Alto Douro, 42 canine cutaneous melanocytic tumours and 5 normal skin samples were obtained. These tumours were excised from dogs presented for treatment at the Veterinary Teaching Hospital of the University of Trás-os-Montes and Alto Douro and several other veterinary private clinics. The anonymity of the sample sources was respected.

The samples were fixed in 10% buffered formalin and paraffin embedded. For the histopathologic study, 4-μm-thick tissue sections were stained with hematoxylin and eosin, with and without melanin blanching, depending on the amount of pigment. The blanching was performed by slide incubation in 0,25% potassium permanganate for 30–60 minutes and 0,1% oxalic acid for 5–8 minutes. Each sample was re-examined by two independent pathologists (IP and JP) in order to confirm the diagnosis, according to the World Health Organization International Histological Classification of Tumours of Domestic Animals criteria [63]. All slides were taken into consideration for this study and complete sections of the tumours were fully analysed.

2.2. Histopathological evaluation

The following pathological features were evaluated: histological type - melanocytoma (benign), melanoma (malign); presence of ulceration; presence of necrosis; mitotic index;

nuclear grade; degree of pigmentation, presence of aberrant tumoural cells; stroma; and tumoural vascular invasion. Mitotic index was calculated by counting all the mitosis present in 10 high power fields (HPF) (400x): mitotic index I (<3 mitosis in 10 HPF); mitotic index II (3–5 mitosis in 10 HPF) or mitotic index III (>5 mitosis in 10 HPF). For nuclear grade, the following grades were defined: nuclear grade I when the nuclei had minimal variations in their shape and size compared to normal nuclei; nuclear grade II consisted of moderate alterations of nuclear shape; and nuclear grade III consisted of the nuclei that were irregular and larger than normal [64].The degree of pigmentation was estimated using a subjective scale from scant (pigment in fewer than 30% of cells), moderate (pigmentation in 31–80% of cells), and abundant (pigment in more than 80% of cells). The amount of stroma was categorized in: scant, moderate, and abundant [65].

2.3. Immunohistochemistry

For immunohistochemical studies, 3-μm sections were cut from each specimen and mounted on silane-coated slides. MMP-2 and MMP-9 immunoexpression were carried out by the streptavidin-biotin-peroxidase complex method, with a commercial detection system (Ultra Vision Detection System; Lab Vision Corporation) following the manufacturer's instructions, with and without blanching. All the washes and dilutions were made in phosphate buffered saline (PBS) solution (pH=7.4).

Sections were deparaffinized in xylene and rehydrated in a graded alcohol series, ending in tap water. The blanching was performed with 0,25% potassium permanganate ($KMnO_4$) and 0,1% oxalic acid ($H_2C_2O_4$). For MMP-2, antigens were retrieved by microwave treatment for 20min at 750W in a solution of citrate buffer, in distilled water. No pre-treatment was used for MMP-9 labeling.

After cooling the slides at room temperature, endogenous peroxidase was blocked, through the incubation with 3% hydrogen peroxidase for 30min. Slides were then dried and sections outlined with a hydrophobic pen (Liquid Blocker, Daido),washed in PBS for 5min and applied the blocking serum for 5min (Ultra VBlock, Labvision Corporation). Subsequently the sections were incubated overnight at 4 ∘C, with the primary antibodies: MMP-2 (Neomarkers) diluted 1:150 and MMP-9 diluted 1:200 (Neomarkers) in phosphate buffered saline (PBS; pH 7,4; 0,01 M). On the following day, sections were washed in PBS for 5min, at room temperature, and then applied biotinylated serum and streptavidine peroxidase for 10min each (both included in the kit Ultravision Detection System, Labvision Corporation), with intermediate washings in PBS, for 5min. Immunolabeling was observed by incubation with 3,3-diaminobenzidine tetrahydrochloride (DAB; SIGMA) 0,05% with 0,01% H_2O_2 for 5min. After washing in distilled water, the sections were counterstained with Gill haematoxylin, dehydrated, cleared and mounted. Each set of staining included a known positive control. The primary antibody was replaced by PBS and by an irrelevant antibody for negative controls

2.4. Immunohistochemistry evaluation

Positivity was indicated by the presence of distinct brown cytoplasmic labeling. Each specimen was evaluated in a blinded manner by 2 independent investigators (IP e FLQ). The interobserver variability was low; in case of discrepancy, a consensus was reached among 3 observers. The number of malignant cells expressing MMP-2 and MMP-9 was assessed using a semi-quantitative scale by estimating the percentage of positive tumoural cells (labeling extension). A 4-grade scale was used: negative,0,<5%; 1, 5-20% of positive cells; 2, 21–49%; and 3, over 50% of positive cells (adapted from [57]). The labeling intensity was recorded as: negative (0); weak (+); moderate (++) and strong (+++).

2.5. Statistical analysis

Statistical analyses were made to determine correlation between MMPs immunoexpression (labeling extension and intensity) and tumor diagnosis (benign or malignant), and between MMPs immunoexpression in malignant melanomas and the pathological variables under study. The statistical software SPSS (Statistical Package for Social Sciences, IL, USA), version 12.0, was used for statistical analysis. We performed a chi-square test (χ^2) for studying categorical variables. In all statistical comparisons, $p< 0.05$ was accepted as denoting significant differences.

3. Results

3.1. Tumours

The studied canine cutaneous melanocytic tumours were originated from dogs of different breeds. Undefined breed (n=13/42), Boxer (n=11/42), Rottweiller (n=5) and Cocker Spaniel (n=2) were most commonly represented. The age of the animals ranged from 9 months to 15 years, with an average of 10 years. Twenty dogs were female and 22 were male.

The lesions occur as nodules solitaries, occasionally ulcerated, varying in size between 0,4-9 cm (average of 2,7cm).

From the 42 tumours included in the study, 11 cases were classified as melanocytomas (benign tumours) and 21 cases as malignant melanomas.

3.2. MMP-2 and MMP-9 expression in canine cutaneous melanocytic tumours

Five samples of normal skin and 42 melanocytic tumours were examined (Table 1). Occasional dermal fibroblasts and macrophages were positive for both MMP-2 and MMP-9 in normal skin and tumours.

Intracytoplasmic immunostaining for MMP-2 and MMP-9 immunoreactive protein was found in epidermal and dermal nests of tumoural cells, both centrally and peripherally. Positive cells were homogeneously distributed without any constant increase in invasive fronts.

http://dx.doi.org/10.5772/54878

Sample nº	Histological Classification	MMP-2		MMP-9	
		Extension	Intensity	Extension	Intensity
1	Melanoma	3	+++	1	+
2	Melanocytoma	3	++	2	++
3	Melanocytoma	2	+++	0	0
4	Melanoma	3	+++	1	+
5	Melanocytoma	3	+++	3	+
6	Melanocytoma	3	++	0	0
7	Melanoma	2	+	2	++
8	Melanoma	1	++	1	+
9	Melanoma	1	++	2	++
10	Melanoma	3	+	3	+++
11	Melanoma	2	+	3	+
12	Melanoma	2	+	3	+++
13	Melanoma	3	++	2	++
14	Melanoma	1	+	3	++
15	Melanoma	1	+	3	++
16	Melanocytoma	3	++	0	0
17	Melanocytoma	3	++	3	+
18	Melanoma	1	+	3	+++
19	Melanoma	2	++	2	++
20	Melanoma	3	+	3	++
21	Melanoma	2	+	1	+++
22	Melanocytoma	3	++	0	0
23	Melanocytoma	3	++	2	+
24	Melanocytoma	3	++	2	+

Sample nº	Histological Classification	MMP-2		MMP-9	
		Extension	Intensity	Extension	Intensity
25	Melanoma	1	++	2	++
26	Melanoma	3	++	2	++
27	Melanoma	2	++	1	+
28	Melanocytoma	3	+++	2	+
29	Melanocytoma	3	+++	2	+
30	Melanoma	2	++	1	+
31	Melanoma	1	+	1	+
32	Melanoma	3	+	3	+++
33	Melanoma	1	+	1	++
34	Melanoma	2	+	1	+
35	Melanoma	2	+	3	++
36	Melanoma	1	+	3	+
37	Melanoma	1	++	3	++
38	Melanoma	2	+	1	++
39	Melanoma	3	++	3	+++
40	Melanoma	3	++	3	++
41	Melanoma	3	+	3	+
42	Melanoma	2	+	1	+

Extension – <5 (0), 5–20% (1), 21–50% (2), >51% of positive cells (3); Intensity - negative (0), weak (+), moderate (++), strong (+++)

Table 1. MMP-2 and MMP-9 immunoexpression in canine cutaneous melanocytic tumours.

The expression of MMP-2 was observed in all tumours. The percentage of labeled cells ranged from (1) isolated cells (n=10; 23.8%), to (2) foci of labeled cells (n=12; 28,6%), to (3) diffuse labeled cells (n=20; 47,6%). With respect to labeling intensity, there was weak positivity (+) in 18 cases (42,9%), moderate intensity (++) of labeling in 18 cases (42.9%) and strong intensity (+++) in 6 cases (14,3%), which is represented in Figures 1 and 2.

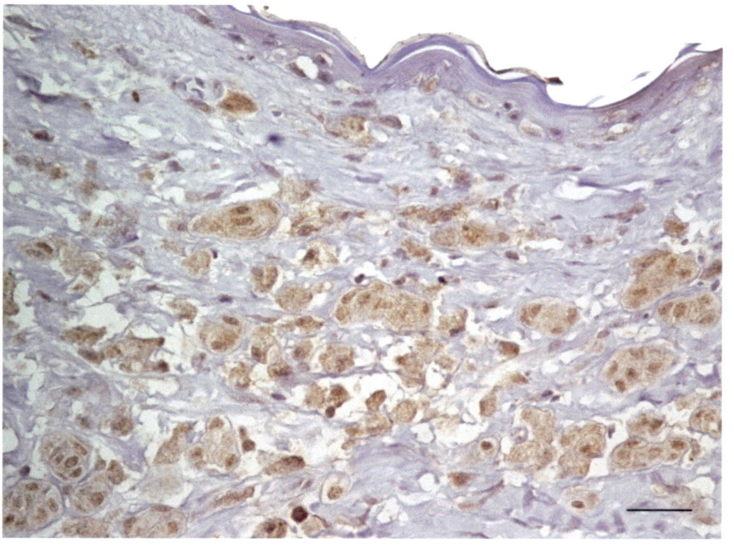

Figure 1. MMP-2 expression in canine cutaneous melanocytoma: difuse (3) and moderate labelling intensity (++). IHC. Bar, 30 μm

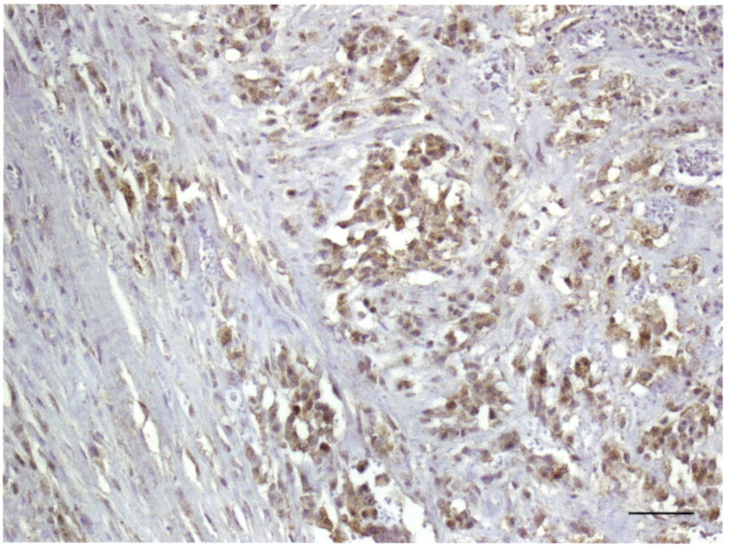

Figure 2. MMP-2 expression in canine cutaneous malignant melanoma. The positivity is moderate in a 2 extension of positive cells IHC. Bar, 60 μm

For MMP-9 immunolabeling extension, 16 melanocytic tumours showed a diffuse (3) immunolabeling (36.1%), and 22 an intermediate labeling (2) pattern represented in Figure 3. Only 4 tumours were negative (9,5%). For labeling intensity, the weak (+) and moderate (++) labeling pattern (Figure 3) was most frequently observed (n=17 and n=15 respectively). Six cases showed a strong (+++) reaction to MMP-9 (Figure 4).

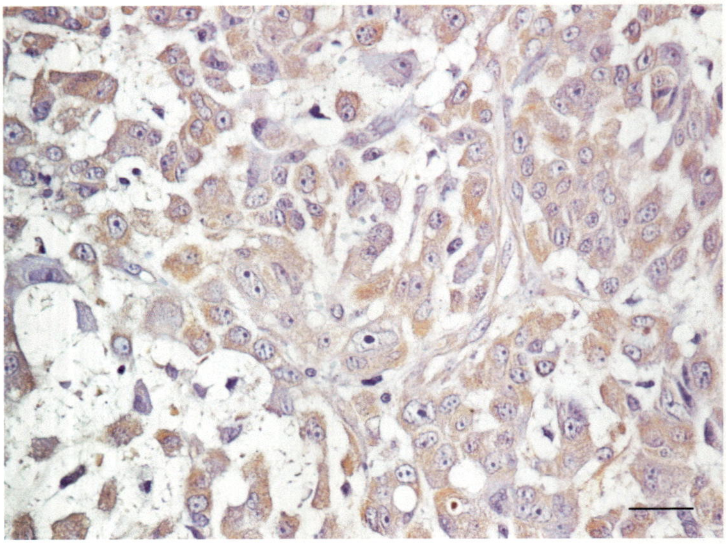

Figure 3. Difuse (3) MMP-9 expression in canine malignant melanoma, with a moderate intensity (++). IHC. Bar, 30 μm

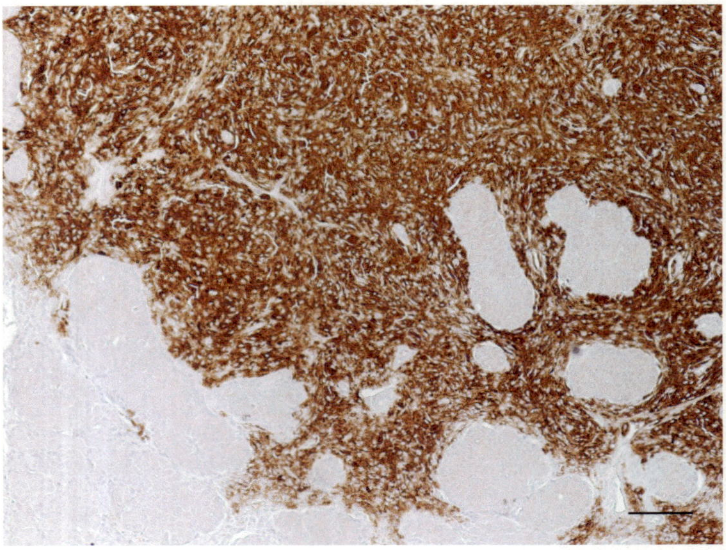

Figure 4. MMP-9 expression in canine malignant melanoma, with a difuse (3) and strong (+++) labelling intensity. The tumoural cells invades hepatoid perianal gland. IHC. Bar, 120 μm

http://dx.doi.org/10.5772/54878

3.3. Association between MMP-2 and MMP-9 expression and tumour malignancy

The percentage of MMP-2 positive cells and the intensity of reaction were significantly different between benign and malignant tumours. Benign tumours (melanocytomas) showed a higher expression of MMP-2 [both for extension (p=0,003) and intensity (p=0,02)] than malignant melanomas (Table 2).

Regarding MMP-9, the differences observed between benign and malignant tumours were statistically significant both for the extension of positive cells (p<0,0001) and for the labeling intensity (p=0,001). Malignant melanomas generally showed a higher number of positive cells than benign tumours The melanocytomas did not show MMP-9 or, when present, the immunoexpression was generally weak (Table 2).

		Melanocytoma		Melanoma		Total		p
		n	%	n	%	n	%	
MMP-2								
Extension	**1**	0	0%	10	40,7%	10	23,8%	0,003
	2	1	9,1%	11	40,7%	12	28,6%	
	3	10	90,9%	10	18,6%	20	47,6%	
Intensity	**+**	0	0%	18	58,1%	18	42,9%	0,002
	++	7	63,6%	11	35,5%	18	42,9%	
	+++	4	36,4%	2	6,5%	6	16,3%	
MMP-9								
Extension	**0**	4	36,4%	0	0%	4	9,5%	<0,0001
	1	0	0%	11	35,5%	11	26,2%	
	2	5	45,5%	6	19,4%	11	26,2%	
	3	2	18,2%	14	45,2%	16	38,1%	
Intensity	**0**	4	36,4%	0	0%	4	9,5%	0,001
	+	6	54,5%	11	35,5%	17	40,5%	
	++	1	9,1%	14	45,2%	15	35,7%	
	+++	0	0%	6	19,4%	6	14,3%	

Table 2. MMP-2 and MMP-9 immunoexpression in benign and malignant canine cutaneous melanocytic tumours.

3.4. Association between MMP-2 and MMP-9 and pathological features in canine cutaneous melanoma

The association analysis between MMP-2 immunoexpression (for labeling extension and intensity) in malignant melanomas (n=31) and the pathological criteria showed that the differences observed in labeling extension and intensity were not associated with any parameter (p>0,05), except for MMP-2 intensity and nuclear grade (p=0,049). Table 3 presents the pathological variables analyzed and their association with MMP-2 expression in canine cutaneous malignant melanomas.

Pathological features	MMP-9 Extension				MMP-9 Intensity			
	1	2	3	p	+	++	+++	p
Ulceration								
Absent	6	3	5	0,30	10	4	0	0,25
Present	4	8	5		8	7	2	
Necrosis								
Absent	6	6	6	0,96	10	7	1	0,89
Present	4	5	4		8	4	1	
Mitotic index								
I	0	0	1		0	1	0	
II	4	3	5	0,44	7	4	1	0,74
III	6	8	4		11	6	1	
Nuclear grade								
I	3	1	2		2	11	5	
II	3	7	5	0,61	4	6	1	0,049
III	4	3	3		0	0	2	
Degree of pigmentation								
Scant	5	4	1		6	3	1	
Moderate	4	4	7	0,31	8	6	1	0,92
Abundant	1	3	2		4	2	0	
Aberrant cells								
Absent	7	9	7	0,77	14	8	1	0,69
Present	3	2	3		4	3	1	
Stroma								
Scarse	4	5	5		8	6	0	
Moderate	6	6	4	0,62	10	4	2	0,35
Abundant	0	0	1		0	1	0	
Vascular invasion								
Absent	8	7	7	0,71	14	8	0	0,07
Present	2	4	3		4	3	2	

Table 3. Association of pathological variables with MMP-2 expression in canine cutaneous malignant melanomas.

MMP-9 labeling intensity presented a statistical significant association with the presence of necrosis (p=0,032), nuclear grade (p=0,09), and degree of pigmentation (p=0,008). Canine melanocytic tumours without necrosis, with a lower nuclear grade and more pigmented, showed a higher MMP-9 labeling intensity. In respect to MMP-9 extension, a positive association is observed with the degree of pigmentation (p=0,003), where the percentage of MMP-9 positive cells is higher in malignant melanomas with abundant amounts of melanin (Table 4).

Pathological features	**MMP-2 Extension**				**MMP-2 Intensity**			
	1	**2**	**3**	**p**	**+**	**++**	**+++**	**p**
Ulceration								
Absent	3	2	9	0,15	2	8	4	0,08
Present	8	4	5		9	6	2	
Necrosis								
Absent	5	6	7	0,07	3	10	5	0,032
Present	6	0	7		8	4	1	
Mitotic index								
I	0	1	0		0	1	0	
II	5	2	5	0,34	5	5	2	0,82
III	6	3	9		6	8	4	
Nuclear grade								
I	1	5	5		1	3	7	
II	3	3	0	0,12	4	9	1	0,009
III	2	9	3		6	5	0	
Degree of pigmentation								
Scant	8	0	2		8	2	0	
Moderate	2	3	10	0,003	3	8	4	0,008
Abundant	1	3	2		0	4	2	
Aberrant cells								
Absent	7	5	11	0,59	6	12	5	0,18
Present	4	1	3		5	2	1	
Stroma								
Scarse	7	2	5		7	5	2	
Moderate	4	3	9	0,17	4	8	4	0,50
Abundant	0	1	0		0	1	0	
Vascular invasion								
Absent	6	4	12	0,23	6	11	5	0,32
Present	5	2	2		5	3	1	

Table 4. Association of pathological variables with MMP-9 expression in canine cutaneous malignant melanomas.

4. Discussion

Cutaneous melanoma is one of the most frequent malignant tumours in younger age people and is characterized by its high capacity for invasion and metastasis. The incidence of human cutaneous melanoma is increasing in the U.S.A., Australia, and Europe [66,67]. Among canine population, the incidence of melanocytic tumours is also increasing. Cutaneous canine melanocytic neoplasms are usually benign. However, when malignant they could be highly aggressive metastasizing both locally as in distant organs [2,68-70].

Human cutaneous melanoma may develop *de novo* from normal melanocytes or from potential precursor lesions, such as atypical dysplastic nevi or congenital nevi [66,67] but in the dog this evolution is not well established.

Canine malignant melanoma is resistant to most current therapeutic regimens. The search of novel therapeutic tools is crucial in the fight against this disease. Furthermore, the similarities between human and canine melanoma make spontaneous canine melanoma an excellent disease model for studying the corresponding human disease [14,71].

Much work is currently underway in order to identify specific tumour markers, associated with malignancy [71-73]. However, more studies are needed to differentiating benign from malignant canine melanocytic neoplasms or predicting survival times.

The involvement of ECM-degrading enzymes, such as MMPs and serine proteases, during tumour progression and metastasis is well established [28,30]. During the last few decades, in both human and veterinary oncology there has been considerable interest in studying MMPs activity as a possible independent prognostic marker and target for therapeutic options [19,27,29,31,32]. However, the biological significance of expression of MMP-2 and MMP-9 expression in melanocytic tumours is still poorly understood, presenting conflicting results regarding the relation of MMP expression and the invasiveness of melanoma cells both *in vitro* and *in vivo* [11,74-76].

In canine melanocytic tumours, studies concerning MMP-2 and MMP-9 expression are very scarce [49,51], and as far as we know, only one study was performed in cutaneous melanocytic tumours [49] until present.

Here, we analyzed the expression patterns of MMP-2 and MMP-9 in benign and malignant canine cutaneous melanocytic tumors and its relation with classical parameters of aggressiveness in malignant melanoma.

In our study, both benign and malignant lesions express MMP-2, according to human analogous studies [60]. However, MMP-2 labeling was significantly higher in benign melanocytic tumours than in malignant counterpart, contrarily to a previous human study, in wich MMP-2 expression was higher in malignant lesions [60]. Indeed, *in vitro* and *in vivo* studies suggests that MMP-2 activity could be related to the progression of melanoma and may be required for melanoma cell invasion and metastasis formation [59,77-79]. In canine cutaneous melanocytic tumours, Docampo et al. [49] did not observe any differences in MMP-2 expression between benign and malignant neoplasias.

We also observed that, in canine cutaneous malignant melanoma, a higher intensity of the MMP-2 labeling appears to be associated, in a statistical significant way, with nuclear grade (p=0,049) but not with other histological features. Interestingly, in dogs, this characteristic seems to be very accurate in predicting overall behavior in these tumours [80]. Being this, MMP-2 could be implied in canine melanoma aggressiveness. These data are in agreement with previous human studies, where the expression of MMP-2 increased notably with architectural disorder, atypia, and progression to melanoma [81,82]. Additionally, some of these studies observed a correlation between MMP-2 expression and human melanoma metastization and prognosis [60,83-86]. Indeed, active MMP-2 regulates VEGF-A in melanoma cells on a transcriptional level via an integrin $\alpha v\beta 5$/phosphoinositide-3-kinase-dependent pathway. In that context, MMP-2 plays a pivotal role in the autocrine regulation of VEGF-A expression in melanoma cells, and consequently in angiogenesis [87]. However, in our study, in spite of the association of MMP-2 and nuclear grade, we observed a lack of a association with vascular tumoural embolus, that needs to be clarified.

With respect to MMP-9, in our samples, all melanomas expressed this MMP, like described in human ciliary body melanomas [88]. We also observed significant differences in MMP-9 labeling extension (p<0,0001) and intensity (p=0,001) between benign and malignant tumours. Malignant tumours had a higher MMP-9 expression as described in a previous study in canine melanocytic tumours [49]. The differences found in MMP-9 immunoreactivity between benign and malignant lesions were also similar to the previously described in human melanocytic neoplasms [89] and lead us to speculate that MMP-9 might be involved in the neoplastic transformation of canine melanocytic tumours. In human benign pigment cell lesions, MMP-9 was expressed in cellular blue nevi whereas all other benign lesions, including common blue nevi, were negative. In malignant melanomas MMP-9 was variably expressed in the pure and invasive radial growth phase but not in the vertical growth phase [90].

Analyzing MMP-9 expression and the pathological parameters, we observed that MMP-9 presented a statistical significant association between its labeling intensity and the presence of necrosis (p=0,032), nuclear grade (p=0,09) and degree of pigmentation (p=0,008). Additionally, MMP-9 extension was significantly associated with the degree of pigmentation (p=0,003). These characteristics are classically linked to higher tumoural aggressiveness and poor clinical prognosis in these neoplasias. However, contrarily to the expected, the less aggressive tumours, without necrosis, with a lower nuclear grade and elevated pigmentation degree, showed a higher MMP-9 labeling. Even non consensual, some previous studies in melanoma suggest the opposite [91-93]. *In vitro*, MMP-9 expression was present or could be induced only in cell lines derived from advanced primary melanomas, and was absent in cell lines derived from early stage primary lesions [94]. In other study, the authors showed that less aggressive cell lines were unable to produce MMP-9 after treatment with either interleukin-1β (IL-1β) or tumour necrosis factor α(TNF-α) [93]. In murine, integrin receptor $\alpha 5\beta 1$ and extracellular matrix fibronectin ligand interaction induce the invasive potential of B16F10 cells and MMP-9 induction is the downstream effectors in the process [95].

In skin human melanoma, an involvement of MMP- 9 in invasion and metastatic growth, as in the regulation of tumour growth and progress has been suggested, by modulation of the levels of N-cadherin and PCNA [96]. Also, in human uveal melanomas, MMP-9 was associated with the presence of necrosis, a high mitotic rate [62] and with metastization [11]. In opposition, no correlation was found between MMP-9 immunoreactivity occurrence of metastases in cases of human ocular melanomas [88]. It has been proposed that not the melanoma cells themselves, but the tumour-surrounding host cells secrete MMP-9 *in vivo*, indicating that host-derived MMP-9 plays an important role in melanoma metastasis formation [97].

In canine cutaneous melanocytic tumours, according to our results, early invasion seems to be associated with *de novo* expression of MMP-9 by neoplastic melanocytes. The lack of association with aggressiveness in malignant lesions could suggest that other factors are involved in tissue degradation during later stages of tumour progression, as proposed in human melanocytic tumours [90].

Summarizing, in our study, malignancy is associated with an increase of MMP-9 and a decrease of MMP-2 expression. In malignant lesions, however, the aggressiveness, evaluated by nuclear grade, seems to be associated with a decrese of MMP-9 and an increase of MMP-2 expression. These results suggest that might occurs a switch in the MMP expression profile during tumour progression, involving not only emergence of MMP expression but also its downregulation, as described in human melanoma [93].

Nevertheless, further studies involving MMPs, their tissue inhibitors, and other regulation factors and their correlation with prognostic are needed to clarify this subject in canine melanocytic tumours.

5. Conclusion

Both MMP-2 and MMP-9 were expressed in the majority of tumours. Our results showed a close relationship between their expression and tumour behavior. The differences observed between benign and malignant melanocytic tumours may suggest that MMP-2 and MMP-9 could be implicated in the progression of melanocytic precursor lesions to malignant melanoma, although in an inverse manner, since MMP-2 is mainly found in melanocytomas and MMP-9, on the other hand, is frequently absent in benign lesions. Therefore, our study suggests that malignancy is associated with an increase of MMP-9 and a decrease of MMP-2 expression. The association of MMP-2 with nuclear grade could indicate its role in tumour agressiveness.

Understanding MMPs regulation in melanoma provides new platforms to develop efficient therapies. For that reason, more studies concerning MMPs and their regulators are needed in order to deepen the knowledge about this enzymes, regarding their potential as prognostic markers and future therapeutic targets in several cancers, including melanoma.

http://dx.doi.org/10.5772/54878

Acknowledgements

The authors thank to Mrs. Lígia Bento for expert technical assistance. he work was supported by the strategic research project PEst-OE/AGR/UI0772/2011 financed by the Foundation for Science and Technology (FCT).

Author details

Isabel Pires[1*], Joana Gomes[2], Justina Prada[1], Dinora Pereira[1] and Felisbina L. Queiroga[1]

*Address all correspondence to: ipires@utad.pt

1 CECAV, Department of Veterinary Sciences, University of Trás-os-Montes and Alto Douro, Vila Real, Portugal

2 ECVA, Department of Genetics and Biotechnology, University of Trás-os-Montes and Alto Douro, Vila Real, Portugal

References

[1] Modiano JF, Ritt MG, Wojcieszyn J. The Molecular Basis of Canine Melanoma: Pathogenesis and Trends in Diagnosis and Therapy. Journal of Veterinary Internal Medicine 1999;13(3): 163-74.

[2] Smith SH, Goldschmidt MH, McManus PM. A Comparative Review of Melanocytic Neoplasms. Veterinary Pathology 2002;39(6): 651-78.

[3] Sulaimon SS, Kitchell BE, Ehrhart EJ. Immunohistochemical Detection of Melanoma-specific Antigens in Spontaneous Canine Melanoma. Journal of Comparative Pathology 2002;127(2–3): 162-8.

[4] Malaponte G, Zacchia A, Bevelacqua Y, Marconi A, Perrotta R, Mazzarino MC, Cardile V, Stivala F. Co-regulated expression of matrix metalloproteinase-2 and transforming growth factor-beta in melanoma development and progression. Oncology Reports 2010;24(1): 81-7.

[5] Hofmann UB, Houben R, Bröcker E-B, Becker JC. Role of matrix metalloproteinases in melanoma cell invasion. Biochimie 2005;87(3–4): 307-14.

[6] Kondratiev S, Gnepp DR, Yakirevich E, Sabo E, Annino DJ, Rebeiz E, Laver NV. Expression and prognostic role of MMP2, MMP9, MMP13, and MMP14 matrix metalloproteinases in sinonasal and oral malignant melanomas. Human Pathology 2008;39(3): 337-43.

[7] Koenig A, Wojcieszyn J, Weeks BR, Modiano JF. Expression of S100a, Vimentin, NSE, and Melan A/MART-1 in Seven Canine Melanoma Cell Lines and Twenty-nine Retrospective Cases of Canine Melanoma. Veterinary Pathology 2001;38(4): 427-35.

[8] Aina OH, Maeda Y, Harrison M, Zwingenberger AL, Walker NJ, Lam KS, Kent MS. Canine malignant melanoma alpha-3 integrin binding peptides. Veterinary Immunology and Immunopathology 2011;143(1–2): 11-9.

[9] Hofmann UB, Westphal JR, Waas ET, Zendman AJ, Cornelissen IM, Ruiter DJ, van Muijen GN. Matrix metalloproteinases in human melanoma cell lines and xenografts: increased expression of activated matrix metalloproteinase-2 (MMP-2) correlates with melanoma progression. British Journal of Cancer 1999;81(5): 774-82.

[10] Moretti RM, Montagnani Marelli M, Mai S, Limonta P. Gonadotropin-releasing hormone agonists suppress melanoma cell motility and invasiveness throught the inhibition of a3 integrin and MMP-2 expression and activity. International Journal of Oncology 2008;33(2): 405-13.

[11] El-Shabrawi Y, Ardjomand N, Radner H, Ardjomand N. MMP-9 is predominantly expressed in epithelioid and not spindle cell uveal melanoma. The Journal of Pathology 2001;194(2): 201-6.

[12] Todoroff RJ, Brodey RS. Oral and pharyngeal neoplasia in the dog: a retrospective survey of 361 cases. Journal of the American Veterinary Medical Association 1979;175(6): 567-71.

[13] Vail DM, Thamm DH. Spontaneously Occurring Tumors in Companion Animals as Models for Drug Development. In: Teicher BA, Andrews PA. (eds.) Cancer Drug Discovery and Development:Anticancer Drug Development Guide: Preclinical Screening, Clinical Trials, and Approval. Totowa, NJ: Humana Press Inc.; 2004. p 259-84.

[14] Bergman PJ, Camps-Palau MA, McKnight JA, Leibman NF, Craft DM, Leung C, Liao J, Riviere I, Sadelain M, Hohenhaus AE, Gregor P, Houghton AN, Perales MA, Wolchok JD. Development of a xenogeneic DNA vaccine program for canine malignant melanoma at the Animal Medical Center. Vaccine 2006;24(21): 4582-5.

[15] Paoloni M, Khanna C. Translation of new cancer treatments from pet dogs to humans. Nature Reviews Cancer 2008;8(2): 147-56.

[16] Chaudhary A, Singh M, Bharti A, Asotra K, Sundaram S, Mehrotra R. Genetic polymorphisms of matrix metalloproteinases and their inhibitors in potentially malignant and malignant lesions of the head and neck. Journal of Biomedical Science 2010;17(10).

[17] Gialeli C, Theocharis AD, Karamanos NK. Roles of matrix metalloproteinases in cancer progression and their pharmacological targeting. FEBS Journal 2011;278(1): 16-27.

[18] Kessenbrock K, Plaks V, Werb Z. Matrix Metalloproteinases: Regulators of the Tumor Microenvironment. Cell 2010;141(1): 52-67.

[19] Björklund M, Koivunen E. Gelatinase-mediated migration and invasion of cancer cells. Biochimica et Biophysica Acta (BBA) - Reviews on Cancer 2005;1755(1): 37-69.

[20] Handsley MM, Edwards DR. Metalloproteinases and their inhibitors in tumor angiogenesis. International Journal of Cancer 2005;115(6): 849-60.

[21] Joyce JA, Pollard JW. Microenvironmental regulation of metastasis. Nature Reviews Cancer 2009;9(4): 239-52.

[22] Foda HD, Zucker S. Matrix metalloproteinases in cancer invasion, metastasis and angiogenesis. Drug Discovery Today 2001;6(9): 478-82.

[23] Szabo KA, Ablin RJ, Singh G. Matrix metalloproteinases and the immune response. Clinical and Applied Immunology Reviews 2004;4(5): 295-319.

[24] Cauwe B, Van den Steen PE, Opdenakker G. The biochemical, biological, and pathological kaleidoscope of cell surface substrates processed by matrix metalloproteinases. Critical Reviews in Biochemistry and Molecular Biology 2007;42: 113-85.

[25] Yoon S-O, Park S-J, Yun C-H, Chung A-S. Roles of matrix metalloproteinases in tumor metastasis and angiogenesis. Journal of Biochemistry and Molecular Biology 2003;36(1): 128-37.

[26] Mannello F, Medda V. Nuclear localization of Matrix metalloproteinases. Progress in Histochemistry and Cytochemistry 2012;47(1): 27-58.

[27] López-Otín C, Palavalli LH, Samuels Y. Protective roles of matrix metalloproteinases: From mouse models to human cancer. Cell Cycle 2009;8(22): 3657-62.

[28] Sternlicht MD, Werb Z. How matrix metalloproteinases regulate cell behavior. Cell and Developmental Biology 2001;17: 463-516.

[29] Bergman RL. Matrix Metalloproteinases 2 and 9 in Normal Canine Cerebrospinal Fluid. Master thesis. Faculty of the Virginia Polytechnic Institute and State University; 2001.

[30] Tonti Ga, Mannello F, Cacci E, Biagioni S. Neural stem cells at the crossroads: MMPs may tell the way. The International Journal of Developmental Biology 2009;53(1): 1-17.

[31] Folgueras AR, Pendás AM, Sánchez LM, López-Otín C. Matrix metalloproteinases in cancer: from new functions to improved inhibition strategies. The International Journal of Developmental Biology 2004;48(5-6): 411-24.

[32] Loukopoulos P, Mungall B, Straw R, Thornton J, Robinson W. Matrix metalloproteinase-2 and -9 involvement in canine tumors. Veterinary Pathology 2003;40(4): 382 - 94.

[33] Aresu L, Giantin M, Morello E, Vascellari M, Castagnaro M, Lopparelli R, Zancanella V, Granato A, Garbisa S, Arico A, Bradaschia A, Mutinelli F, Dacasto M. Matrix metalloproteinases and their inhibitors in canine mammary tumors. BMC Veterinary Research 2011;7: 33.

[34] Biljana E, Boris V, Cena D, Veleska-stefkovska D. Matrix metalloproteinases (with accent to collagenases). Journal of Cell and Animal Biology 2011;5(7): 113-20.

[35] Visse R, Nagase H. Matrix Metalloproteinases and Tissue Inhibitors of Metalloproteinases. Circulation Research 2003;92(8): 827-39.

[36] Morelli C, Campioni K, Parolin C, Palù G, Tognon M. Activity of the matrix metalloproteinase-9 promoter in human normal and tumor cells. Journal of Cellular Physiology 2004;199(1): 126-33.

[37] Kerkelä E, Saarialho-Kere U. Matrix metalloproteinases in tumor progression: focus on basal and squamous cell skin cancer. Experimental Dermatology 2003;12(2): 109-25.

[38] Stamenkovic I. Extracellular matrix remodelling: the role of matrix metalloproteinases. The Journal of Pathology 2003;200(4): 448-64.

[39] Fingleton B. Matrix metalloproteinases as valid clinical targets. Current pharmaceutical design 2007;13(3): 333-46.

[40] Kallakury BVS, Karikehalli S, Haholu A, Sheehan CE, Azumi N, Ross JS. Increased Expression of Matrix Metalloproteinases 2 and 9 and Tissue Inhibitors of Metalloproteinases 1 and 2 Correlate with Poor Prognostic Variables in Renal Cell Carcinoma. Clinical Cancer Research 2001;7(10): 3113-9.

[41] Van den Steen PE, Dubois B, Nelissen I, Rudd PM, Dwek RA, Opdenakker G. Biochemistry and Molecular Biology of Gelatinase B or Matrix metalloproteinase-9 (MMP-9). Critical reviews in biochemistry and molecular biology 2002;37(6): 375-536.

[42] Johansson N. Matrix metalloproteinases in tumor invasion. Cellular and Molecular Life Sciences 2000;57(1): 5-15.

[43] Deryugina E, Quigley J. Matrix metalloproteinases and tumor metastasis. Cancer and Metastasis Reviews 2006;25(1): 9-34.

[44] Stamenkovic I. Matrix metalloproteinases in tumor invasion and metastasis. Seminars in Cancer Biology 2000;10(6): 415-33.

[45] Gentilini F, Calzolari C, Turba ME, Agnoli C, Fava D, Forni M, Bergamini PF. Prognostic value of serum vascular endothelial growth factor (VEGF) and plasma activity of matrix metalloproteinase (MMP) 2 and 9 in lymphoma-affected dogs. Leukemia Research 2005;29(11): 1263-9.

[46] Bergers G, Brekken R, McMahon G, Vu TH, Itoh T, Tamaki K, Tanzawa K, Thorpe P, Itohara S, Werb Z, Hanahan D. Matrix metalloproteinase-9 triggers the angiogenic switch during carcinogenesis. Nature Cell Biology 2000;2(10): 737-44.

[47] Kawai K, Uetsuka K, Doi K, Nakayama H. The Activity of Matrix Metalloproteinases (MMPs) and Tissue Inhibitors of Metalloproteinases (TIMPs) in Mammary Tumors of Dogs and Rats. Journal of Veterinary Medical Science 2006;68(2): 105-11.

[48] Turpeenniemi-Hujanen T. Gelatinases (MMP-2 and -9) and their natural inhibitors as prognostic indicators in solid cancers. Biochimie 2005;87(3-4): 287-97.

[49] Docampo M-J, Cabrera J, Rabanal RM, Bassols A. Expression of matrix metalloproteinase-2 and -9 and membrane-type 1 matrix metalloproteinase in melanocytic tumors of dogs and canine melanoma cell lines. American Journal of Veterinary Research 2011;72(8): 1087-96.

[50] Miya K, Misumi K, Miyoshi N, Arai K, Fujiki M, Kubota C, Sakamoto H. Interpreting Gelatinase Activity in Tumor Tissue and Serum as a Prognostic Marker of Naturally Developing Canine Tumors. Journal of Veterinary Medical Science 2005;67(8): 769-75.

[51] Nakaichi M, Yunuki T, Okuda M, Une S, Taura Y. Activity of matrix metalloproteinase-2 (MMP-2) in canine oronasal tumors. Research in Veterinary Science 2007;82(2): 271-9.

[52] Loukopoulos P, O'Brien T, Ghoddusi M, Mungall BA, Robinson WF. Characterisation of three novel canine osteosarcoma cell lines producing high levels of matrix metalloproteinases. Research in Veterinary Science 2004;77(2): 131-41.

[53] Hofmann UB, Westphal JR, van Muijen GNP, Ruiter DJ. Matrix Metalloproteinases in Human Melanoma. Journal of Investigative Dermatology 2000;115(3): 337-44.

[54] Li N, Mangini J, Bhawan J. New prognostic factors of cutaneous melanoma: a review of the literature. Journal of Cutaneous Pathology 2002;29(6): 324-40.

[55] Redondo P, Lloret P, Idoate M, Inoges S. Expression and serum levels of MMP-2 and MMP-9 during human melanoma progression. Clinical and Experimental Dermatology 2005;30(5): 541-5.

[56] Simonetti O, Lucarini G, Brancorsini D, Nita P, Bernardini ML, Biagini G, Offidani A. Immunohistochemical expression of vascular endothelial growth factor, matrix metalloproteinase 2, and matrix metalloproteinase 9 in cutaneous melanocytic lesions. Cancer 2002;95(9): 1963-70.

[57] Väisänen AH, Kallioinen M, Turpeenniemi-Hujanen T. Comparison of the prognostic value of matrix metalloproteinases 2 and 9 in cutaneous melanoma. Human Pathology 2008;39(3): 377-85.

[58] Béliveau A, Bérubé M, Rousseau A, Pelletier G, Guérin SL. Expression of Integrin alpha5beta1 and MMPs Associated with Epithelioid Morphology and Malignancy of Uveal Melanoma. Investigative Ohpthalmology & Visual Science 2000;41(8): 2363-72.

[59] Bérubé M, Deschambeault A, Boucher M, Germain L, Petitclerc E, Guérin SL. MMP-2 expression in uveal melanoma: differential activation status dictated by the cellular environment. Molecular Vision 2005;11: 1101-11.

[60] Kim HK, Chae SW, Woo KI, Kim YD. Expression of matrix metalloproteinase (MMP)-2, MMP-9, and tissue inhibitor of MMP (TIMP)-1 in conjunctival melanomas and clinical implications. Japanese Journal of Ophthalmology 2010;54(3): 221-6.

[61] Lai K, Conway RM, Crouch R, Jager MJ, Madigan MC. Expression and distribution of MMPs and TIMPs in human uveal melanoma. Experimental Eye Research 2008;86(6): 936-41.

[62] Sahin A, Kiratli H, Soylemezoglu F, Tezel GG, Bilgic S, Saracbasi O. Expression of Vascular Endothelial Growth Factor-A, Matrix Metalloproteinase-9, and Extravascular Matrix Patterns and Their Correlations with Clinicopathologic Parameters in Posterior Uveal Melanomas. Japanese Journal of Ophthalmology 2007;51(5): 325-31.

[63] Goldschmidt MH, Dunstan R, Stannard, A. Histological classification of epithelial and melanocytic tumors of the skin of domestic animals. Washington: American Registry of Pathology; 1998.

[64] Queiroga FL, Pires I, Parente M, Gregorio H, Lopes CS. COX-2 overexpression correlates with VEGF and tumour angiogenesis in canine mammary cancer. The Veterinary Journal 2010;189(1): 77-82.

[65] Ramos-Vara JA, Beissenherz ME, Miller MA, Johnson GC, Pace LW, Fard A, Kottler SJ. Retrospective study of 338 canine oral melanomas with clinical,

histologic, and immunohistochemical review of 129 cases. Veterinary Pathology 2000;37(6): 597-608.

[66] Herlyn M, Clark WH, Rodeck U, Mancianti ML, Jambrosic J, Koprowski H. Biology of tumor progression in human melanocytes. Laboratory Investigation 1987;56(5): 461-74.

[67] Clark WH, Jr., Elder DE, Guerry Dt, Epstein MN, Greene MH, Van Horn M. A study of tumor progression: the precursor lesions of superficial spreading and nodular melanoma. Human Pathology 1984;15(12): 1147-65.

[68] Marino DJ, Matthiesen DT, Stefanacci JD, Moroff SD. Evaluation of dogs with digit masses: 117 cases (1981-1991). Journal of the American Veterinary Medical Association 1995;207(6): 726-8.

[69] Theon AP, Rodriguez C, Madewell BR. Analysis of prognostic factors and patterns of failure in dogs with malignant oral tumors treated with megavoltage irradiation. Journal of the American Veterinary Medical Association 1997;210(6): 778-84.

[70] Bergman PJ. Canine oral melanoma. Clinical Techniques in Small Animal Practice 2007;22(2): 55-60.

[71] Gomes J, Queiroga FL, Prada J, Pires I. Study of c-kit immunoexpression in canine cutaneous melanocytic tumors. Melanoma Research 2012;22(3): 195-201.

[72] Pires I, Garcia A, Prada J, Queiroga FL. COX-1 and COX-2 expression in canine cutaneous, oral and ocular melanocytic tumours. Journal of Comparative Pathology 2010;143(2-3): 142-9.

[73] Pires I, Prada J, Coelho L, Garcia A, Queiroga FL. Tumour-Associated Macrophages (TAMs) and Cox-2 Expression in Canine Melanocytic Lesions. In: Murph M. (ed.) Melanoma in the Clinic - Diagnosis, Management and Complications of Malignancy. Rijeka: InTech; 2011.

[74] Banerji A, Chakrabarti J, Mitra A, Chatterjee A. Effect of curcumin on gelatinase A (MMP-2) activity in B16F10 melanoma cells. Cancer Letters 2004;211(2): 235-42.

[75] Banerji A, Das S, Chatterjee A. Culture of human A375 melanoma cells in the presence of fibronectin causes expression of MMP-9 and activation of MMP-2 in culture supernatants. Journal of Environmental Pathology, Toxicology and Oncology 2008;27(2): 135-45.

[76] Akhavan MM, Karimi M, Ghodrati M, Falahtpishe H. AT1 receptors activation enhances the expression of MMP-2, MMP-13 and VEGF but not MMP-9 in B16F10 melanoma cells. Pakistan Journal of Biological Sciences 2011;14(17): 821-30.

[77] Hofmann UB, Westphal JR, Zendman AJ, Becker JC, Ruiter DJ, van Muijen GN. Expression and activation of matrix metalloproteinase-2 (MMP-2) and its co-localization with membrane-type 1 matrix metalloproteinase (MT1-MMP) correlate with melanoma progression. The Journal of Pathology 2000;191(3): 245-56.

[78] Ohnishi Y, Tajima S, Ishibashi A. Coordinate expression of membrane type-matrix metalloproteinases-2 and 3 (MT2-MMP and MT3-MMP) and matrix metalloproteinase-2 (MMP-2) in primary and metastatic melanoma cells. Eur J Dermatol 2001;11(5): 420-3.

[79] Ohnishi Y, Tajima S, Ishibashi A. Coordinate expression of membrane type-matrix metalloproteinases-2 and 3 (MT2-MMP and MT3-MMP) and matrix metalloproteinase-2 (MMP-2) in primary and metastatic melanoma cells. European Journal of Dermatology 2001;11(5): 420-3.

[80] Spangler WL, Kass PH. The histologic and epidemiologic bases for prognostic considerations in canine melanocytic neoplasia. Veterinary Pathology 2006;43(2): 136-49.

[81] Vaisanen A, Tuominen H, Kallioinen M, Turpeenniemi-Hujanen T. Matrix metalloproteinase-2 (72 kD type IV collagenase) expression occurs in the early stage of human melanocytic tumour progression and may have prognostic value. The Journal of Pathology 1996;180(3): 283-9.

[82] Redondo P, Lloret P, Idoate M, Inoges S. Expression and serum levels of MMP-2 and MMP-9 during human melanoma progression. Journal of Clinical & Experimental Dermatology 2005;30(5): 541-5.

[83] Vaisanen A, Kallioinen M, Taskinen PJ, Turpeenniemi-Hujanen T. Prognostic value of MMP-2 immunoreactive protein (72 kD type IV collagenase) in primary skin melanoma. The Journal of Pathology 1998;186(1): 51-8.

[84] Vaisanen A, Kallioinen M, von Dickhoff K, Laatikainen L, Hoyhtya M, Turpeenniemi-Hujanen T. Matrix metalloproteinase-2 (MMP-2) immunoreactive protein--a new prognostic marker in uveal melanoma? The Journal of Pathology 1999;188(1): 56-62.

[85] Baltazar-Rodriguez L, Anaya-Ventura A, Andrade-Soto M, Monrroy-Guizar E, Bautista-Lam J, Jonguitud-Olguin G. Polymorphism in the matrix metalloproteinase-2 gene promoter is associated with cervical neoplasm risk in Mexican women. Biochemical Genetics 2008;46(3-4): 137-44.

[86] Chen T, Zhu J. Evaluation of EMMPRIN and MMP-2 in the prognosis of primary cutaneous malignant melanoma. Medical Oncology 2010;27(4): 1185-91.

[87] Desch A, Strozyk EA, Bauer AT, Huck V, Niemeyer V, Wieland T, Schneider SW. Highly Invasive Melanoma Cells Activate the Vascular Endothelium via

an MMP-2/Integrin alphavbeta5-Induced Secretion of VEGF-A. American Journal of Pathology 2012;181(2): 693-705.

[88] Sahin A, Kiratli H, Tezel GG, Soylemezoglu F, Bilgic S. Expression of vascular endothelial growth factor a, matrix metalloproteinase 9 and extravascular matrix patterns in iris and ciliary body melanomas. Ophthalmic Research 2007;39(1): 40-4.

[89] Chen Y, Huang L, Yu J. Evaluation of heparanase and matrix metalloproteinase-9 in patients with cutaneous malignant melanoma. Journal of Dermatology 2012;39(4): 339-43.

[90] van den Oord JJ, Paemen L, Opdenakker G, de Wolf-Peeters C. Expression of gelatinase B and the extracellular matrix metalloproteinase inducer EMMPRIN in benign and malignant pigment cell lesions of the skin. American Journal of Pathology 1997;151(3): 665-70.

[91] Kong L, Fang W, Zhong H, Heng W, Li Y, Wu B. Controlled expression of matrix metalloproteinase 9 promotes expression of invasive phenotype of human melanoma cells. Beijing Da Xue Xue Bao 2003;35(1): 7-11.

[92] Bodey B, Bodey B, Jr., Siegel SE, Kaiser HE. Matrix metalloproteinase expression in malignant melanomas: tumor-extracellular matrix interactions in invasion and metastasis. In Vivo 2001;15(1): 57-64.

[93] MacDougall JR, Bani MR, Lin Y, Muschel RJ, Kerbel RS. 'Proteolytic switching': opposite patterns of regulation of gelatinase B and its inhibitor TIMP-1 during human melanoma progression and consequences of gelatinase B overexpression. British Journal of Cancer 1999;80(3-4): 504-12.

[94] MacDougall JR, Bani MR, Lin Y, Rak J, Kerbel RS. The 92-kDa gelatinase B is expressed by advanced stage melanoma cells: suppression by somatic cell hybridization with early stage melanoma cells. Cancer Research 1995;55(18): 4174-81.

[95] Sil H, Sen T, Chatterjee A. Fibronectin-integrin (alpha5beta1) modulates migration and invasion of murine melanoma cell line B16F10 by involving MMP-9. Oncology Research 2011;19(7): 335-48.

[96] Aksenenko MB, Gyrylova SN, Ruksha TG. Changes in the Levels of N-Cadherin and PCNA in Skin Melanoma Cells Are Mediated through Matrix Metalloproteinase 9. Bulletin of Experimental Biology and Medicine 2012;153(3): 364-6.

[97] Mehrotra R, Pandya S, Chaudhary A, Kumar M, Singh M. Prevalence of oral pre-malignant and malignant lesions at a tertiary level hospital in Allahabad, India. Asian Pacific Journal of Cancer Prevention 2008;9(2): 263-65.

Chapter 8

Glutamate Signaling in Human Cancers

Brian A. Wall, Seung-Shick Shin and Suzie Chen

Additional information is available at the end of the chapter

http://dx.doi.org/10.5772/55174

1. Introduction

G-protein coupled receptors (GPCRs) represent a class of therapeutic targets that have been widely exploited for drug designs and development. Metabotropic glutamate receptors (mGluRs) belong to Class C GPCRs and are predominantly involved in maintaining cellular homeostasis in the central nervous system (CNS). The natural ligand of mGluRs, glutamate, interacts with receptor proteins leading to the activation of multiple signaling pathways. More recently, aberrant glutamate signaling has been shown to play a role in the transformation and maintenance of various cancer types, including melanoma. Glutamate secretion from these cells has been found to stimulate regulatory pathways that control tumor growth, proliferation and survival. In addition to synaptic transmissions, accumulating evidence suggesting other functional roles of glutamatergic signaling in human malignancies has presented intriguing possibilities to make mGluRs putative, novel targets for human cancer treatments. To this end, the aberrant expression of metabotropic glutamate receptor 1 (mGluR1) was found as the driving force in inducing melanomagenesis in transgenic mouse models. Since then, other subtypes of mGluRs have been implicated in the pathogenesis of various cancer types such as malignant gliomas and medulloblastomas. As such, increased efforts have been generated to elucidate the mechanisms by which mGluRs confer oncogenic potentials. This chapter summarizes our current knowledge on the participation of glutamate signaling in human cancers. Given that mGluRs are "druggable" members of the GPCR superfamily and their oncogenic implications in cancer, further understanding on anti-mGluR signaling pathways will be beneficial.

2. Glutamate and cancer

The amino acid L-glutamine is a precursor for peptide and protein synthesis, amino sugar synthesis, and nucleotide synthesis. The amide of glutamate, glutamine, is the most abundant free amino acid with a concentration ranging from 500-900 μmol/L. In the majority of cell types, the glutamine is rapidly converted to L-glutamate (we will refer to as glutamate), which is the most abundant intracellular amino acid. Glutamate is a key component in cellular metabolism contributing as a metabolic fuel for intermediates in energy producing pathways as well as an important component in the body's disposal of excess, or waste, nitrogen. Glutamate is a principal excitatory neurotransmitter in the mammalian central nervous system where it is involved in cognitive functions such as learning and memory. In an attempt to appease the insatiable needs that transformed cell types require to sustain their energy expenditure and biosynthetic requirements, tumor cells become major consumers of glutamine.

2.1. The role of glutamate in normal and cancer cells

The uncontrolled proliferation that represents the hallmark of neoplastic disease not only involves deregulated cell proliferation but also requires adjustments in the energy metabolism that fuels the cells growth. Normal eukaryotic cells process the conversion of glucose to pyruvate via the metabolic pathway glycolysis in the cytosol, then to carbon dioxide in the mitochondria under aerobic conditions through the process of cellular respiration. In oxygen deprived environments, or hypoxic conditions, glycolysis is the preferred energy-generating pathway resulting in a decrease in the amount of pyruvate available to the oxygen-consuming mitochondria. It has been observed that even in the presence of physiological relevant levels of oxygen cancer cells have the ability to reprogram their glucose metabolism allowing them to preferentially produce energy via the glycolysis while maintaining the same level of respiration. This "anaerobic respiration" is a process known as the Warburg Effect [1, 2, 3]. Although aerobic metabolism including oxidative phosphorylation is up to 15 times more efficient then anaerobic metabolism. However, the metabolism of cancer cells occurs at an increased glycolytic rate up to 200 times than those of their normal surrounding tissues. Cellular ATP production during such high rates of glycolytic flux can easily exceed the ATP produced via oxidative phosphorylation. This high consumption of glucose requires much more nicotinamide adenine (NAD+), which is consecutively regenerated from the conversion of pyruvate to lactate by increased expression of lactate dehydrogenase making glycolysis self-sufficient [8].

Glutamine serves as a major respiratory fuel of tumor cells and has been shown to be the absolute requirement over glucose for many malignant cell types [4]. The importance of glutamine in tumor cell metabolism is derived from its ability to satisfy the bioenergetic needs of tumor cells as well as providing intermediates for macromolecular synthesis [5]. During periods of rapid growth, the cellular demand for glutamine surpasses its supply. At this time glutamine becomes essential and it is this reason that glutamine has been designated a 'conditionally' essential amino acid. Traditionally, the role of glutamine has been viewed to function as storage for excess nitrogen and to traffic the nitrogen within, and between, various organs. Metabolically, glutamine is used directly for reactions that require its γ-nitrogen, such as nucleotide and hexosamine synthesis, or indirectly in reactions that utilize the α-nitrogen (amino nitrogen) or its carbon skeleton for energy production and biosynthesis. These indirect reactions are necessary to generate the metabolic intermediates required for cell growth, which begin with the conversion of glutamine into glutamate. Being an abundant extracellular nutrient, glutamine is regularly converted into glutamate by phosphate-dependent glutaminase (GLS), an enzyme found within the inner mitochondrial membrane that has been shown to be overexpressed in both solid tumors and many tumor cell lines. In fact, the majority of glutamine consumption in cancer cells is owed to mitochondrial GLS activity. Consequentially, tumor cells have large intracellular pools of glutamate; through increased GLS activity, the abundantly available amino acid glutamine is converted to less abundant glutamate, there-by maintaining the cells' increasing demand for glutamate metabolism. This is the initial step in glutaminolysis, a series of biochemical reactions by which glutamine is degraded to glutamate, aspartate, pyruvate, alanine, citrate and carbon dioxide thereby providing metabolic intermediates to feed and maintain cells in which aerobic respiration is the biosynthetic hub.

Glycolysis and glutaminolysis both share the capacity to generate NADPH and the secretion of lactate (Figure 1). As mentioned previously, the initial step of glutaminolysis is the conversion of glutamine to glutamate, which is used, intracellularly, as a primary source of energy for proliferating cells. This rate-limiting step of glutamine metabolism is the deamidation reaction catalyzed by GLS. The products formed from this reaction, glutamate and ammonia, are released into the cytosolic compartment of the inner mitochondrial membrane. Glutamate is then further metabolized by conversion to α-ketoglutarate via either oxidative deamination by glutamate dehydrogenase (GIDH) or alanine transaminase (ALT). The deamination reaction is localized to the mitochondrial matrix compartment and yields both α-ketoglutarate and ammonium. The transamination can occur in either the cytosolic and mitochondrial compartments and produces α-ketoglutarate and alanine. Alpha-ketoglutarate is a key intermediate in the citric acid cycle where it is metabolized to regenerate oxaloacetate (OAA) through the production of malate. Mitochondrial metabolism of α-ketoglutarate into malate also generates NADPH via oxidation into pyruvate in the cytosol [6]. The NADPH produced is used by the rapidly metabolizing cell as a required electron donor in lipid synthesis and nucleotide metabolism as well as in antioxidant defense by maintaining glutathione (GSH) in its reduced state. GSH is the major thiol-containing endogenous antioxidant used by the cell to protect against various sources of oxidative stress. Maintaining a supply of GSH is critical for tumor cell survival since the elevated metabolic demand of the rapidly growing cell generates DNA-damaging byproducts that lead to oxidative stress [7].

Proliferating cancer cells consume vast amounts of glucose but only a small portion of which undergoes oxidative phosphorylation, even in the presence of sufficient oxygen [1]. It has been established that these rapidly dividing cells prefer to utilize glycolysis, which yields less net ATP molecules per glucose molecule. However, glycolysis can occur in hypoxic conditions that are usually associated with the highly necrotic regions of rapidly proliferating tumor masses. The end-product of glycolysis, pyruvate, can then enter the TCA cycle or is reduced into lactate by lactate dehydrogenase A, which is then excreted in the interstitial fluid. Within a tumor mass is a composition of genetically heterogeneous subpopulations of cancer cells that differ in their energy production pathways. It is possible that these subpopulations have the ability to function symbiotically within the tumor mass; one subpopulation of cells, consisting of hypoxic, glucose-dependent cells, secretes lactate as waste while the other subpopulation, located in a region that is more oxygenated, preferentially imports and utilizes the lactate

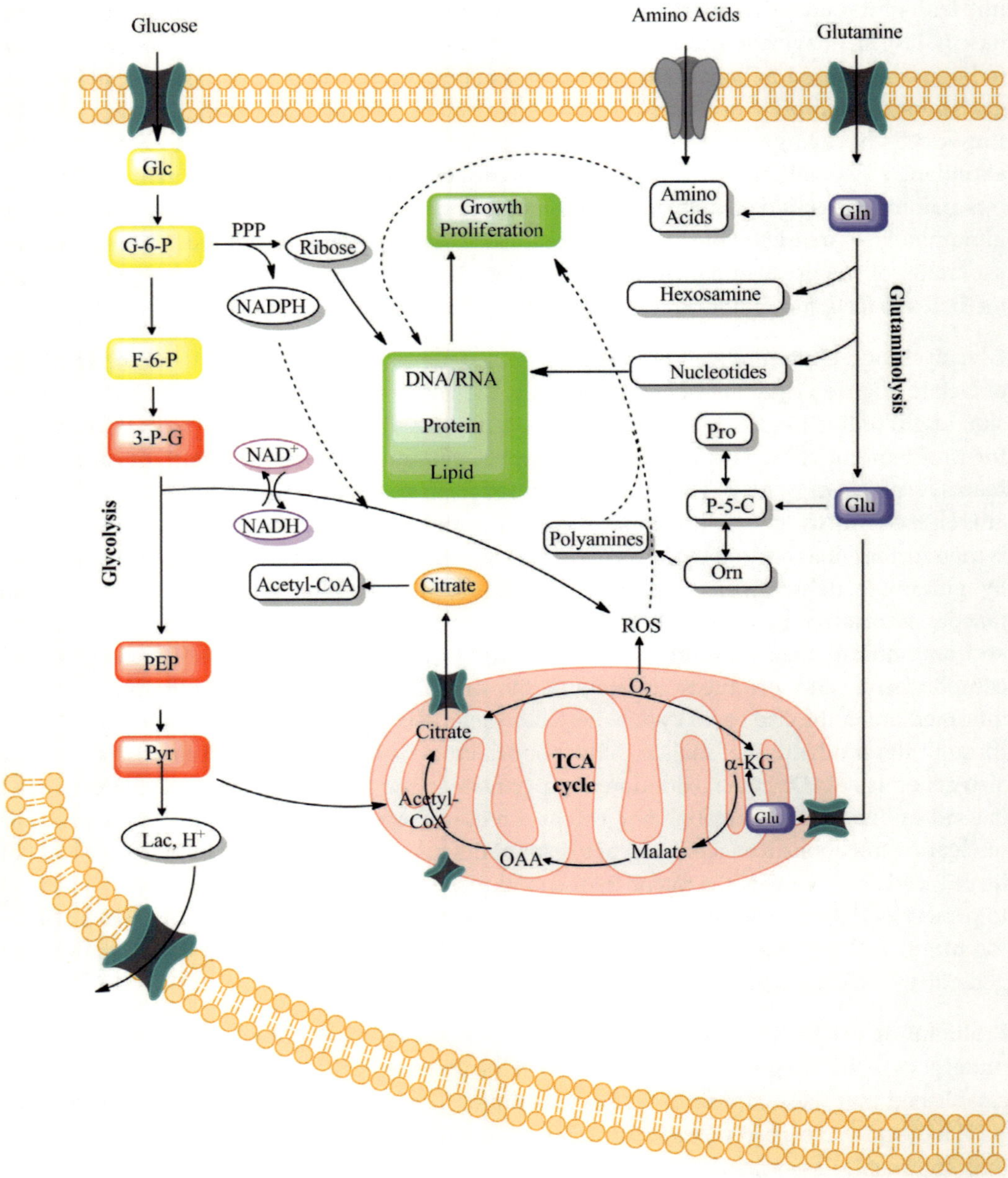

Figure 1. Metabolic pathways including glycolysis and glutaminolysis. Glycolysis produces NADPH and 5-carbon ribose via the pentose phosphate pathway (PPP) at glucose-6-phosphate (G-6-P) and detours toward lactate production (aerobic glycolysis) at pyruvate. The carbons of glucose are further diverted into various synthetic pathways to generate the precursors of hexosamines, amino acids and lipids. Mitochondria are fueled by the anapleurotic substrate, α-ketoglutarate (α-KG), generated from glutamate. Depending on the oxygen supply, α-ketoglutarate metabolizes through the tricarboxylic acid (TCA) cycle to malate and oxaloacetate (OAA) providing energy and a carbon resource for lipids.

produced by the first subpopulation to be used in the citric acid cycle [8, 9]. The idea of "metabolic symbiosis" that exists between hypoxic and aerobic cells in which lactate produced by hypoxic cells and taken up by aerobic cells to be used in oxidative support the bioenergetic needs of rapidly proliferating cancer cells within a solid tumor mass.

Cancer cells utilize TCA cycle intermediates to provide proliferating tumor cells with biosynthetic precursors (cataplerosis) as well as the production of ATP. The influx of metabolic intermediates in an attempt to maintain the mitochondrial TCA cycle (anaplerosis) is due to, in large part, glutaminolysis in which the first step is the conversion of glutamine to glutamate. Beyond its role in intermediary metabolism and biomass production, glutamate is also involved in influencing signal transduction pathways involved in promoting cellular proliferation, survival, and tumorigenesis. In the next section, we will review glutamate signaling and its role in the process of cellular transformation.

3. Aberrant expression of G-protein coupled receptors in neoplastic transformation

GPCRs are able to transduce extracellular signals into the cell via the activation of heterotrimeric G proteins. Malignant cells have been shown to appropriate the normal physiological functions of GPCR and utilize them to upregulate cell proliferation, invade surrounding tissue, increase blood supply, and evade cell death. In this section we will address the roles of GPCRs in tumor progression and metastasis.

3.1. G-Protein coupled receptors

Guanine nucleotide binding-protein coupled receptors (GPCRs; G-protein coupled receptors) comprise a large and diverse family of seven-pass membrane helix proteins found in most eukaryotic organisms. Members of the GPCR superfamily are diverse in their primary structure. The principal function of GPCRs is to transmit information about the extracellular environment via recognition of a variety of ligands including peptide and non-peptide hormones and neurotransmitters, chemokines, prostanoids and proteinases, biogenic amines, nucleosides, lipids, growth factors, odorant molecules and light to the interior of the cell by interacting with G-proteins. G-proteins are heterotrimeric subunits, G_α, G_β and G_γ, associated with the inner surface of the plasma membrane where they function as dimers. These G-proteins regulate the activity of small molecules that act as second messengers. Most of the human GPCRs can be found divided into five families based on phylogenetic criteria: *Glutamate, Rhodopsin, Adhesion, Frizzled/Taste2 and Secretin* (GRAFS classification system) [10]. The total number of known and verified human GPCRs consists of over 800 members. The Glutamate family consists of 22 human proteins categorized into ionotropic receptors (iGluRs) and metabotropic receptors (mGluRs). The iGluR family consists of *N*-methyl-D-aspartate receptors (NMDAR, α-amino-3-hydroxy-5-methyl-4-isoazolepropionic acid receptors (AMPAR), and kainite receptors (KAR). The mGluR family consists of eight different subtypes (mGluR1-8) [11]. The mGluRs are coupled to G-proteins, which distinguishes them from iGluRs, which contain ligand-gated ion-channels. The mGluRs are key receptors in the modulation of excitatory synaptic transmission in the central nervous system (CNS). The eight subtypes of mGluRs are further classified into three groups (I, II, III) based on sequence homology, signal transduction pathways, and agonist selectivity. mGluR1 and 5 belonging to subgroup I; mGluR2 and 3 belonging to subgroup II; and mGluRs 6, 7, and 8 belonging to subgroup III. The structures of mGluRs are composed of a heterotrimeric extracellular region, a seven-α helical transmembrane region and a cytoplasmic region. The extracellular region is further divided into the ligand-binding region (LBR) and the cysteine–rich region. The LBR has a sequence homologous with the extracellular regions of both iGluR and the γ-amino butyric acid (GABA) receptor [12, 13]. Table 1 lists the expression of mGluRs in non-neuronal cells.

Cell Type	GPCR	Reference
Melanocytes	mGluR5	*Frati et al.,2000*
Kerotinocytes	mGluR1, 2	*Genever et al.,1999*
Osteoclasts	mGluR8	*Morimoto et al.,2006*
Pancreatic Islets/β cells	mGluR5,8	*Storto et al.,2006* *Tong et al.,2002*
Hepatocytes	mGluR5	*Storto et al.,2000b*
Myocytes	mGluR1,2,3,5	*Gill et al.,1999*
Thymocytes	mGluR1,2,3,5	*Storto et al.,2000a*
Embryonic Stem Cells	mGluR4,5	*Melchiorri et al.,2007*

Table 1. Expression of mGluRs in select non-neuronal cells

3.2. GPCR signaling

The two principal signal transduction pathways involving GPCRs are the cAMP signaling pathway and the phosphatidylinositol signaling pathway. Glutamate-stimulated activation causes a conformational change in the extracellular domains, which catalyze the exchange of a GTP for a GDP on the Gα subunit of the intracellularly coupled G-protein. This exchange decreases the affinity of the Gα subunit for the G$\beta\gamma$ monomer at which time they either dissociate or rearrange [14, 15]. The dissociated Gα and G$\beta\gamma$ subunits interact with and modulate downstream signaling targets including adenylyl cyclases, phosphodiesterases, phosphlipases, tyrosine kinases, and ion channels.[16, 17]. Group I mGluRs are coupled to $G_{\alpha q}/G_{\alpha/11}$ G-proteins that, upon glutamate-mediated activation, result in stimulation of phospholipase C beta (PLC_{β}). Activation of PLC_{β} causes hydrolytic cleavage of phosphatidylinositol-4, 5-diphosphate (PIP_2) resulting in the formation of diacyl glycerol (DAG) and inositol 1, 4, 5-triphosphate (IP_3). DAG remains bound to the membrane while IP3 is released as a soluble structure into the cytosol. Release of these secondary messengers results in increased calcium release from the endoplasmic reticulum and activation of protein kinase C

(PKC) which phosphorylates other molecules, leading to altered cellular activity (Figure 2). Group II and III mGluRs are coupled to $G_{\alpha i/o}$ G-proteins that, upon activation prevent the formation of cyclic adenosine monophosphate (cAMP). Upon activation, group II mGluRs couple to $G_{\alpha i/o}$ subunit. $G_{\alpha i/o}$ G-proteins can inhibit adenylyl cyclase activity. Activation of the $G_{\alpha i/o}$ results in $G_{\alpha i/o}$ -mediated inhibition of adenylyl cyclase causing a reduced production of cyclic adenosine monophosphate (cAMP).

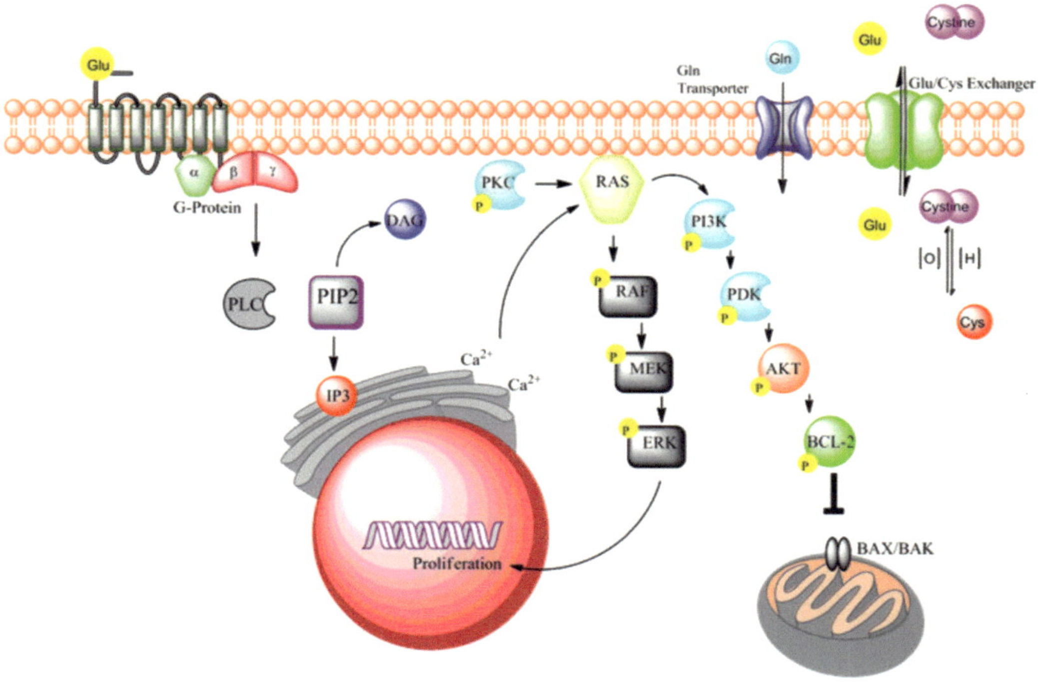

Figure 2. Signal transduction pathways activated by mGluR1 stimulation. Activation of mGluR1 by its ligand, glutamate, results in the activation of signaling pathways that upregulate cell proliferation (MAPK) and promotes cell survival (PI3K/AKT).

3.3. G-protein coupled receptors and cellular transformation

GPCRs comprise the largest known family of cell surface receptors that mediate cellular responses to a diverse array of signaling molecules including hormones, neurotransmitters, and chemokines. In addition, potent mitogens such as thrombin, bombesin, lysophosphatidic acid (LPA), gastrin-releasing peptide (GRP), endothelin and prostaglandins can stimulate cell proliferation by interacting with their cognate GPCR in various homologous cell types [18, 19, 20, 21, 22].

A fundamental trait of cancer cells involves their ability to sustain chronic proliferation. In normal cells, the production and release of growth-promoting signals that allow entry and progression through the cell cycle are tightly regulated. This regulation maintains cellular homeostasis promoting normal tissue structure and function and is controlled, in part, by growth factors that bind cell-surface receptors, which usually transmit signals through branched signaling pathways. By deregulating these signals, cancer cells are able to bypass regulatory control allowing them to proliferate and grow unconditionally. Cancer cells can acquire the ability to sustain proliferative signaling by producing these growth factors themselves in which the cells respond through the expression of cognate receptors resulting in autocrine proliferative stimulation. Alternatively, cancer cells may send signals to the surrounding tissue in a paracrine-like manner causing them to release various growth factors that promote growth of the cancer cells [23]. Activation of the surface receptors may also cause the constitutive activation of downstream signaling pathways.

Overexpression of GPCRs is detected in various cancer types, contributing to tumor cell growth once activated by circulating or locally produced ligands. The oncogenic potential of G protein-coupled receptors was revealed with the discovery of the *MAS* receptor in 1986, which provided a direct link between misregulated cell growth and GPCRs [24]. In contrast to most oncogenes identified at that time, *MAS* did not harbor genetic mutations resulting in its constitutive activation. Subsequent to its discovery, studies demonstrated that wild-type GPCRs have the ability to become tumorigenic when exposed to an excess of locally produced or circulating ligands and agonists while other GPCRs harboring mutations in key conserved residues can have transforming activity even in the absence of their ligands [14, 16, 17, 25, 26, 27, 28]. It has also been found that the level of expression of GPCRs is not as imperative to oncogenesis as is the receptor simply being expressed [28]. Since then, abnormal functioning of GPCR pathways have been shown to be the cause of several human diseases, and a large body of evidence links aberrant G-protein signaling to the development and progression of certain cancers [17].

The oncogenic transformation of cell types by way of GPCRs occurs, in part, by the establishment of autocrine or paracrine feedback in which the cell releases the ligand which binds and activates the receptor, maintaining its activation, as well as that of downstream effector proteins leading to enhanced cell proliferation [29, 30]. mGluRs are members of GPCR with glutamate as the natural ligand [31, 32]. Glutamate is the predominant excitatory neurotransmitter in the central nervous system and stimulates both ionotropic (ligand-gated ion channels) and metabotropic (G-protein-coupled) glutamate receptors [33]. Previously, glutamate signaling was believed to be exclusive to the central nervous system (CNS). It has since become apparent that various peripheral, non-neuronal cells express different types of glutamate receptors and these receptors are required for normal physiological function [34]. Studies have demonstrated that not only are mGluRs involved in the normal maintenance and regulation of physiological homeostasis, but they can also be involved in the progression of a variety of human malignancies. Initially, because of prior implications of GPCR expression being exclusive to the CNS, the first speculations of mGluRs in human cancers were in neuronal tumors such as neuroblastoma, medulloblastoma and glioma [35, 36, 37]. It was found that among these neuronal tumors that released excess amount of glutamate into the surrounding microenvironment were growing at a much-increased rate compared to neuronal tumors that were not secreting glutamate into their surroundings [38]. Subsequent studies revealed that

http://dx.doi.org/10.5772/55174

inhibition of glutamate release correlated with a decrease in the proliferation of not only neuroblastoma, rhabdomyosarcoma, brain astrocytoma, but also thyroid carcinoma, lung carcinoma, colon adenocarcinoma and breast carcinoma while having no effect on the growth rates of normal human fibroblast or bone marrow stromal cells [37].

	Subclass	Malignancy	Reference
Group I	mGluR1	Melanoma	*Chen et al 1996* *Pollock et al.,2003* *Ohtani et al 2008*
		Glioma Breast	*Aronica et al.,2003* *Albasanz et al.,1997* *Shinno et al.,1994* *Speyer et al 2011*
	mGluR5	Osteosarcoma Oral squamous cell carcinoma Melanoma	*Kalariti et al.,2007* *Park et al.,2007* *Choi et al 2011*
Group II	mGluR2	Glioma	*D'Onofrio et al.,2003*
	mGluR3	Glioma	*D'Onofrio et al.,2003,* *Aronica et al , 2003* *Arcella et al 2005*
		Melaonma	*Prickett et al 2011*
Group III	mGluR4	Colorectal adenocarcinoma	*Chang et al.,2005*
		Malignant Melanoma	
		Squamous cell carcinoma	
		Breast carcinoma	
		Medulloblastoma	*Lacovelli et al.,2006*
	mGluR6	-	
	mGluR7	-	
	mGluR8	Melanoma	*Prickett et al 2011*

Table 2. Implications of mGluRs in human cancer

3.4. Ectopic expression of mGluR1

Our group has previously described an unknown mechanism of melanoma pathogenesis in which the expression of an otherwise normal receptor, metabotropic glutamate receptor 1 (mGluR1) in an unnatural cellular environment (melanocytes) is able to upregulate cell proliferation and tumor development *in vitro* and *in vivo*. Chen and colleagues have established a transgenic mouse line (TG-3) that spontaneously develops melanoma with 100%

penetrance that was constructed using a 2-kb genomic fragment, termed clone B, which was previously shown to commit fibroblasts to undergo adipocyte differentiation [39, 40]. In an attempt to establish an animal model of obesity, five founder animals were established using clone B DNA: TG-1 through -5. Instead of the expected obese phenotype, one of the five founders, TG-3, developed heavily pigmented lesions on the ears, around the eyes, and the perianal region at approximately eight months of age. Upon histological analyses these pigmented lesions were identified as melanoma, Further examination shown these lesions were metastatic as evident by detecting these pigmented lesions in distant organs including the lymph nodes, brain, bone, lung and muscle. Using physical mapping we identified a single insertion of clone B in mouse chromosome 10, region A2, which is orthologous to human chromosome 6q23-24. Further molecular mapping found a concurrent insertion of clone B in a head-to-head, head-to-tail, tail-to-tail configuration and a deletion of approximately 70-kb of the host sequences located in intron 3 of the gene encoding mGluR1. Assessment of mGluR1 at both the protein and mRNA levels revealed the expression of the murine form of metabotropic glutamate receptor 1 only in the pigmented lesion but not normal counterpart. These results suggested that ectopic expression of mGluR1 in melanocytes might be the driving basis for melanoma development [41]. To verify this hypothesis, we engineered a new transgenic mouse line [TG(Grm1)EPv] directing mGluR1 expression in melanocytes under the control of a melanocyte-specific promoter, dopachrome tautomerase (DCT). This new transgenic line displays a melanoma susceptibility phenotype and progression very similar to the TG-3 line [42]. It was concluded that *in vivo,* aberrant mGluR1 expression in melanocytes is sufficient to induce spontaneous melanoma development with 100% penetrance. Progeny that are heterozygous at the transgenic integration site develop melanotic lesions as soon as 4 months post-natal while those homozygous at the integration site develop lesions within 30 days after birth. Ohtani and co-workers confirmed our observation with an inducible mGluR1 transgenic mouse model, when the expression of mGluR1 is conditionally activated in adult mice melanoma develops in these animals 100% of the time [43]. The results that mGluR1 has a role in melanocytic neoplasia in the murine system prompted our group to examine human melanoma for ectopic expression of the human form of metabotropic glutamate receptor 1. Examination of numerous melanoma biopsies and cell lines demonstrated aberrant expression of the receptor in approximately 60% of the samples suggesting that mGluR1 may be involved in the oncogenesis of a subset of human melanomas [41, 44]. These findings as well as those by others prompted our group to explore the underlying mechanisms of mGluR1- mediated melanocytic transformation. In a set of studies we confirmed that mGluR1 expression in melanocytes confers oncogenic activities *in vitro* and is sufficient to cause malignant phenotype *in vivo* [45].

In both the murine and human melanoma cell lines, stimulation of mGluR1 by glutamate results in similar if not identical formation of second messengers as described above for the CNS. One of the second messengers, DAG, stimulates PKC. PKC plays a key role in a multitude of cellular processes including apoptosis, malignant transformation, and metastasis [46] and once it is activated it in turn can activate the MAPK and PI3K/AKT pathways [47, 48, 49, 50, 51]. It is well known that the RAS-RAF-MEK-ERK module of the MAPK signaling cascade regulates cell proliferation and inhibits apoptosis. PI3K/AKT pathway activation is important for tumor cell survival, epithelial-mesenchymal transition (EMT), and angiogenesis [52]. In addition, gain-of-function mutations causing constitutive activation in G-proteins also result in the activation of downstream effector pathways leading to uncontrolled cell proliferation and cell survival. This is often a consequence of specific amino acid substitutions in the GTP binding region of the Gα subunit resulting in defective GTPase activity. The inability for GTP to be cleaved to GDP allows constitutive activation of downstream effector molecules. Such hypermorphic mutant G proteins in melanocytes were initially found to cause increased dermal pigmentation in transgenic mice. It was later found that the two functionally related G protein subunits, GNAQ and GNA11 encoding the stimulatory Gα_q and Gα_{11} subunits of heterotrimeric G-proteins respectively, are genetic hotspots for somatic mutations found in early uveal melanoma pathogenesis [53]. These mutations were also detected in benign intradermal melanocytic tumors as well as primary and metastatic ocular melanocytic tumors. Therefore, activation of ectopically expressed metabotropic glutamate receptors in human cells upregulate signaling pathways known to be important in the pathogenesis of human cancers associated with increased growth and angiogenesis while interruption of such pathways would result in a decrease in cell proliferation and survival.

The acquisition of tumor phenotypes is dependent not on one, but on successive alterations in the genomes of neoplastic cells. Specific genotypes confer selective advantages on subclones of cells enabling them to outgrow, and eventually dominate, the local tissue environment. This idea of multistage tumor progression can be viewed as a succession of clonal expansion each triggered by chance acquisition of mutant genotypes transitioning a cell from normal through pre-malignant and eventually cancer. One stage involved in malignant transformation of cell types is the ability of a cell to maintain its capacity to spread and divide in the absence of a stable or inter surface to attach. In a study performed by Prickett et al, exon capture sequencing of GPCRs in malignant melanoma specimens identified activating mutations within a region encoding for a member of the group II metabotropic glutamate receptors, mGluR3. The mutations were found throughout the coding region and affected the extracellular domains as well as the seven-transmembrane domain with two mini-hotspots located proximal to the transmembrane domains. Four somatic mutations (mGluR3^{E767K}, mGluR3^{S610L}, mGluR3^{G561E}, and mGluR3^{E870K}) were found to selectively regulate the phosphorylation of MEK1/2 kinase *in vivo* and induce micro metastasis *in vivo*. This activation resulted in the increased migration and anchorage independence growth of melanoma cells. These studies suggest the existence of a melanoma tumor type in which activating mutations in mGluR3 can lead to hypersensitivity to agonist stimulation of the MEK-MAPK pathway that bypasses the RAF/RAS genotypes.

In addition to melanoma, inappropriate glutamatergic signaling has been shown to be sufficient in the dysregulating growth leading to the transformation of other cell types. The ectopic expression of mGluR1 alone was able to induce the neoplastic transformation of immortalized baby mouse epithelial cells (iBMK) *in vitro* and promote tumor cell proliferation *in vivo* [54, 55]. The iBMK cell model was engineered to be immortal but not tumorigenic while also retaining normal epithelial characteristics. It was shown that full-length wild-type mGluR1 is tumorigenic when ectopically expressed in epithelial cells via stimulated MAPK and AKT signaling pathways. Additionally, studies performed by Speyer and colleagues (2011) described mGluR1 expression in several triple-negative breast cancer cell lines (TNBC) in which shRNA-mediated knockdown of mGluR1 expression as well as antagonists to the receptor inhibited cell proliferation in TNBC lines. Malignancies involving other mGluRs include mGluR4 first reported by Chang and colleagues that mGluR4 is overexpressed in more than 40% of colorectal adenocarcinomas, malignant melanomas, laryngeal squamous cell carcinomas, and breast carcinomas tested [56]. Among these cancers, there was a correlation with mGluR4 overexpression and increased mortality rate in patients with colorectal carcinoma. mGluR5 overexpression was found to induce melanoma in transgenic mice [57]. The increased expression in mGluR5 in the mouse melanocytes was correlated with enhanced levels of MAPK activation. These studies suggested that glutamatergic signaling plays a significant role in the initiation, progression and maintenance in human malignancies.

4. mGluR1 expression is required to maintain transformed phenotype

In an attempt to maintain tumor phenotypes, cancer cells are able to limit or bypass apoptotic cell response. In addition to manipulating cellular signals that control proliferation, oncogenic mutations have a profound effect in the disruption of apoptosis. These disruptions cause evasion of death response signals and have been shown to promote tumor initiation and progression leading to multistage carcinogenesis [58, 59, 60]. Indeed, defects in apoptotic pathways contribute to a number of human disease phenotypes from neurodegeneration to malignancy. The phosphatidylinositol 3-kinase (PI3K), phosphatase and tensin homolog deleted on chromosome 10 (PTEN) have critical roles in the transmission of signals that control multiple functions such as cell metabolism, proliferation, cell-cycle progression, and survival. PI3Ks are divided into three types (type I, II and III) with type I being further divided into two sub classes, class IA and IB. PI3Ks belonging to class IA are activated by receptor tyrosine kinases (RTKs) and those classified in class IB are activated by GPCRs [61]. All type I PI3Ks catalyze the conversion of the lipid phosphatidylinositol-4,5-bisphosphate (PIP2) to phosphatidylinositol-3,4,5-triphosphate (PIP3) from activation of upstream receptors such as epidermal growth factor receptor (EGFR), fibroblast growth factor receptor (FGFR), platelet-derived growth factor receptor (PDGFR) and insulin-like growth factor 1 receptor (IGF-1R), which interact with the p85 regulatory subunit of PI3K [62, 63]. The Ras protein interacts by directly activating p110 catalytic subunit of PI3K in a GTP-dependent manner. The activation of Ras is regulated by the extracellular stimuli that interact with cell surface receptors of the tyrosine kinase or seven transmembrane-spanning families [64]. Once activated Ras phosphorylates MEK, the mitogen activated protein (MAP) kinase kinase, which in turn activates MAP kinase. This cascade stimulates the MAP kinase pathway leading to phosphorylation of transcription factor that promote cellular proliferation and survival.

4.1. PI3K/AKT/PTEN

The serine-threonine protein kinase, AKT (also known as protein kinase B or PKB) and phosphoinositide-dependent kinase 1 (PDK1) are important downstream targets of PI3K. The

http://dx.doi.org/10.5772/55174

main biological consequences of AKT activation are cell survival and increased cell growth. AKT activation is known to involve in both mitogenic signaling and cell survival in a number of human cancer types. Human AKT exists in three isoforms: AKT1, AKT2 and AKT3. PI3K mediates cleavage of PIP_2,which produce PIP_3 at the inner surface of the plasma membrane. PIP which acts as a second messenger to recruit AKT through interaction of its pleckstrin homology (PH) domain, a domain conserved in signaling proteins that accumulate at sites of PI3K activation. Phosphorylation of AKT is dependent on phosphorylation, in part, by PDK1 [61, 65]. Activated AKT in turn mediates signaling through the phosphorylating inactivation of a multitude of downstream targets involved in apoptosis, including the phosphorylation of cyclic AMP response element--binding protein (CREB) as well as IκB kinase (IKK), which further activates central regulators of cell death: nuclear factor –κB (NF-κB) and p53. AKT-mediated induction of NF-κB occurs via activation of IκB which induces degradation of the NF-κB inhibitor IκB leading to release of NF-κB from the cytoplasm and translocation to the nucleus leading to the expression of survival genes such as IAP that promotes survival by inhibiting downstream activation of caspase-9 and -3 [66, 67, 68, 69, 70]. AKT influences p53 activity through phosphorylation of the p53-binding protein, MDM2. MDM2 regulates p53 function by targeting p53 for degradation by its E3 ubiquitin ligase. AKT phosphorylation of MDM2 allows increased translocation of the proteasome to the nucleus where it binds p53 resulting in its degradation [70, 71]. In addition, the oncological significance of amplified AKT expression has been well documented in gastric carcinoma, ovarian, pancreatic and breast tumors [72, 73, 74]. AKT phosphorylation of the apoptosis-inducing protein, Bad, prevents binding of Bad to the antiapoptotic Bcl-2-type proteins, Bcl-2 and Bcl- x_L. Bad promotes cell death by forming a non-functional hetero-dimer with the survival factor Bcl-x_L. Upregulation of Bcl-x_L promotes survival by regulating coupled respiration through supporting ATP/ADP exchange across the outer mitochondrial membrane [75]. Phosphorylation of Bad by AKT prevents heterodimerization with Bcl- x_L restoring its antiapoptotic function. In addition, it has also been implicated that PI3K-AKT has effects on tumor-induced angiogenesis, mediated in part through hypoxia-induced factor-1α and NF-κB induced expression of the proangiogenic growth factor, vascular endothelial growth factor (VEGF) and suppression the endogenous antiangiogenic molecule, thrombospondin-1 (TSP-1). VEGF and its receptor, VEGFR are major angiogenesis inducers associated with tumor angiogenesis in numerous malignancies [76].

The PTEN tumor suppressor is a dual-specificity phosphatase, which has protein phosphatase activity and lipid phosphatase activity that antagonizes the PI3K-AKT pathway and is found to contain inactivating mutations in many human cancers. PTEN negatively regulates PIP_3-mediated signaling cascades by hydrolyzing the 3-phosphate to generate PIP_2 making PTEN critical in phosphatidylinositol homeostasis and regulating the proliferation and invasion of many cancer cells [77].

AKT is an important regulator of cell growth and apoptosis that activate downstream from PI3K and is inhibited by the actions of the tumor suppressor PTEN. The ability to promote cell growth and suppress cell death suggests the PI3K/AKT /PTEN pathways are critical participants in tumorigenesis. As previously stated, the ectopic expression of mGluR1 was detected in approximately 60% of human melanoma biopsies and cell lines examined while its expression was not found in in normal skin or benign nevi [42, 44]. Stimulation of mGluR1 by an agonist of the receptor, L-quisqualate, results in the activation of MAPK in mouse and human melanoma cell lines independent of the presence of the most common NRAS/BRAF-activating mutations [46]. Constitutively activated MAPK pathway is common in many human cancers including melanoma, frequently due to mutations in the BRAF and RAS genes. In melanomas, mutation rates for BRAF is ~60% and NRAS is ~20% [44, 78, 79]. Treatment of human melanoma cells with a competitive antagonist of mGluR1, LY367385, which binds to the same catalytic site as glutamate, showed dose-dependent inhibition of cell proliferation via suppression of ERK activation [80]. In addition, a noncompetitive mGluR1 antagonist which binds to the transmembrane domain of the receptor resulting in stabilization of inactive conformation, BAY36-7620, suppressed cell growth and promoted apoptosis in cultured melanoma cells that express mGluR1 [81]. Both LY367385 and BAY36-7620 were shown to result in a decrease in the levels of the secondary messengers, IP_3 and DAG, in these studies. Further investigation of mGluR1 functionality and activity using dominant-negative mGluR1 (dn-mGluR1) mutant yielded in an increase in the number of apoptotic cells as demonstrated by the increased cleavage of poly-ADP ribose polymerase (PARP), a well-known marker of apoptosis. The dn-mGluR1 mutants derived from small deletions or single base substitutions in the intracellular loop 2 or 3, which have been shown previously to be essential in mGluR1 signaling [44, 46, 82]. These studies demonstrated that ablation of the functionality of mGluR1 in melanoma cells, we were able to reduce cell proliferation and induce cell death *in vitro* without affecting normal cell types [44].

5. Inhibition of mGluR1

Targeting strategies for cancer therapy differ from chemotherapy and radiotherapy in their potential to provide tumor specificity. Preclinical studies have demonstrated that inhibition of glutamatergic signaling results in decreased tumor cell growth and increased cell death. Identifying key upstream molecular targets that lead to the activation of proliferation and survival pathways is important in cancer drug discovery. Gene-targeting techniques that selectively inactivate gene expression assist in the validation of novel proteins involved in disease pathogenesis.

5.1. Suppression of mGluR1 by siRNA

Gene silencing by short-interfering RNAs (siRNAs) has been used to investigate their roles in different cell types and in various organisms. However, constitutive suppression the expression of a gene could have deleterious consequences therefore, inducible silencing RNA approaches could be useful by relying on small molecules that act as inducers to modify synthetic transcription factors thereby regulating the expression of a target gene [83-87]. The tetracycline operon based tetracycline inducible system and the non-mammalian steroid based ecdysone inducible system are two complementary approaches we have used. Previous attempts to inhibit mGluR1 expression in human melanoma cells using constitutively ex-

http://dx.doi.org/10.5772/55174

pressed mGluR1 specific siRNAs resulted in the cells exhibiting a dormancy-like state prior to dying. Employing the inducible knock-down of mGluR1 was shown to result in suppression of MAPK as evident by a decrease in the phosphorylated form of ERK as well as inhibition of the PI3/AKT cell survival pathway seen by the reduced form of activated AKT [84]. Our previous studies on mouse melanoma cells as well as mouse melanocytic clones that stably expressed mGluR1 showed elevated levels of glutamate were released into their surroundings compared to normal mouse melanocytes or vector controls [85]. This finding correlated with earlier works in rats in which suppression of glutamate uptake coupled with stimulation of group I mGluRs results in an increase in the accumulation of extracellular glutamate. It was implicated that these mGluRs may work systematically with cystine-glutamate exchangers to regulate extracellular glutamate concentrations [86, 87]. From this discovery, Chen and co-workers hypothesized that instead of inhibiting mGluR1 directly, if they were able to interrupt the autocrine/paracrine activity by limiting the amount of free ligand this would result in a similar decrease in cell proliferation/survival.

5.2. Suppression of mGluR1 using an inhibitor of glutamate release

Glutamate is a major excitatory neurotransmitter in the CNS. The over activation of neurons by excessive glutamate stimulation is excitotoxic, resulting in neuronal death [88]. Interestingly, the brain is one of the most common sites of metastatic melanoma. It is possible the excessive glutamate found in the brain promotes tumor growth while inducing excitotoxicity to the surrounding neuronal tissue. Because of this, Chen and co-workers took advantage of using an inhibitor of glutamate release, riluzole, a Food and Drug Administration (FDA)-approved drug for the treatment of amyotrophic lateral sclerosis (ALS or Lou Gehrig's disease). ALS is a degenerative motor neuron disease of the upper and lower motor neurons that progressively causes weakness, muscle atrophy and fasciculation. Riluzole is known to inhibit the release of glutamate from the presynapse resulting in a decrease of the molecule in the synaptic cleft resulting in a decrease in excitotoxicity caused by the neurotransmitter. This leads to a decreased progression of ALS [89]. Riluzole treated melanoma cells showed a reduction in the levels of glutamate in the surroundings *in vitro,* which correlated with a decrease in cell growth *in vivo* when compared to normal cells exposed to the drug. Additionally, melanoma cells treated with relatively low concentrations of riluzole were shown to undergo apoptosis by an increase in the levels of the cleaved form of PARP after riluzole treatment. The therapeutic potential of riluzole was validated *in vivo* using a human melanoma cell xenograft model where animals were treated with a human equivalent of the maximally allowed daily amount of riluzole per body weight per day via p.o. gavage for 18 days. The use of riluzole as a putative antagonist of mGluR1 to inhibit glutamate signaling resulted in a reduction in tumor volume in treated animals vs. control. These results were translated to the clinic.

5.3. Translational study in patients

Clinical trials involving new compounds are classified into four phases: Phase 0, I, II and III. Phase 0 is the designation for exploratory, first-in-human trials conducted with the U.S.

FDA's guidelines on Exploratory Investigational New Drug Studies (IND). Phase 0 trials are designed to speed-up the development of promising drugs or imaging agents by establishing very early on whether the drug or agent behaves in human subjects as was anticipated from preclinical studies. Based on results from previous findings in preclinical studies using riluzole, a phase 0 trial using the compound in patients with stage III and IV melanoma was performed to see if in itds presence the target, glutamatergic signaling, is reduced. The trial resulted in a significant short-term response rate of 34% of patients. Tumors from patients that displayed shrinkage of tumors showed an inhibition of signaling through both the MAPK and PI3K/AKT pathways, reflecting results that were previously observed in preclinical studies [44, 90]. Positron Emission tomography (PET) documented complete resolve of multiple nodal and cutaneous metastases in several patients. One patient having six different tumors measured by PET/CT demonstrated shrinkage of the lesions by 10% to 20%. Out of eleven patients that completed the study, only two had shown progression of the disease after treatment [90]. The tumor samples were a composed of patients harboring both V600E BRAF as well as Q61K NRAS mutations. In addition all the patients admitted into the trial expressed mGluR1, although mGluR1 expression status was not a requirement for entry. It is possible that, from this observation, that more advanced tumors, those found in stage III and IV metastases, have a higher frequency of mGluR1 expression and that ectopic mGluR1 occurs and is more frequent in more progressed stages of the disease.

6. Conclusion

Melanoma is a genetically diverse disease owing to the dysfunction of multiple regulatory pathways. As such, it is important to test the therapeutic potential of agents that reflect the genetic diversity of this disease. In addition to ectopic expression of mGluR1, mutations in BRAF have been identified in more than 60% of melanomas, most of these due to the substitution of a single amino acid at residue 600 in the B-RAF kinase domain resulting in constitutive activation of the RAF/MAP/ERK kinase signaling pathway [91]. Melanoma cells with aberrant glutamate receptor signaling also exhibit hyperactive PI3K/AKT and MEK/MAPK pathways [44, 92, 93]. Additionally, a recent examination of a publicly available gene expression data bank identified a variety of GPCRs that are over-expressed in diverse types of cancer tissues [94]. These findings illustrate the role that glutamate receptors and transporters play in the cellular signaling somatic cell types. The molecular physiology of GPCRs allow them to be regulated by many agonists and antagonists and are the target, directly and indirectly, of approximately 50% of pharmaceutical agents used to treat various human diseases. GPCRs have been shown to have a role in both normal and aberrant mitogenic signaling in functions that regulate cell migration in tumor metastasis and angiogenesis as well as key molecular events implicated in cancer progression and invasion. Based on these findings, it is perhaps not surprising that interruption of the glutamatergic signaling pathway by targeting GPCRs in cancers could result in more effective the treatment of this devastating disease.

http://dx.doi.org/10.5772/55174

Author details

Brian A. Wall[1,2], Seung-Shick Shin[3] and Suzie Chen[1,2,3]

1 Susan Lehman Cullman Laboratory for Cancer Research, Ernest Mario School of Pharmacy, Rutgers University, NJ, USA

2 Joint Graduate Program of Toxicology, Rutgers, the State University, Piscataway, NJ, USA

3 The Cancer Institute of New Jersey, Little Albany Street, New Brunswick, NJ, USA

References

[1] Warburg, O. On the origin of cancer cells. *Science* (1956). Feb 24;, 123(3191), 309-14.

[2] Warburg, O. On respiratory impairment in cancer cells. *Science* (1956). Aug 10;, 124(3215), 269-70.

[3] Warburg, O, Wind, F, & Negelein, E. The Metabolism of Tumors in the Body. *J Gen Physiol* (1927). Mar 7;, 8(6), 519-30.

[4] Moreadith, R. W, & Lehninger, A. L. The pathways of glutamate and glutamine oxidation by tumor cell mitochondria. Role of mitochondrial NAD(P)+-dependent malic enzyme. *J Biol Chem* (1984). May 25;, 259(10), 6215-21.

[5] Deberardinis, R. J, Sayed, N, Ditsworth, D, & Thompson, C. B. Brick by brick: metabolism and tumor cell growth. *Curr Opin Genet Dev* (2008). Feb;, 18(1), 54-61.

[6] Deberardinis, R. J, Mancuso, A, Daikhin, E, Nissim, I, Yudkoff, M, Wehrli, S, et al. Beyond aerobic glycolysis: transformed cells can engage in glutamine metabolism that exceeds the requirement for protein and nucleotide synthesis. *Proc Natl Acad Sci U S A* (2007). Dec 4;, 104(49), 19345-50.

[7] Estrela, J. M, Ortega, A, & Obrador, E. Glutathione in cancer biology and therapy. *Crit Rev Clin Lab Sci* (2006). , 43(2), 143-81.

[8] Feron, O. Pyruvate into lactate and back: from the Warburg effect to symbiotic energy fuel exchange in cancer cells. *Radiotherapy and oncology : journal of the European Society for Therapeutic Radiology and Oncology* (2009). Sep;, 92(3), 329-33.

[9] Semenza, G. L. Tumor metabolism: cancer cells give and take lactate. *J Clin Invest* (2008). Dec;, 118(12), 3835-7.

[10] Fredriksson, R, Lagerstrom, M. C, Lundin, L. G, & Schioth, H. B. The G-protein-coupled receptors in the human genome form five main families. Phylogenetic analysis, paralogon groups, and fingerprints. *Mol Pharmacol* (2003). Jun;, 63(6), 1256-72.

[11] Bjarnadottir, T. K, Fredriksson, R, & Schioth, H. B. The gene repertoire and the common evolutionary history of glutamate, pheromone (taste(1) and other related G protein-coupled receptors. *Gene* (2005). Dec 5;362:70-84., 2R

[12] Hara, O, Sheppard, P. J, Thogersen, P. O, Venezia, H, Haldeman, D, & Mcgrane, B. A. V, et al. The ligand-binding domain in metabotropic glutamate receptors is related to bacterial periplasmic binding proteins. *Neuron* (1993). Jul;, 11(1), 41-52.

[13] Kaupmann, K, Huggel, K, Heid, J, Flor, P. J, Bischoff, S, Mickel, S. J, et al. Expression cloning of GABA(B) receptors uncovers similarity to metabotropic glutamate receptors. *Nature* (1997). Mar 20;, 386(6622), 239-46.

[14] Hamm, H. E. The many faces of G protein signaling. *J Biol Chem* (1998). Jan 9;, 273(2), 669-72.

[15] Bunemann, M, Frank, M, & Lohse, M. J. Gi protein activation in intact cells involves subunit rearrangement rather than dissociation. *Proc Natl Acad Sci U S A* (2003). Dec 23;, 100(26), 16077-82.

[16] Lappano, R, & Maggiolini, M. G protein-coupled receptors: novel targets for drug discovery in cancer. *Nat Rev Drug Discov* (2011). Jan;, 10(1), 47-60.

[17] Lee, H. J, & Wall, B. Chen S. G-protein-coupled receptors and melanoma. *Pigment Cell Melanoma Res* (2008). Aug;, 21(4), 415-28.

[18] Rozengurt, E, Guha, S, & Sinnett-smith, J. Gastrointestinal peptide signalling in health and disease. *Eur J Surg Suppl* (2002). , 587, 23-38.

[19] Teerawattananon, Y, Tangcharoensathien, V, Tantivess, S, & Mills, A. Health sector regulation in Thailand: recent progress and the future agenda. *Health Policy* (2003). Mar;, 63(3), 323-38.

[20] Marinissen, M. J. Gutkind JS. G-protein-coupled receptors and signaling networks: emerging paradigms. *Trends Pharmacol Sci* (2001). , 22(7), 368-76.

[21] Dorsam, R. T. Gutkind JS. G-protein-coupled receptors and cancer. *Nat Rev Cancer* (2007). Feb;, 7(2), 79-94.

[22] Rzeski, W, Turski, L, & Ikonomidou, C. Glutamate antagonists limit tumor growth. *Proc Natl Acad Sci U S A* (2001). May 22;, 98(11), 6372-7.

[23] Cheng, N, Chytil, A, Shyr, Y, Joly, A, & Moses, H. L. Transforming growth factor-beta signaling-deficient fibroblasts enhance hepatocyte growth factor signaling in mammary carcinoma cells to promote scattering and invasion. *Mol Cancer Res* (2008). Oct;, 6(10), 1521-33.

[24] Young, D, Waitches, G, Birchmeier, C, Fasano, O, & Wigler, M. Isolation and characterization of a new cellular oncogene encoding a protein with multiple potential transmembrane domains. *Cell* (1986). Jun 6;, 45(5), 711-9.

[25] Li, F, Wang, Y, Zeller, K. I, Potter, J. J, Wonsey, D. R, & Donnell, O. KA, et al. Myc stimulates nuclearly encoded mitochondrial genes and mitochondrial biogenesis. *Mol Cell Biol* (2005). Jul;, 25(14), 6225-34.

[26] Lundstrom, K. Latest development in drug discovery on G protein-coupled receptors. *Curr Protein Pept Sci* (2006). Oct;, 7(5), 465-70.

[27] Knox, W. E, Horowitz, M. L, & Friedell, G. H. The proportionality of glutaminase content to growth rate and morphology of rat neoplasms. *Cancer Res* (1969). Mar;, 29(3), 669-80.

[28] Van Raamsdonk, C. D, Bezrookove, V, Green, G, Bauer, J, Gaugler, L, & Brien, O. JM, et al. Frequent somatic mutations of GNAQ in uveal melanoma and blue naevi. *Nature* (2009). Jan 29;, 457(7229), 599-602.

[29] Burger, M, Burger, J. A, Hoch, R. C, Oades, Z, Takamori, H, & Schraufstatter, I. U. Point mutation causing constitutive signaling of CXCR2 leads to transforming activity similar to Kaposi's sarcoma herpesvirus-G protein-coupled receptor. *J Immunol* (1999). Aug 15;, 163(4), 2017-22.

[30] Takayama, H. LaRochelle WJ, Sharp R, Otsuka T, Kriebel P, Anver M, et al. Diverse tumorigenesis associated with aberrant development in mice overexpressing hepatocyte growth factor/scatter factor. *Proc Natl Acad Sci* (1997). , 94, 701-6.

[31] Pin, J. P, & Duvoisin, R. The metabotropic glutamate receptors: structure and functions. *Neuropharmacology* (1995). Jan;, 34(1), 1-26.

[32] Hermans, E, & Challiss, R. A. Structural, signalling and regulatory properties of the group I metabotropic glutamate receptors: prototypic family C G-protein-coupled receptors. *Biochem J* (2001). Pt 3):465-84.

[33] Ozawa, S, Kamiya, H, & Tsuzuki, K. Glutamate receptors in the mammalian central nervous system. *Prog Neurobiol* (1998). Apr;, 54(5), 581-618.

[34] Haas, H. S, Pfragner, R, Siegl, V, Ingolic, E, Heintz, E, Schraml, E, et al. The non-competitive metabotropic glutamate receptor-1 antagonist CPCCOEt inhibits the in vitro growth of human melanoma. *Oncol Rep* (2007). Jun;, 17(6), 1399-404.

[35] Naarala, J, Nykvist, P, Tuomala, M, & Savolainen, K. Excitatory amino acid-induced slow biphasic responses of free intracellular calcium in human neuroblastoma cells. *FEBS Lett* (1993). Sep 13;, 330(2), 222-6.

[36] Iacovelli, L, Fulceri, F, De Blasi, A, Nicoletti, F, Ruggieri, S, & Fornai, F. The neurotoxicity of amphetamines: bridging drugs of abuse and neurodegenerative disorders. *Exp Neurol* (2006). Sep;, 201(1), 24-31.

[37] Shin, S. S, Martino, J. J, & Chen, S. Metabotropic glutamate receptors (mGlus) and cellular transformation. *Neuropharmacology* (2008). Sep;, 55(4), 396-402.

[38] Takano, T, Lin, J. H, Arcuino, G, Gao, Q, Yang, J, & Nedergaard, M. Glutamate release promotes growth of malignant gliomas. *Nat Med* (2001). Sep;, 7(9), 1010-5.

[39] Chen, S, Zhu, H, Wetzel, W. J, & Philbert, M. A. Spontaneous melanocytosis in transgenic mice. *J Invest Dermatol* (1996). May;, 106(5), 1145-51.

[40] Zhu, H, Reuhl, K, Zhang, X, Botha, R, Ryan, K, Wei, J, et al. Development of heritable melanoma in transgenic mice. *J Invest Dermatol* (1998). Mar;, 110(3), 247-52.

[41] Pollock, P. M, Cohen-solal, K, Sood, R, Namkoong, J, Martino, J. J, Koganti, A, et al. Melanoma mouse model implicates metabotropic glutamate signaling in melanocytic neoplasia. *Nat Genet* (2003). May;, 34(1), 108-12.

[42] Pollock, P. M, Cohen-solal, K, Sood, R, Namkoong, J, Martino, J. J, Koganti, A, et al. Melanoma mouse model implicates metabotropic glutamate signaling in melanocytic neoplasia. *Nat Genet* (2003). May;, 34(1), 108-12.

[43] Ohtani, Y, Harada, T, Funasaka, Y, Nakao, K, Takahara, C, Abdel-daim, M, et al. Metabotropic glutamate receptor subtype-1 is essential for in vivo growth of melanoma. *Oncogene* (2008). Sep 8;, 27, 7162-70.

[44] Namkoong, J, Shin, S. S, Lee, H. J, Marin, Y. E, Wall, B. A, Goydos, J. S, et al. Metabotropic glutamate receptor 1 and glutamate signaling in human melanoma. *Cancer Res* (2007). Mar 1;, 67(5), 2298-305.

[45] Shin, S. S, Namkoong, J, Wall, B. A, Gleason, R, Lee, H. J, & Chen, S. Oncogenic activities of metabotropic glutamate receptor 1 (Grm1) in melanocyte transformation. *Pigment cell & melanoma research* (2008). Jun;, 21(3), 368-78.

[46] Marin, Y. E, Namkoong, J, Cohen-solal, K, Shin, S. S, Martino, J. J, Oka, M, et al. Stimulation of oncogenic metabotropic glutamate receptor 1 in melanoma cells activates ERK1/2 via PKCepsilon. *Cell Signal* (2006). Aug;, 18(8), 1279-86.

[47] Marin, Y. E, & Chen, S. Involvement of metabotropic glutamate receptor 1, a G protein coupled receptor, in melanoma development. *J Mol Med* (2004). Nov;, 82(11), 735-49.

[48] Busca, R, Abbe, P, Mantoux, F, Aberdam, E, Peyssonnaux, C, Eychene, A, et al. Ras mediates the cAMP-dependent activation of extracellular signal-regulated kinases (ERKs) in melanocytes. *Embo J* (2000). Jun 15;, 19(12), 2900-10.

[49] Ferraguti, F, Baldani-guerra, B, Corsi, M, Nakanishi, S, & Corti, C. Activation of the extracellular signal-regulated kinase 2 by metabotropic glutamate receptors. *Eur J Neurosci* (1999). Jun;, 11(6), 2073-82.

[50] Thandi, S, Blank, J. L, & Challiss, R. A. Group-I metabotropic glutamate receptors, mGlu1a and mGlu5a, couple to extracellular signal-regulated kinase (ERK) activation via distinct, but overlapping, signalling pathways. *J Neurochem* (2002). Dec;, 83(5), 1139-53.

[51] Choe, E. S, & Wang, J. Q. Regulation of transcription factor phosphorylation by metabotropic glutamate receptor-associated signaling pathways in rat striatal neurons. *Neuroscience* (2002). , 114(3), 557-65.

[52] Stepulak, A, Luksch, H, Gebhardt, C, Uckermann, O, Marzahn, J, Sifringer, M, et al. Expression of glutamate receptor subunits in human cancers. *Histochem Cell Biol* (2009). Oct;, 132(4), 435-45.

[53] Onken, M. D, Worley, L. A, Long, M. D, Duan, S, Council, M. L, Bowcock, A. M, et al. Oncogenic mutations in GNAQ occur early in uveal melanoma. *Invest Ophthalmol Vis Sci* (2008). Dec;, 49(12), 5230-4.

[54] Degenhardt, K, & White, E. A mouse model system to genetically dissect the molecular mechanisms regulating tumorigenesis. *Clin Cancer Res* (2006). Sep 15;, 12(18), 5298-304.

[55] Martino, J. J, Wall, B. A, Mastrantoni, E, & Wilimczyk, B. J. La Cava SN, Degenhardt K, et al. Metabotropic glutamate receptor 1 (Grm1) is an oncogene in epithilial cells. *Oncogene* (2012). Accepted, September 2012.

[56] Chang, H. J, Yoo, B. C, Lim, S. B, Jeong, S. Y, Kim, W. H, & Park, J. G. Metabotropic glutamate receptor 4 expression in colorectal carcinoma and its prognostic significance. *Clin Cancer Res* (2005). May 1;, 11(9), 3288-95.

[57] Choi, K. Y, Chang, K, Pickel, J. M, & Badger, J. D. nd, Roche KW. Expression of the metabotropic glutamate receptor 5 (mGluR5) induces melanoma in transgenic mice. *Proc Natl Acad Sci U S A* (2011). Sep 13;, 108(37), 15219-24.

[58] Wyllie, A. H, Carder, P. J, Clarke, A. R, Cripps, K. J, Gledhill, S, Greaves, M. F, et al. Apoptosis in carcinogenesis: the role of *Cold Spring Harb Symp Quant Biol* (1994). , 53.

[59] Wyllie, A. H, Kerr, J. F, & Currie, A. R. Cell death: the significance of apoptosis. *Int Rev Cytol* (1980). , 68, 251-306.

[60] Thompson, C. B. Apoptosis in the pathogenesis and treatment of disease. *Science* (1995). Mar 10;, 267(5203), 1456-62.

[61] Engelman, J. A, Luo, J, & Cantley, L. C. The evolution of phosphatidylinositol 3-kinases as regulators of growth and metabolism. *Nat Rev Genet* (2006). Aug;, 7(8), 606-19.

[62] Cantley, L. C. The phosphoinositide 3-kinase pathway. *Science* (2002). May 31;, 296(5573), 1655-7.

[63] Hu, P, Margolis, B, Skolnik, E. Y, Lammers, R, Ullrich, A, & Schlessinger, J. Interaction of phosphatidylinositol 3-kinase-associated with epidermal growth factor and platelet-derived growth factor receptors. *Mol Cell Biol* (1992). Mar;12(3):981-90., 85.

[64] Rodriguez-viciana, P, Marte, B. M, Warne, P. H, & Downward, J. Phosphatidylinositol 3′ kinase: one of the effectors of Ras. *Philos Trans R Soc Lond B Biol Sci* (1996). Feb 29;discussion 31-2., 351(1336), 225-31.

[65] Jiang, B. H, & Liu, L. Z. PI3K/PTEN signaling in tumorigenesis and angiogenesis. *Biochim Biophys Acta* (2008). Jan;, 1784(1), 150-8.

[66] Du, K, & Montminy, M. CREB is a regulatory target for the protein kinase Akt/PKB. *J Biol Chem* (1998). Dec 4;, 273(49), 32377-9.

[67] Zhou, H, Li, X. M, Meinkoth, J, & Pittman, R. N. Akt regulates cell survival and apoptosis at a postmitochondrial level. *J Cell Biol* (2000). Oct 30;, 151(3), 483-94.

[68] Romashkova, J. A, Makarov, S. S, & Is, N. F-k. a. p. p. a. B. a target of AKT in anti-apoptotic PDGF signalling. *Nature* (1999). Sep 2;, 401(6748), 86-90.

[69] Kane, L. P, Shapiro, V. S, Stokoe, D, & Weiss, A. Induction of NF-kappaB by the Akt/PKB kinase. *Curr Biol* (1999). Jun 3;, 9(11), 601-4.

[70] Mayo, L. D, & Donner, D. B. A phosphatidylinositol 3-kinase/Akt pathway promotes translocation of Mdm2 from the cytoplasm to the nucleus. *Proc Natl Acad Sci U S A* (2001). Sep 25;, 98(20), 11598-603.

[71] Zhou, B. P, Liao, Y, Xia, W, Zou, Y, Spohn, B, & Hung, M. C. HER-2/neu induces ubiquitination via Akt-mediated MDM2 phosphorylation. *Nat Cell Biol* (2001). Nov; 3(11):973-82., 53.

[72] Staal, S. P. Molecular cloning of the akt oncogene and its human homologues AKT1 and AKT2: amplification of AKT1 in a primary human gastric adenocarcinoma. *Proc Natl Acad Sci U S A* (1987). Jul;, 84(14), 5034-7.

[73] Bellacosa, A, De Feo, D, Godwin, A. K, Bell, D. W, Cheng, J. Q, Altomare, D. A, et al. Molecular alterations of the AKT2 oncogene in ovarian and breast carcinomas. *Int J Cancer* (1995). Aug 22;, 64(4), 280-5.

[74] Cheng, J. Q, Ruggeri, B, Klein, W. M, Sonoda, G, Altomare, D. A, Watson, D. K, et al. Amplification of AKT2 in human pancreatic cells and inhibition of AKT2 expression and tumorigenicity by antisense RNA. *Proc Natl Acad Sci U S A* (1996). Apr 16;, 93(8), 3636-41.

[75] Schwartz, P. S, Manion, M. K, Emerson, C. B, Fry, J. S, Schulz, C. M, Sweet, I. R, et al. Methoxy antimycin reveals a unique mechanism for Bcl-x(L) inhibition. *Mol Cancer Ther* (2007). Jul;, 6(7), 2073-80.

[76] Okumura, N, Yoshida, H, Kitagishi, Y, Murakami, M, Nishimura, Y, Matsuda, S, & Akt, P. I3K. PTEN Signaling as a Molecular Target in Leukemia Angiogenesis. *Adv Hematol* (2012).

[77] Maehama, T, & Dixon, J. E. The tumor suppressor, PTEN/MMAC1, dephosphorylates the lipid second messenger, phosphatidylinositol 3,4,5-trisphosphate. *J Biol Chem* (1998). May 29;, 273(22), 13375-8.

[78] Huntington, J. T, & Shields, J. M. Der CJ, Wyatt CA, Benbow U, Slingluff CL, Jr., et al. Overexpression of collagenase 1 (MMP-1) is mediated by the ERK pathway in inva-

sive melanoma cells: role of BRAF mutation and fibroblast growth factor signaling. *J Biol Chem* (2004). Aug 6;, 279(32), 33168-76.

[79] Satyamoorthy, K, Li, G, Gerrero, M. R, Brose, M. S, Volpe, P, Weber, B. L, et al. Constitutive mitogen-activated protein kinase activation in melanoma is mediated by both BRAF mutations and autocrine growth factor stimulation. *Cancer Res* (2003). Feb 15;, 63(4), 756-9.

[80] Clark, B. P, Baker, S. R, Goldsworthy, J, Harris, J. R, & Kingston, A. E. methyl-4-carboxyphenylglycine (LY367385) selectively antagonises metabotropic glutamate mGluR1 receptors. *Bioorg Med Chem Lett* (1997). Nov 4;, 7(21), 2777-80.

[81] Carroll, F. Y, Stolle, A, Beart, P. M, Voerste, A, Brabet, I, Mauler, F, et al. BAY36-7620: a potent non-competitive mGlu1 receptor antagonist with inverse agonist activity. *Mol Pharmacol* (2001). May;, 59(5), 965-73.

[82] Francesconi, A, & Duvoisin, R. Role of the second and third intracellular loops of metabotropic glutamate receptors in mediatic dual signal transduction activation. *J biol Chem* (1998). , 273, 5615-24.

[83] Saez, E, Nelson, M. C, Eshelman, B, Banayo, E, Koder, A, Cho, G. J, et al. Identification of ligands and coligands for the ecdysone-regulated gene switch. *Proc Natl Acad Sci U S A* (2000). Dec 19;, 97(26), 14512-7.

[84] Wangari-talbot, J, Wall, B. A, Goydos, J. S, & Chen, S. Functional Effects of GRM1 Suppression in Human Melanoma Cells. *Mol Cancer Res* (2012). Jul 13.

[85] Marin, Y. E, Namkoong, J, Shin, S. S, Raines, J, Degenhardt, K, White, E, et al. Grm5 expression is not required for the oncogenic role of Grm1 in melanocytes. *Neuropharmacology* (2005). Suppl , 1, 70-9.

[86] Melendez, R. I, & Kalivas, P. W. Metabotropic glutamate receptor regulation of extracellular glutamate levels in the prefrontal cortex. *Ann N Y Acad Sci* (2003). Nov;, 1003, 443-4.

[87] Melendez, R. I, Vuthiganon, J, & Kalivas, P. W. Regulation of extracellular glutamate in the prefrontal cortex: focus on the cystine glutamate exchanger and group I metabotropic glutamate receptors. *J Pharmacol Exp Ther* (2005). Jul;, 314(1), 139-47.

[88] Van den Bosch LThe causes and mechanism of selective motor neuron death in amyotrophic lateral sclerosis]. *Verh K Acad Geneeskd Belg* (2006). , 68(4), 249-69.

[89] Van Den Bosch LVan Damme P, Bogaert E, Robberecht W. The role of excitotoxicity in the pathogenesis of amyotrophic lateral sclerosis. *Biochim Biophys Acta* (2006). Nov-Dec;1762(11-12):1068-82.

[90] Yip, D, Le, M. N, Chan, J. L, Lee, J. H, Mehnert, J. A, Yudd, A, et al. A phase 0 trial of riluzole in patients with resectable stage III and IV melanoma. *Clin Cancer Res* (2009). Jun 1;, 15(11), 3896-902.

[91] Davies, H, Bignell, G. R, Cox, C, Stephens, P, Edkins, S, Clegg, S, et al. Mutations of the BRAF gene in human cancer. *Nature* (2002). Jun 27;, 417(6892), 949-54.

[92] Prickett, T. D, Wei, X, Cardenas-navia, I, Teer, J. K, Lin, J. C, Walia, V, et al. Exon capture analysis of G protein-coupled receptors identifies activating mutations in GRM3 in melanoma. *Nat Genet* (2011). Nov;, 43(11), 1119-26.

[93] Ohtani, Y, Harada, T, Funasaka, Y, Nakao, K, Takahara, C, Abdel-daim, M, et al. Metabotropic glutamate receptor subtype-1 is essential for in vivo growth of melanoma. *Oncogene* (2008). Dec 4;, 27(57), 7162-70.

[94] Li, S, Huang, S, & Peng, S. B. Overexpression of G protein-coupled receptors in cancer cells: involvement in tumor progression. *Int J Oncol* (2005). Nov;, 27(5), 1329-39.

Section 3

Therapeutics

Chapter 9

Current Therapies and New Pharmacologic Targets for Metastatic Melanoma

Claudriana Locatelli,
Fabíola Branco Filippin-Monteiro and
Tânia Beatriz Creczynski-Pasa

Additional information is available at the end of the chapter

http://dx.doi.org/10.5772/55192

1. Introduction

Malignant melanoma is a tumor that originates from the melanocytes and manifests mainly on the skin. Melanomas are usually strongly pigmented, however amelanotic forms have been observed. Relative to the tumor mass, melanomas have an early tendency to metastasize; the prognosis is therefore poor. Malignant melanoma is responsible for about 90% of skin cancer related mortality [1]. Several risk factors for the development of melanoma have been identified. Ethnic origin is particularly important with a disease that mostly affects people of European origin. Epidemiological studies have shown that exposure to the sun, especially in childhood, is a major environmental cause of melanoma, and that up to 65% of the cases of melanoma are frequently related to sunburn [2,3].

While it is easy for cancer prevention, the incidence of melanoma has increased dramatically over the last four decades and melanoma is now one of the most common forms of cancer, with significant morbidity and high mortality due to its propensity to metastasize. It has a high propensity for haematogenous and lymphatic dissemination to regional and distant sites and is poorly responsive to most systemic therapies. The 5-year survival rate for metastatic melanoma is dismal, ranging from 5% to 10% with a median survival of less than eight months with treatment [4,5].

The therapies used in advanced cases, such as chemotherapy, radiotherapy, biochemotherapy and vaccine, seem unable to provide a cure or improved survival of becoming a melanoma tumors most refractory to treatment [6,7]. Although surgery and radiation therapy are very important in the treatment of metastatic disease, systemic treatment remains the basis of therapy for the majority of patients, including chemotherapy, immunotherapy, or a combination of approaches such as biochemotherapy [8]. Many compounds have been investigated for antitumor activity in melanoma, but the current treatment options for patients with metastatic disease are limited and non-curative in the majority of cases.

Chemotherapy with cytotoxic agents has been used for the treatment of metastatic melanoma for over three decades. Among the antitumoral agents, efficacy is modest in metastatic melanoma including alkylating agents (dacarbazine, temozolomide, nitrosoureas), analogues of platinum (cisplatin, carboplatin) and microtubular toxins (vincas and taxanes), which have been used alone or in combination [8]. Specifically in relation to cytotoxic chemotherapy, dacarbazine used as a chemotherapeutic agent still represents the single most common option [8]. It was demonstrated that combinations of cytotoxic agents can produce low response rates, although higher than monotherapy with dacarbazine, which are associated with increased toxicity and do not extend significantly the survival of patients [8]. Although of limited therapeutic effect, dacarbazine cannot be dismissed as standard therapy for disseminated melanoma, as in evidence-based analysis no other regimen had greater benefits for the patients' survival [9]. By 2011, only two drugs for metastatic melanoma therapy had been approved by the Food and Drug Administration (FDA), which were dacarbazine and a high dose of interleukin 2 (IL-2). In 2011, the FDA approval of vermurafenib (chemotherapy agent) and ipilimumab (monoclonal antibody) for clinical studies raised optimism for the treatment of metastatic melanoma, since the therapies used until then had had serious limitations, and thus the use of novel strategies for melanoma treatment seemed promising. However, the use of these drugs is limited [10]. The strategies to increase the responsiveness of new therapies are the association with other drugs currently in clinical use, such as dacarbazine, although these therapies are under investigation in vitro and in vivo models.

Other new chemotherapies, including drugs that target biological receptors, are currently in development. Among these are bevacizumab, an endothelial growth factor antibody, and sorafenib, a cellular pathway inhibitor [11]. These agents have shown some efficacy in early clinical trials. The lenalidomide is a thalidomide derivative designed to be more effective and less toxic [12]. In a phase I trial, it was found to be well tolerated by patients with metastatic melanoma and to produce immune activation. Another agent of interest that has shown promising results are the anti Bcl-2 antisense (oblimersen), tested in metastatic melanoma. A combination of Bcl-2 antisense and dacarbazine showed better response than dacarbazine alone, although no significant improvement in overall survival was observed [13,14].

Several clinical trials are being carried out to investigate the antitumor efficacy of new agents as well as diverse immunosuppressive therapeutic strategies, including the use of dendritic cells, high-doses of interferon-α (IFN-α) and/or IL-2 and anti-cytotoxic T lymphocyte-associated antigen 4 (CTLA-4) antibody, alone or in combination with current therapies for treating locally advanced, metastatic and recurrent melanomas [15].

Significant advancements made in the last few years have provided important information on the molecular signalling pathways and gene products, which are frequently deregulated in melanoma stem/progenitor cells and their progenies during melanoma formation and progression to locally advanced and metastatic disease states. Consequently, the combination

http://dx.doi.org/10.5772/55192

of different molecular biomarkers or cytotoxic agents targeting distinct gene products altered during melanoma development may constitute more promising therapeutic strategies. Several other signal transduction pathways have been found to be constitutively active or mutated in other subsets of melanoma tumors that are potentially targetable with new agents. Among these, NF-kB is another pathway that melanoma tumors use to achieve survival, proliferation, resistance to apoptosis and metastasis. In fact, it has been demonstrated that up regulation of the NF-kB levels is involved in both the progression of melanoma and an increase of its metastatic potential. Therefore, inhibition of NF-kB activation seems to be a promising target for anti-cancer therapies [16,17].

Recent studies have shown that proteasome inhibitors such as bortezomib represent a new class of anticancer agents by degradation inhibition of cell cycle regulatory proteins, such as cyclin-dependent kinase inhibitors and I-kB protein. The efficacy of bortezomib was recently explored in another 2-stage phase 2 clinical trials in combination with other chemotherapeutic agents, including paclitaxel and carboplatin, in patients with advanced solid tumors. The results from these studies evidenced narrow clinical benefit and significant toxicity, hindrances that limit the use of bortezomib [18].

Another compound known to exert numerous pharmacological properties - mostly antioxidant, anti-inflammatory and antiproliferative - is curcumin, a polyphenol present in in *Curcuma longa,* a species belonging to the ginger family (Zingiberaceae). With regard to antiproliferative activity, it showed pro-apoptotic activity in a variety of tumors in vitro. To achieve these results, curcumin was used in experiments based on melanoma either in vitro or in vivo models. The importance of curcumin also lies in the fact that this drug seems to reduce the metastatic potential of melanoma, which is the main cause of death [19].

Understanding and overcoming resistance pathways by combining current and future agents, identifying biomarkers to improve therapy and discover new therapeutic targets are promising advances in the treatment of melanoma. In light of this, the purpose of this chapter is to summarize the recent advances in the treatment of metastatic melanoma and to describe the current limitations, as well as to comment on promising future strategies to overcome the limitations.

2. Single agent chemotherapy

Melanoma is considered a chemotherapy-resistant tumor, but in fact several chemotherapeutic agents show single-agent activity at the level of 10% to 15%, similar to the efficacy of the chemotherapeutic armamentarium used against other tumor types. Several combination chemotherapy regimens have been tested, but no survival benefit has been demonstrated. Few of these trials have been compared with standard dacarbazine (DTIC) in an adequately powered randomized trial, and even the most extensive of these trials only aimed to detect unrealistically large improvements in overall survival [20]. For the systemic monotherapy of advanced melanoma, several substances are available whose clinical efficacy is comparable. Palliative monochemotherapy can shrink tumors and thus achieve a reduction in tumor-related symptoms. The more active agents are the alkylants (dacarbazine, temozolomide, fotemustine, carmustine, semustine), platinum drugs (cisplatin and carboplatin), vinca alkaloids (vindezine and vinblastine), taxanes (docetaxel and paclitaxel), and tamoxifen [7,21]. Table 1 shows the drugs and dosages for monotherapy to melanoma.

Drugs	**Dosage**	**Overall response**
Dacarbazine	250 mg/m^2/day for 5 days every 3-4 weeks	5.3 – 25%
Temozolomide	150-200 mg/m^2/day for 5 days every 4 weeks	13.5-21%
Carmustine	75-110 mg/m^2	13-18%
Semustine	130 mg/m^2	16%
Fotemustine	100 mg/m^2/day every 3 weeks	7.4-25%
Cisplatin	60-150 mg/m^2	15%
Carboplatin	400 mg/m^2 every 4 weeks	19%
Vindezine	3 mg/m^2 every 14 days	12-26%
Vinblastine	6-8 mg/m^2 every 1 week	13%
Docetaxel	100 mg/m^2 every 21 days	14%
Paclitaxel	125-275 mg/m^2	15%
Tamoxifen	20 mg/day	4-13%
Interferon α	9m-18m IU/m^2 3x/week continuous administration	13-25%
Interleukin-2	600 000 IU/Kg as 15 minute short infusion i.v. every 8 hours on days 1-5 (maximum 14 individual doses) repeat cycle day 14	16-21.6%

Adapted by Garbe et al. (2008) [21] and Mouawad et al. (2010) [7].

Table 1. Single drugs, dosage and their activity in melanoma.

2.1. Alkylants agents

2.1.1. Triazenes

The alkylating agent dacarbazine (DTIC, dimethyltriazeno imidazole carboxamide) was first introduced some 30 years ago, and it is considered to be the reference of single agent for the management of advanced melanoma. This compound was initially designed as an antimetabolite because it is an analogue of 5-aminoimidazole-4-carboxamide, an intermediate in purine biosynthesis. However, it presented cytotoxicity that is related to the generation of methyldiazonium, which methylates DNA during its metabolism [22]. Methyldiazonium has a half-life of about 0.4 s in aqueous solution, sufficient time to allow it to reach its target. In 1975 this carboxamide was approved by the Food and Drug Administration (FDA), and has since been considered the standard of metastatic melanoma care. Single-agent DTIC has remained the standard of care for 3 decades, with response rates of 8% to 20% and mean duration of response of approximately four to six months. Several studies of dacarbazine in the management of metastatic melanoma were published in the early 1970s [23,24]. The first of these trials demonstrated a 19% response rate in 110 evaluable patients who received dacarbazine in 3-weekly cycles, most frequently at a dose of 250 mg/m^2 daily for five days [25]. A second study showed an overall response rate of 28% in 115 evaluable patients receiving dacarbazine 2.5 or 4.5 mg/kg daily for ten days of a thirty-day cycle, and another showed response rates approaching 20% with dacarbazine 150 mg/m^2 daily for five days of a thirty-day cycle in 112 evaluable patients [24]. The typical dacarbazine dose is 850 to 1,000 mg/m^2 every three weeks [26].

Among the randomized trials in which dacarbazine was used as a comparator arm, the patients treated with dacarbazine with an overall response rate of 13.4% and median survivals ranging from about six months to eleven months. Given the low response rate, it is unrealistic to expect dacarbazine to have an effect on median survival [27].

Studies suggest that less than 5% of patients achieve a complete response to therapies with dacarbazine alone or in combination, and less than 2% of patients survive five years more. The majority of previous reports suggest that long-term survival is restricted to patients with favourable clinical features, such as nodal, cutaneous or pulmonary metastasis [28].

Although dacarbazine presents a relatively small therapeutic response, it is still considered the standard drug for the treatment of melanoma, whereas the drug combination and the use of other drugs do not show effect as monotherapy.

Another problem with associated dacarbazine is the high toxicity. The major toxic effects associated with dacarbazine are the development of neutropenia, thrombocytopenia, alopecia, nausea or vomiting, fatigue and liver damage [29].

Besides its toxicity, dacarbazine has several drawbacks because of its hydrophilicity, which leads to slow and incomplete oral absorption, and therefore the alternative is intravenous administration. Another disadvantage is its high photosensitivity, with a very short half-life (about 30 min), decomposing to 2-azah hypoxanthine via an intermediate diazonium species. For this reason, intravenous infusion bags of dacarbazine must be protected from light. These problems have stimulated the synthesis of dacarbazine analogues, the most important of which is temozolomide [20].

Temozolomide is an oral alkylated compound similar to dacarbazine (the most active single agent in primary melanoma), which has 100% of oral bioavailability and considerable penetration in Central Nervous System tissue, mainly due to its lipophilic character [30]. Moreover, for its acid-stability the molecule remains in cerebro-spinal fluid, where it reaches 30–40% of plasmatic concentration [31]. For this reason, differently from dacarbazine, temozolomide is employed in the treatment of primitive [32] and metastatic brain tumors [31]. Although the FDA has not approved it for melanoma, temozolomide is widely used and has response rates similar to dacarbazine in melanoma [26,33].

Despite the absence of approval, temozolomide is also used "off-label" in patients with malignant melanoma after standard treatment. Temozolomide has been proven to have an equal efficacy (with a 10–20% response rate) to that of dacarbazine, the most commonly used chemotherapy agent in metastatic melanoma, in a randomized phase III trial [34,35]. However, TMZ administered in monotherapy did not show significant improvement in the overall response rate or median survival time. Nonetheless, the works of Biswas et al. (2006) [36], Chang et al. (2007) [37], Platta et al. (2007) [38] and Mehta et al. (2010) [39] show the efficacy and modest side effects of single-agent TMZ in patients with recurrent or progressive brain metastases.

In a randomized trial comparing temozolomide given for five days every month with dacarbazine given once every 3 weeks, there was no difference in response rate or survival [26]. Despite this, temozolomide offers two potential advantages over dacarbazine. Temozolomide readily crosses the intact blood-brain barrier, which provides enhanced activity against brain metastases. Unfortunately, the objective response rate of melanoma brain metastases to temozolomide is low [37], although there is some indication that treatment with temozolomide is associated with a lower incidence of disease progression in the brain [38,39]. Another potential advantage of temozolomide is that, as an oral agent, continuous dosing is feasible. An extended-dosing schedule of 75 mg/m^2/day for 42 days followed by 14 days off has been used in several clinical trials. This schedule provides six weeks of continuous drug exposure and delivers 50% more drug over two months compared with the standard schedule of five days every month. However, a phase II trial using extended-dosing temozolomide showed only a 12.5% response rate [40], which is not different from what would be expected with standard-dosing of temozolomide or of dacarbazine.

Patients that received oral temozolomide at a starting dosage of 200 mg/m^2/d for five days every 28 days showed median survival time of about eight months, while patients treated with dacarbazine of about seven months. These results showed that treatment with temozolomide presented significantly longer survival, nevertheless no major difference in drug safety was observed. Temozolomide was well tolerated and produced a noncumulative, transient myelosuppression late in the 28-day cycle. The most common nonhematologic toxicities observed were mild to moderate nausea and vomiting, which were easily managed. Temozolomide therapy improved health-related life quality [26].

The most common hematologic side-effect of temozolomide is myelosuppression (similar to that produced by dacarbazine), particularly neutropenia and thrombocytopenia (dose-limiting toxicity). In contrast, nausea and vomiting are limited (10–15%), whereas the same side effects are remarkably severe and very frequent (i.e. of the order of 90%) in patients treated with dacarbazine. Both drugs can induce headache, fatigue, liver toxicity and constipation [34].

Nevertheless, the development of resistance against the treatment is very common. There are likely multiple mechanisms of chemotherapy resistance specifically for dacarbazine or temozolomide, such as DNA repair of the adduct formation (O6-guanine) with the O6-methylguanine-DNA methyltransferase [26,41]. Other mechanisms of resistance include Bcl-2 overexpression, silencing of *apoptotic protease activating factor-1* gene (a key mediator of apoptosis), and activation of proliferative and antiapoptotic signalling pathways, including the mitogen-activated protein kinase and phosphoinositide 3-kinase/Akt pathways [34,35,42-44]. In addition, NF-κB activation of its down-stream target genes (angiogenesis, adhesion, antiapoptosis, and chemokine growth factors) likely plays a central role in the proliferation and chemotherapy resistance observed in melanoma [45-47]. It is well established that chemotherapy itself can induce NF-κB activation in cancer cells [46,47]. Any number of these or other biological processes are likely important to chemotherapy resistance in melanoma.

In an attempt to reduce resistance to chemotherapy in patients with melanoma, new therapies are introduced including the combination of temozolomide and dacarbazine with other chemotherapeutic drugs that have similar mechanism of action or act in different ways. Alternatives used in polychemotherapy in treating melanoma or as monotherapy are the nitrosoureas such as fotemustine.

2.1.2. Nitrosoureas

The nitrosoureas (carmustine, lomustine, semustine and fotemustine) all have single agent activity in melanoma because they cross the blood-brain barrier, thus enabling its use in the treatment of metastatic melanoma. However, at conventional doses, little or no activity was observed against melanoma brain metastases, and overall response rates were low, with only a few complete remissions and short response durations [7,48]. Fotemustine is probably the most active nitrosourea against metastatic melanoma, and especially against cerebral metastasis; its efficacy has been widely demonstrated through several phase II studies.

In patients without brain metastasis treated with fotemustine, the median time for the development of brain metastasis was longer as compared to patients treated with dacarbazine (22.7 months vs. 7.2 months) [49]. It has been widely tested in Europe and has shown overall response of 20-25%, including 5-8% of complete response rates, and it was the first drug to show significant efficacy in brain metastases [50,51].

A multicenter trial of monotherapy was undertaken in 153 evaluable French patients, in which a response rate of 24.2% was obtained. In phase II studies fotemustine was administered intravenously as a rapid infusion, at a dose of 100 mg/m^2 on days 1, 8, 15, then after four to five weeks every three weeks for maintenance. These studies showed response rates between 16% and 47% in non-visceral metastasis, and long-term survival without metastasis was reported [50,52,53].

In a phase III clinical trial of fotemustine (100 mg/m^2 weekly for three weeks) versus dacarbazine (250 mg/m^2/ day for five days every four weeks), the response rate for fotemustine was 15.2% versus 6.8% for dacarbazine [49].

Previous preclinical studies have indicated that fotemustine inhibits enzymes involved in the ribonucleotide reduction pathway (i.e. DNA synthesis), whereby responding patients appeared to favour the thioredoxin reductase/thioredoxin electron transfer to ribonucleotide reductase, whereas non-responders expressed the alternate glutathione reductase/glutaredoxin mechanism. The 47% response rate obtained in these studies vs. the 24% reported previously for fotemustine may reflect variations in enzymes in the ribonucleotide reduction pathway in different patients. However, the efficacy of fotemustine against advanced melanoma warrants more extensive trials of this drug, especially because the quality of life of the patients during and after chemotherapy was not severely affected [54].

Fotemustine was well tolerated by the patients, with the only mild side effects being thrombocytopenia, leukocytopenia in 40% patients, and easily controlled nausea/vomiting [55].

2.2. Platinum derivatives

Cisplatin and carboplatin have shown modest activity as single agent therapy in patients with metastatic melanoma. Cisplatin and carboplatin showed good activity against human melanoma cell line, but during in vivo study it did not improve the response comparing with other drugs used in monoterapy of melanoma treatment. It has been shown that cisplatin induced a 15% response rate with a short median duration of three months [8]. Evidence that the activity of cisplatin may be dose-dependent has come from single institution studies. Cisplatin is also used as a palliative in selected patients with malignant melanoma and central nervous system metastases. It was shown that cisplatin can be administered alone via intracarotid infusion in doses varying from 40 to 75mg/m^2, but the response is not satisfactory, as only about 13% of the patients presented stabilization of the disease [56]. With regard to carboplatin, in a study on 26 chemotherapy naive metastatic melanoma patients, a response rate of 19% with five partial responses has been reported, and thrombocytopenia was the dose-limiting toxicity [57]. Oxaliplatin is a platinum analogue, which cytotoxic activity observed in an in vitro assay appears to be significantly superior to that of carboplatin. Its activity becomes comparatively closer to that of cisplatin as exposure time increases. Indeed, at a 24 h exposure oxaliplatin appears to be significantly more active than cisplatin [58]. Preclinical data have confirmed its non-overlapping spectrum of activity with cisplatin, including acquired and intrinsic platinum resistant cell lines [59]. In a small phase II trial by Evans et al. (1987) [60], no objective response was observed from 10 patients who had previously failed to respond to chemotherapy.

2.3. Vinca alkaloids

The vinca alkaloids, especially vindesine and vinblastine, are usually used in melanoma treatment. A phase II study by Mohammed et al. (2000) [61] with vinorelbine 30mg/m^2/week by intravenous bolus with 21 patients no complete or partial response was observed. The estimated median progression-free survival was two months, and the estimated median overall survival was six months. Patients received vinorelbine at a dose of 30 mg/m^2 on days one and eight of a 21-day cycle, on an outpatient basis. Thirteen patients were included in the study, and received 64 cycles. All patients were assessable for response, toxicity and survival. The median progression-free survival was 3.3 months and the estimated median overall survival was 8.1 months. Vinorelbine as a single agent on days one and eight of a 21-day cycle has a favourable toxicity profile, but seems to have no relevant clinical activity in patients with metastatic melanoma [62] Vindesine is frequently included in combination regimens for the treatment of malignant melanoma and head and neck cancer, although its single-agent activity in these diseases is modest (average of 14 and 12% response rates, respectively) [63]. Similarly, another study that investigated the usefulness of vindesine monotherapy as salvage therapy in stage IV melanoma patients who had previously failed to respond to chemotherapies also failed; the treatment with vindesine 3mg/m^2 given to the patients every two weeks in a median of three treatments was stopped due to the disease progression. The median survival after starting vindesine therapy was four months. In this study the authors concluded that vindesine monotherapy is ineffective in stage IV melanoma patients [64]. A phase II study by Retsas et al. (1979) [68] showed a 30% rate response in 25 patients' treatment with vindesine, but with pronounced side effects. Apart from a low rate response the vinorelbine showed significant toxicity, including febrile neutropenia, granulocytopenia, leukopenia, asthenia, nausea, neuropathy, myalgia, dyspnea and fatigue [61].

2.4. Taxol

Preclinical studies indicate that taxanes disturb the cytoskeleton architecture and stabilize microtubules, causing mitotic arrest [65]. Taxol is a major new antitumor agent with significant activity against a number of human cancers. Preclinical investigation demonstrated significant activity against B16 melanoma and against cells derived from melanoma in a human stem cell assay [66]. Studies in phases II and III have shown that taxol has activity against melanoma, but the responses were partial with 16.2% rate response and median duration of approximately five months [67]. Another study with paclitaxel administered at a dose of 100mg/m^2 intravenously on day one each week for six weeks, the median survival was 209 days [68]. In a phase I trial with paclitaxel administered at 200 to 275 mg/m^2 over 24 hours every three weeks, there were four partial responses observed in the 12 patients enrolled [69]. A phase II trial with paclitaxel administered at 250 mg/m^2 over 24 hours every three weeks in 25 patients resulted in three partial responses (12%); an additional four patients had durable objective regression although failing to qualify for partial response [74]. An additional 28 evaluated patients were studied in a second phase II study with paclitaxel administered at 250 mg/m^2 over 24 hours. Four patients (14%) had objective responses with three complete responses [70]. In another study phase II clinical trial, patients received paclitaxel at 80 mg/m^2 over one hour, weekly for three weeks, followed by a one-week rest period; the disease status was assessed every other cycle and the treatment was continued until the patients experienced either disease progression or unacceptable toxicity. All patients were considered to be evaluable for toxicity and all patients were included for response assessment in an intention-to-treat analysis. Patients received paclitaxel for a median of two cycles. None of the 27 patients showed a response to treatment; eight patients had stable disease. The median progression-free survival was 1.8 months and the median survival was 7.6 months [76]. A phase II trial achieved with paclitaxel administered at 90 mg/m^2 on days one, five, and nine every three weeks demonstrated a 15.6% response in 5/32 patients [71].

Docetaxel showed an average response rate of 11.4% in three phase II clinical trials. In an assay performed by the Enzig group, they administered 100 mg/m^2 docetaxel every three weeks to chemotherapy naive patients. Two out of 35 (6%) of the patients responded with one complete response. Both these responses lasted longer than two years [65]. In a phase II clinical trial, 38 patients were also treated with 100 mg/m^2 docetaxel every three weeks and evaluated after two cycles; five partial responses were noted in the 30 evaluable patients (17%) [72].

The most common toxicity of taxois is haematological, mainly related with neutropenia. Additional toxicities included hypersensitivity reaction and diarrhoea, peripheral neuropathy, fatigue, fluid retention and oral mucositis [72,73].

2.5. Tamoxifen

In 1976, Fischer and collaborators reported the presence of estrogen receptors on human melanoma cells derived from metastatic tumors [74]. Following a preliminary report, studies were performed with tamoxifen in the treatment of melanoma, either as a single agent or more commonly in combination with other chemotherapeutic agents. In a meta-analysis study it was demonstrated that tamoxifen does not improve the overall response rate, complete response rate or survival rate when administered as chemotherapy regimens. The rate responses ranged from zero to 10% [75]. However, for women 50 years of age or older treated with tamoxifen alone, a response rate of 25% was observed. Despite these promising results, a subsequent phase II trial published in 1992 showed a response rate of only 4.9% in post-menopausal women treated with tamoxifen 40 mg daily (14). In phase II studies the patients treated with tamoxifen 100 mg/m^2 did not show objective response [76,77]. Another study by Aamdal et al. (1994) [78] reported that the enzyme tyrosinase could mimic estrogen receptors binding, leading to the possibility that this or other interfering substances could account for apparent estrogen receptors activity and the failure to correlate this activity with response to tamoxifen. A remaining controversial question is the inclusion of the antiestrogen in different active chemotherapy regimens, because clinical investigations on the role of tamoxifen in single agent of melanoma have produced inconclusive results.

2.6. Immunotherapy

The relationship between melanoma and the immune system has been recognized, spontaneous tumor regression in patients with metastatic melanoma have suggested that immunotherapy might have a greater impact on the outcome of metastatic melanoma than in other cancers [7]. Immune based treatment using biologic response modifiers, especially interleukin-2 and interferon-α, which have important roles in both adjuvant therapy and in the treatment of metastatic melanoma, may became an antimelanoma strategy [7,79]. However, the landscape for late-stage treatment options has changed recently, with FDA approval in March 2011 for a new immunotherapy drug ipilimumab for treatment of metastatic melanoma [80]. The Ipilimumab, a humanized monoclonal antibody against CTLA-4, is actually a unique way of enhancing patients' immune response against tumors [81].

2.6.1. Interferon alpha (IFN-α)

Interferons represent a family of glycoproteins with a broad spectrum of effects including antiviral, immunomodulatory, antiproliferative, prodifferentiating and antiangiogenic [82,83].

Interferon-α (INF-α) has shown antitumor activity in metastatic malignant melanoma, both as single-agent therapy and in combination with chemotherapeutic agents. As a single agent, IFN-α yields an objective response rate of approximately 15% of responses with less than 5%

of complete response rates and median response duration of between six and nine months with a maximum of 12 months for the best studies [84,85]. Patients that received INF-α intravenously for one month and 10 MIU/m^2 subcutaneously three times per week for 48 weeks showed a significantly increased overall survival rate, with a median follow-up of 6.9 years (Kirkwood et al., 1996)

In a controlled trial of two lower doses of IFN-α conducted in patients in observation or in other regimen of treatment, with an intermediate dose of IFN-α (four weeks with 10 MIU/m^2 administered five times per week, followed by 10 MIU/m^2 three times per week for one year or five MIU/m^2 three times per week for two years) for 13 or 25 months, intermediate dose IFN-α did not significantly improve distant metastasis free interval or overall survival outcomes [28]. Low-dose IFN-α also failed to improve survival outcomes versus observation alone when patients were treated with three MIU/m^2 two times weekly for six months or three MIU/m^2 three times weekly for two or three years [86-88]. Clinical data were recorded by IFN-α dose: high (20 MIU/m^2), intermediate (5–10 MIU/m^2), low (3 MIU/m^2), and very low (1 MIU/m^2) doses. Groups were also stratified by duration of treatment (6 months, 12–18 months or 24 months). Although there was a statistically significant overall survival benefit for treatment of patients with IFN-α, this assimilation did not find evidence of a clear difference in overall survival with different dose levels or duration of the treatments [89]. The mechanism of the therapeutic effects of IFN-α is not completely known. Additional data from Håkansson et al. (1998) [95] and Yurkovetsky et al. (2007) [96] revealed significant decreases of serum levels of immunosuppressive and tumor angiogenic/growth stimulatory factors and increased levels of antiangiogenic. This study also demonstrated a profile of pro-inflammatory cytokines that may help to predict response to therapy. A fundamental question has been raised regarding whether the benefit of IFNs such as immunologic, antiangiogenic, or other antitumor effects would persist long-term or if it would require prolonged, and perhaps indefinite, exposure to IFN-α [90]. When using IFN-α in the long term, the tolerability needs to be weighed up. IFN-α induces acute flu like symptoms and widespread haematological and nonhaematological organ toxicity, dose-dependent fatigue/anorexia, and neuropsychiatric side effects that may endanger compliance over the course of several years' therapy [21].

2.6.2. Interleukin-2 (IL-2)

IL-2, a natural product secreted by CD^{4+} T lymphocytes, was described as a T cell growth factor, which plays a central role in immune regulation. However, IL-2 can also modulate immunological effects by stimulating HLA-restricted or non-restricted cytotoxic cell, activate natural killer cells, B lymphocytes, macrophages and induce lymphokine-actived killer cells in vitro as well as the production of other cytokines [7]. The FDA initially approved IL-2 for the treatment of patients with metastatic melanoma in 1998. High-doses of IL-2 (600.000-720.000 IU/Kg every eight hours on days 1-5 and 15-19) produce overall response rates in 15-20% of patients with complete responses in 4-6% [91-93]. In phase II trials in patients with metastatic melanoma, a high-dose regimen of 600.000 U/Kg IL-2 was administered every eight hours for up to 14 doses; only 16% presented objective response and a small percentage of patients (5%) experienced long-term, durable complete response, which has been interpreted as a potential cure [84]. However, this therapy has not been shown to improve overall survival in the patient population and has never been evaluated in a phase III setting [94,95]. In addition, IL-2 treatment-related toxicity is severe, which include hemodynamic toxicity (e.g. hypotension, edema, weight gain and decreased renal function), respiratory insufficiency, and neurotoxicity [96,97]. Based on the available data assessing prognostic factors and patient selection, patients with non-visceral metastases and fewer metastatic sites have a much higher response rate. In these select patients, high dose IL-2 may be considered for first-line therapy [98].

2.6.3. Ipilimumab a new hope for metastatic melanoma

Stimulation of tumor-expressed Cytotoxic T-Lymphocyte Antigen 4 (CTLA-4) with soluble ligands or agonistic mAb triggers the apoptosis [99,100], as well as inhibition of proliferation and secretion of angiogenic cytokines [101]. Preclinical studies showed that blocking CTLA-4 results in anti-tumor activity and tumor regression in many mice tumor models (prostate, breast, lymphoma, melanoma) [102,103]. Two anti-CTLA-4 monoclonal antibodies, generated by different companies, were tested in clinical trials in metastatic melanoma patients: tremelimumab (Pfizer) and ipilimumab/Yervoy (Bristol Myers Squibb), but only the latter was successful in phase III studies. Based on its ability to prolong survival of previously treated as well as untreated metastatic melanoma patients [104,105], ipilimumab received European Union (2010) [106] and FDA (March 2011) approval.

Widely touted as a therapeutic breakthrough, ipilimumab works by enhancing T-cell activity by modifying the function of the CTLA-4 inhibitory receptor. Ipilimumab is directed against the CTLA-4 antigen present on the surface of cytotoxic T-lymphocytes. The presence of the CTLA-4 antigen negatively regulates the activity of T-lymphocytes, ultimately suppressing the immune response [107]. Evidence for ipilimumab offers hope for patients with a clearly lethal disease, but also highlights some of the dangers and relative infancy of immunotherapies in the clinical setting [108].

Blocking the CTLA-4 antigen with ipilimumab will stimulate the patient's own immune response, which will be helpful in destroying cancerous cells [109]. Ipilimumab has been studied in more than 2,000 patients with metastatic melanoma and response patterns showing shrinkage of baseline lesions, a decline of tumor burden with a complete response in few patients. An objective response rate of above 30% was observed in later stages of clinical trials, after failing in the initial stages of the treatment, in which the response rate was 10%. The results of the advanced phase III trials indicate that one third of the patients taking Ipilimumab will receive long-term survival benefits [104]. Objective response rates combining complete response and partial response were in the range of 5–20% [104,110]. Disease control rates were reported averaging 15–30%. In contrast, the two therapies approved by the FDA, high-dose of IL- 2 and dacarbazine, are both associated with response rates of only 10 to 20% and a small percentage of complete response. They are not thought to improve overall survival [104]. Two exciting phase III studies tested the clinical effects of Ipilimumab in advanced metastatic melanoma patients. In the first, 676 participants from 125 different medical centers, who had already been given standard treatments, received Ipilimumab or gp100 vaccine separately, or a combination of both, in a randomized, double-blind manner. Treatment with Ipilimumab improved median overall survival rates (10.0 and 10.1 months in the Ipilimumab-treated groups as compared with 6.4 months in the gp100-only treated group). In the second trial [105], 502 patients who had not previously been treated received either dacarbazine (DTIC, standard care chemotherapy) or Ipilimumab in combination with dacarbazine in a double-blind, placebo-controlled manner. In this experiment, Ipilimumab increased overall survival rates from 9.1 to 11.2 months and 3-year survival from 12.2% to 20.8%. A study of single agent Ipilimumab with intra-patient dose escalation every 2 cycles of therapy also resulted in an increased toxicity with no improvement in the response rates [111]. In this study, patients were initially dosed at 3 mg/kg every three weeks for two doses. If there was no objective response or higher autoimmune toxicity, the dose was increased to 5 mg/kg for two doses and then to 9 mg/kg for two doses. Five out of 46 patients (11%) achieved an objective clinical response at the expense of 35% of patients experiencing significant toxicities. The authors concluded that increasing doses of Ipilimumab to increase autoimmune toxicities did not seem to increase the antitumor activity [111]. Adverse effects, mainly immune related in the skin and gastro-intestinal track, were experienced by nearly all patients in the two trials, with about half of the patients suffering from severe adverse effects in the second trial and several severe immune effects-related deaths in the first trial. Therefore, these exciting results also demonstrate the complicity of specifically manipulating immune responses.

3. Multi-drugs combinations

The disappointing results with single agent chemotherapy led to the evaluation of multi-drug combinations regimens in the 1980s in an effort to improve outcome and enhance response rates in patients with metastatic disease. The combinations of different chemotherapeutic drugs)or cytotoxic agents with cytokines occasionally yield substantially higher remission rates without prolonging overall survival [7,21]. The therapeutic schemes that have become established for melanoma are listed in Table 2. The toxicity of combined chemotherapeutics regimes is significantly higher than with monotherapy. Multi-drug combinations can, however, be of palliative use in individual cases and can provide effective treatment for tumor related symptoms. Since regimes are potentially toxic, intensive supportive treatment is crucial for the patient's quality of life [7].

Many of the combination regimens tested in melanoma (see Table 2) have combined dacarbazine with immunologic agents (e.g., IFN, IL-2), hormones (e.g., tamoxifen) or novel biologic agents, each of which individually has shown little single-agent activity. Some of the common combinations of cytotoxic chemotherapeutic regimens used in melanoma are discussed and the few phase III randomized trials that have been published are highlighted.

Historically, promising combination regimens like BOLD (bleomycin, vincristine, lomustine and DTIC) and CVD (cisplatin, vinblastine and DTIC) have induced responses on metastatic lesions in the liver, bone and brain, commonly unresponsive to DTIC alone, even though they have failed to have an impact on patient survival. Several other studies have suggested a significant enhancement of antitumor effect associated with the addition of tamoxifen to various cytotoxic regimens [112]. The other drug combinations have been observed and some authors recommend the combination of cisplatin, carmustine, dacarbazine and tamoxifen as reference therapy, even though recently presented results of a randomized phase III trial of this combination versus dacarbazine alone show no statistical difference in survival between the two groups. While a survival benefit from dacarbazine based chemotherapy or dacarbazine alone has never been shown in metastatic melanoma patients and, therefore, the survival has remained unchanged over the past 30 years, some long term survivors have been reported after receiving the "Dartmouth regimen" (Dacarbazine /Carmustine /Cisplatin /Tamoxifen) and/or high doses of IL-2 based regimens, whose role is going to be defined in prospective randomized phase III trials [112].

Scheme	Drugs/dosage	Overall response
BHD scheme	BCNU 150 mg/m^2 i.v. day 1, only every 2nd cycle/Hydroxyurea 1500 mg/m^2 oral days 1-5/Dacarbazine 150 mg/m^2 i.v. days 1-5 every 4 weeks	12.7-30.4%
BOLD scheme	Belomycin 15 mg i.v. days 1 + 4/Vincristine 1 mg/m^2 i.v days 1+ 5/CCNU 80 mg/m^2 p.o day 1/Dacarbazine 200 mg/m^2 i.v. days 1-5 every 4-6 weeks	22-40%
DVP scheme	Dacarbazine 250 mg/m^2 i.v. days 1-5/Vindesine 3 mg/m^2 i.v day 1/Cisplatin 100 mg/m^2 i.v day 1 every 3-4 weeks	31.4-45%
DVP scheme	Dacarbazine 450 mg/m^2 i.v. days 1 + 8/Vindesine 3 mg/m^2 i.v day 1 + 8/Cisplatin 50 mg/m^2 i.v day 1 + 8 every 3-4 weeks	24%
CarboTax scheme	Carboplatin AUC6 i.v day 1, after 4 cycles reduce dose to AUC5/Paclitaxel 225 mg/m^2 i.v. day 1 every 3 weeks	12.1% (second-line)
GemTreo scheme	Gemcitabine 1000 mg/m^2 i.v. days1 + 8/Treosulfan 3500 mg/m^2 i.v. days 1 + 8 every 4 weeks	33.3% (partial remission and stable disease)
	Carmustine 150 mg/m^2 i.v. + Vincristine 2 mg/m^2 i.v. on day 1 only	25%
	Cisplatin 20 mg/m^2/day for 4 days starting on day 2 + Vinblastine 1.6 mg/m^2/day x 5 days + Dacarbazine 800 mg/m^2 i.v. on day 1	24%
	Tamoxifen 10 mg twice daily by mouth 1 week before chemotherapy + Carmustine 150 mg/m2 on day 1 + Dacarbazine 220 mg/m^2 i.v. + Cisplatin 25 mg/m^2/days 1–3	18.5%
	Dacarbazine 250 mg/m^2 i.v days 1–4 every 3 weeks + Detorubicin 120 mg/m^2 i.v. every 3 weeks	36%
	Carmustine 150 mg/m^2 i.v. on day 1 + Cisplatin 25 mg/m^{2}i.v./day on days 1–3 + Dacarbazine 220 mg/m^2 i.v./day on days 1–3 + Tamoxifen 160 mg orally/day x 7 days prior to chemotherapy. Treatment cycles repeated every 28 days, BCNU every 2 cycles	26%

Scheme	Drugs/dosage	Overall response
	Dacarbazine 2.5 mg/m² i.v. by means of bolus injection on days 1–4 every 4 weeks + *Corynebacterium parvum* 7mg i.m. 1 week before starting DTIC and at 4-week intervals thereafter	27%
	Dacarbazine 250 mg/m² i.v. x 5 days, every 3-weeks + Tamoxifen 20 mg/m² orally daily	28%
	CCNU 200 mg/m² once every 6 weeks/Dacarbazine 150 mg/m² i.v. x 5 days/3 weeks + CCNU 130 mg/m² 1/6 weeks	15%
	Dacarbazine 250 mg/m² i.v./day on days 1–5 + Epirubicin 90 mg/m² on day 1 every 3 weeks	21%
	Vinblastine 6 mg/m²/day i.v. on days 1–2 + 24-h infusion of Bleomycin 15 units/m² from days 1–5 + Cisplatin 50 mg/m² 1 h i.v. infusion on day 5. After four courses, vinblastine and Cisplatin were given alone. Courses repeated on a cycle of 4 weeks	10%
	Dacarbazine 100 mg/m² 8 h x 6 days every month/ Carmustine 150 mg/m² + Vincristine 2 mg/m² every 30 days	24-29%
	Dacarbazine 250 mg/m²/day i.v. x 5 days every 4 weeks + Vindesine 3 mg/m²/week	25%
	Dacarbazine 220 mg/m² on day 1–3 + Carboplatine AUC 5, day 1, 21 Days	21.3%
	IFN-α 15MU/m²/day i.v. days 1–5 x 3 weeks, then 10MU/m² s.c. 3x/week + Dacarbazine 200 mg/m² daily i.v. days 1–5 starting on day 22, every 28 days	21%
	Tamoxifen 20 mg/day v.o. starting day 1 + Dacarbazine 200 mg/m²/day i.v. days 1–5 every 28 days	18%
	IFN-γ 15MU/m²/day i.v. days 1–5 x 3 weeks, then 10MU/m² s.c. 3x/week + orally Tamoxifen 20 mg/day starting day 1 + Dacarbazine 200 mg/m²/day i.v. days 1–5/28 days	19%
	Dacarbazine 800 mg/m² i.v. days 1 and 21 + daily INF-α i.m. 3 MIU at days 1–3, 6 MIU days 4–6, and 9 MIU daily thereafter. Started concomitantly	28%
	Dacarbazine 800 mg/m² i.v. days 1 and 21 + INF-α i.m. 3MIU 3 x /week. Started concomitantly	23%
	Dacarbazine i.v. escalating dose 200 mg/m², 400 mg/m², 800 mg/m²/3 weeks; IFN-α s.c. starting at 3 MU/day on days 1–3, 9 MU/day on days 4–70, then 9 MU 3 x /week	21%

BCNU = 1,3-bis(chroethyl)-1-nitrosourea (Carmustine) CCNU = Lomustine

Adapted by Garbe et al. (2008) [21] and Mouawad et al. (2010) [7].

Table 2. Multi-drug combinations and their activity in melanoma.

The Dartmouth Regimen was described for the first time in 1984 with the treatment of 20 patients with melanoma. This association showed promising results, with high response rates of 40% to 50% [113,114]. However, another study shows a response rate of 18.5% with this combination [115]. In another randomized phase II trial, Dartmouth Regimen was compared with dacarbazine alone in patients with melanoma, wherein 60 patients were randomly assigned to receive carmustine 150 mg/m^2 intravenously on day one, cisplatin 25 mg/m^2 intravenously daily on days one to three, dacarbazine 220 mg/m^2 intravenously daily on days one to three, and tamoxifen 160 mg orally daily for seven days. The overall response was 26%, complete responses were 2.5%, with median progression-free survival and the median survival four and nine months respectively. These results show that the combination had limited impact on overall survival when compared with dacarbazine alone, with the additional drawback of high toxicity [116].

In a multicenter phase III trial, 240 patients with measurable stage IV melanoma were randomly selected to receive the Dartmouth regimen (dacarbazine 220 mg/m^2 and cisplatin 25 mg/m^2 on days one to three, carmustine 150 mg/m^2 on day one every other cycle and tamoxifen 10 mg orally bid). The treatment was repeated every three weeks. The results showed median survival time from randomization of seven months; response rate was 18.5% when compared with dacarbazine alone this treatment was not better [115]. In addition to the low activity, the Dartmounth Regimen showed high toxicity, mainly bone marrow suppression, nausea, vomiting and fatigue. Although advanced melanoma is often not curable with systemic therapy, the considered use of currently available regimens can induce clinically significant remissions and, possibly, prolong the life of some patients.

Su et al. (2011) [124] evaluated the combination of carmustine (150 mg/m^2, on day one every eight weeks), cisplatin (25 mg/m^2, days one to three every four weeks), dacarbazine (220 mg/m^2 days one to three every four weeks), tamoxifen (10 mg twice a day) and IL-2 18 Million International Units in divided doses by subcutaneous injection three times a week for four weeks. The treatment was repeated for a total of six cycles or until disease progression or unbearable toxicity. The response rate was 32.5% including 5% with a complete response, 27.5% with a partial response and 17.5% with a stable disease. The median progression-free survival was 6.2 months and median overall survival was 11.3 months. The toxicity associated with IL-2 included indurate injection site, fever, chills, itchy skin, bone pain and myalgia and eosinophilia.

The Dartmouth Regimen was associated with IL-2 and IFN-α. In those patients who received sequential immunotherapy, each cycle of chemotherapy was followed by outpatient s.c. IL-2 (10 x 10^6 IU/m^2, on days three to five, week four; 5 x 10^6 IU/m^2, on days one, three and five, week five) and s.c. IFN-α (5 x 10^6 IU/m^2, on day one, week four; on days one, three and five, week five). The overall response rate of patients treated with the combination of chemotherapy and IL-2/IFN-α was 34.3% with complete responses (10.9%) and partial responses (23.4%). In patients treated with chemotherapy only, the overall response rate was 29.9% with complete responses (13.3%) and partial responses (16.6%). There was no significant difference in median progression-free survival (zero months vs. four months) and in median overall survival (12 months vs. 13 months) for combined chemoimmunotherapy and for chemotherapy, respectively [117].

A prospective randomized phase III clinical trial was performed to assess whether the addition of tamoxifen to the Dartmounth Regimen would ameliorate the responses. The median survival observed was 6.9 months, but the progression-free survival as well as the overall survival was not different from the treatment with Dartmounth Regimen alone [118].

Other chemotherapeutic agents have also been combined with tamoxifen for the treatment of metastatic melanoma. Bajetta et al. (1993) [119] treated two groups of patients sequentially; the first group received carboplatin and cytarabine alone and for the second group, tamoxifen 40 mg was added daily throughout the cycle. Of 21 evaluable patients in the first group, 19% responded. In contrast, 8% of patients responded in the tamoxifen-treated group. All patients had received prior chemotherapy and/or immunotherapy. In an attempt to confirm synergism between tamoxifen and cisplatin and to overcome clinically established cisplatin resistance, McClay et al. (1995) [120] treated 24 metastatic melanoma patients with cisplatin 100 mg/m^2 every three weeks; 13% of patients responded. Those who failed to respond clinically (cisplatin resistant) were then treated with the same dose of cisplatin plus tamoxifen 160 mg on day one, followed by 20 mg daily throughout the three-week cycle. In 19 assessable patients, 16% achieved a complete response or partial response as conventionally defined; however, when the authors included mixed responses, the overall response rate (32%) was statistically significantly. In a phase I study, McClay et al. (1995) [120] treated successive groups of patients with escalating doses of tamoxifen and weekly cisplatin 80 mg/m^2. Patients received up to 320 mg/m^2 at the time of the report and none of the patients responded at doses less than 240 mg/m^2.

Studies have combined chemotherapy, immunomodulators and tamoxifen. Antoine et al. (1995) [121] added tamoxifen to a regimen of cisplatin, IL-2, and IFN-γ. The response rate with tamoxifen (41%) was lower than the response rate observed without tamoxifen (54%). Rixe et al. (1994) [122] treated 91 patients with high-dose cisplatin, IL-2, IFN-α and tamoxifen. The trial was stopped prematurely due to an increased frequency of sepsis and because the response rates were similar to those observed in historical controls that did not receive tamoxifen.

Fierro et al. (1993) [123] treated 32 patients with a combination including carmustine, cisplatin, dacarbazine and tamoxifen, which showed an overall response rate of 47%, complete response of 16%, partial response of 31% and median survival of 10 months. The pretreatment with INF-α did not modify the survival or the response rate.

In a phase II trial with a high dose of tamoxifen and cisplatin administered weekly were used; tamoxifen was started on day one with a dose of 240 mg/day. Cisplatin (80 mg/m^2) was started on day two and repeated weekly for a total of three weeks. During week four, the patient was not treated with cisplatin but was evaluated for response. If disease stabilization or regression was documented, the patient received a second three-week cycle of cisplatin and was then re-evaluated for response. Patients with progressive disease at any evaluation were removed from the study. In 28 consecutive patients, the overall response rate was 32%. Toxicity was primarily nausea and vomiting. While this combination presented activity, the overall response rate was not significantly better that that observed with the original Dartmouth regimen and besides, the toxicity is substantial [128].

The cisplatin, vinblastine and bleomycin were combined in the treatment of 51 patients with metastatic melanoma; among these patients only 22% had complete or partial response. However, the response durations were brief and the toxicity was substantial. The authors concluded that such a combination was not sufficiently beneficial to warrant its use in metastatic melanoma [132] Bajetta et al. (1982) [133] treated 22 patients with metastatic melanoma with vinblastine, bleomycin and cisplatin. In this study, the survival rate was 10 months and the results showed that this combination did not exceed the treatment with dacarbazine. Nathanson et al. (1981) [134] also studied this combination and the patients showed a median duration of response of 26 weeks associated with significant toxicity, marrow suppressive, gastrointestinal, pulmonary and mucocutaneous.

The BOLD scheme (bleomycin, vincristine, lomustine plus dacarbazine) included bleomycin at 7.5 units subcutaneously in the first course and 15 units in subsequent courses on days one and four; vincristine at 1mg/m^2 intravenously on days one and five; lomustine at 80 mg/m^2 on day one and dacarbazine 200 mg/m^2 intravenously on days one through five. These treatments showed 9% complete response, 31% partial response and 17% stabilization of disease and overall median survival of 31 weeks. The authors concluded that the BOLD scheme was an effective alternative treatment for metastatic melanoma, because the overall toxicity was moderate [135]. Several other works that used the BOLD scheme in combination with IFN-α showed better results with response rates from 13 to 24%, which is not significant when compared with the treatment with the BOLD scheme alone, but patients with soft tissue or lung metastases may achieve more complete response [124]. Another study reported the treatment of twenty-two patients with metastatic melanoma with the BOLD scheme every four weeks, together with IFN-α 3 x 10^6 IU daily for six weeks, followed by 6 x 10^6 IU three times per week. This treatment showed median progression-free survival of four months and median overall survival of 12 months, associated with moderate toxicity [137]. A similar scheme was used in a study reported by Atzpodien et al. (2002) [125], in which the median progression-free survival was 1.9 months and overall survival 10.6 months, but the scheme showed more toxicity in 13% of the patients (alopecia and neurotoxicity). The regimen of BOLD plus interferon is active in the treatment of metastatic uveal melanoma. The precise role of the regimen has to be defined in light of its toxicity, particularly the unpredictable pulmonary toxicity. The pattern of occurrence of these pulmonary events is most consistent with either an acquired hypersensitivity reaction, or a cumulative toxic effect from two or more agents. Patients considered for treatment with this regimen must be judiciously selected. Those with no clear contraindications may benefit from a trial of this regimen, but they must be monitored closely.

Another regimen that has shown good results was the combination of bleomycin 15 mg administered subcutaneously on days one and four, vindesine 3 mg/m^2 administered intravenously on days one and five and lomustine 80 mg/m^2 orally on day one and dacarbazine

200 mg/m² intravenously on days one through five in a phase III study. This combined response rate of 45% is considerably better than that seen in single- or dual-agent chemotherapy. The toxicity was tolerable. The median survival for all treated patients was 43 weeks, and the median follow-up time was now 63 weeks [139]. Stables et al. (1992) [140] evaluated the treatment of 72 patients with melanoma with a regime combination including bleomycin, vindesine, lomustine and dacarbazine. This study showed a complete response in 17.6% of the patients, partial response in 14.7% of the patients and overall median survival of 38 weeks. These results are comparable with other combinations of chemotherapy regimens, which have not yet been supplanted by the newer biological therapies.

Based on the independent activity of cisplatin, vinblastine, and dacarbazine (CVD), a combination of these agents was used in the treatment of patients with advanced melanoma. Different doses are used in this treatment scheme, but the most common combination is vinblastine in a dose of 1.6 $mg/m^2/d$ for five days, dacarbazine in a dose of 800 mg/m^2 intravenously on day one, and cisplatin in a dose of 20 $mg/m^2/d$ for four days starting on day two of chemotherapy or, 3-week cycles of cisplatin 20 $mg/m^2/day$ x 4; vinblastine 2 $mg/m^2/day$ x 4, and dacarbazine 800 mg/m^2 on day one [141]. In a phase II trial with 50 evaluable patients, a response rate of 40% was achieved with an estimated 1-year survival of 50% [141]. In a randomized trial using biochemotherapy, in which CVD was the control arm, the same investigators reported that CVD showed an objective response rate of 27% and an estimated 1-year survival of approximately 40% [142]. The median duration of the response was nine months and the median survival time of the responders was 12 months. The treatment was associated with significant toxicity consisting of nausea, vomiting, diarrhoea and partial hair loss. Additionally, neutropenia with a median nadir granulocyte count of 500/microliters was observed, and significant anaemia required blood transfusions in a majority of the patients after three to four courses of chemotherapy. The dose-limiting toxicity was peripheral neuropathy, which required discontinuation of cisplatin after six to eight courses of chemotherapy [141].

Another study used a combination of dacarbazine 250 $mg/m^2/day$ one to three, cisplatin 30 $mg/m^2/day$ i.v. on days one to three and IFN-α 10 x 10^6 $U/m^2/day$ subcutaneously on days one to five, and one group received the combination mentioned, plus IL-2 as a continuous i.v. infusion in a decreasing schedule starting on day 5 with 18 million U/m^2 over 6 hours followed by 18 million U/m^2 over 12 hours, 18 million U/m2 over 24 hours, and a maintenance dose of 4.5 million $U/m^2/24$ hours for an additional 72 hours. Cycles were repeated every four weeks for a maximum of four cycles. This study showed that the combination was not better than the CVD combination, and was associated with low efficacy and higher toxicity. The authors concluded that the combination neither conferred a clinically meaningful survival benefit for most patients with advanced melanoma, nor conferred an increase in rate response or progression time [94].

Another study has shown results related to the treatment of patients with metastatic melanoma with six concurrent biochemotherapy dose levels. The doses were programed as follows: dacarbazine 800 mg/m^2 or 1000 mg/m^2 (Day 1); cisplatin 25 mg/m^2 or 30 mg/m^2 (Days 1-4); vinblastine 1.6 mg/m^2 or 1.8 mg/m^2 (Days 1-5); interleukin-2 9 million units (MU) per m^2 or 12

MU/m^2 as a 24 h continuous infusion (Days 1-4); and interferon-alpha-2b 5 MU/m^2, 10 MU/m^2, or 15 MU/m^2 (Days 1-5) and 5 MU/m^2 (Days 7, 9, and 11) administered subcutaneously. The dose of IFN-α was reduced in some patients because of thrombocytopenia after five days, and other toxic effects observed included encephalopathy, renal and hepatic dysfunction, pancreatitis and ileus. This treatment showed a median time to disease progression of 6.9 months, and median survival duration of 12.2 months [143]. In a study reported by Legha et al. (1996) [90] e treatment with CVD plus IL-2 or IFN-α reached an overall response rate of 60%, although the duration of partial response was short (median eight months), the median survival of patients receiving sequential biochemotherapy was 13 months compared to nine months observed in the CVD treated group. The treatment with biochemotherapy was associated with severe toxicity including intense myelosuppression, infections; IL-2 induced constitutional toxicity and hypotension. The biochemotherapy regimen produced an apparent increase in the median survival compared to that observed with the CVD regimen.

In a randomized study, 176 patients received cisplatin and dacarbazine with or without carmustine every 21 days, or the same regimen followed by low-dose subcutaneous IL-2 for eight days and IFN-α three times a week, both for six cycles. The regimen without IL-2 and IFN-α resulted in a median overall survival of 9.5 months and the regimen with IL-2 and IFN-α of 11.0 months. The regimen with low-dose immunotherapy did not produce a statistically significant advantage in overall survival, time to progression or overall response when compared with the regimen without immunotherapy. However, the results were not different from the treatment with high dose IL-2 [87].

In a phase III study, 326 patients with metastatic melanoma received the treatment consisting of a combination of dacarbazine (250 mg/m^2 intravenously days one to five every four weeks) and vindesine (3 mg/m^2 intravenously day one weekly), with or without the addition of cisplatin (100 mg/m^2 intravenously day one every four weeks). In this study the authors did not observe a significant difference in overall survival with addition of cisplatin, but the median time to progression was significantly longer in patients treated with dacarbazine, vindesine and cisplatin than patients that did not receive cisplatin (4.2 versus 2.2 months respectively). However, the combination of the three drugs did not change overall survival but did significantly increase toxicity such as leukopenia, alopecia and nausea/vomiting [144]. Similar treatment was used in a phase II study with forty patients with disseminated malignant melanoma. In this study, the authors observed a 38% response rate and median response duration of four months, but the toxicity was intolerable with symptoms such as nephrotoxicity, ototoxicity, hypotonia and nausea/vomiting [126].

Fotemustine has also been used in combination with dacarbazine, in patients with metastatic melanoma. The response rate was 27.2%, confirming the activity of fotemustine. The combination of two drugs showed significant toxicity, mainly haematological with leukopenia and thrombocytopenia. This schedule with sequential dacarbazine and fotemustine had low activity against metastatic melanoma, and the response rate for cerebral metastases was not superior to that shown in other studies with single agent fotemustine, however, the treatment was well tolerated and can be prescribed to outpatients [54].

http://dx.doi.org/10.5772/55192

Preclinical studies have shown some clinical activity against melanoma. It consisted of a combination of carboplatin at an area under the curve (AUC) of 7.5 and paclitaxel at 175 mg/m^2 over three hours administered to 17 patients [127]. There was a 20% response rate with three partial responders in the 15 evaluable patients, with a median survival of nine months. Another phase II study showed results with the administration of paclitaxel either as monotherapy or combined with carboplatin. In the first treatment paclitaxel was administered at a dose of 100 mg/m^2 intravenously on day one each week for six weeks; in the second treatment paclitaxel was administered at a dose of 80 mg/m^2 intravenously followed by carboplatin 200 mg/m^2 on day one each week for six weeks. The next cycle was administered after a two-week intermission. This study showed median survival time of 209 days in patients that received only paclitaxel, and 218 days for those treated with paclitaxel/carboplatin, with overall response rates of less than 10% for both treatments [68]. Paclitaxel at a dose of 100 mg/m^2 and carboplatin of 2 AUC was administered on days one, eight and 15 of a 28 day cycle. This treatment showed 26% partial response and 19% stable disease and a median overall survival of 7.8 months [128].

Kottschade et al. (2011) [148] conducted a study in which the patients were treated with paclitaxel 100 mg/m^2 and carboplatin AUC six administered on days one, eight and 15 every 28 days. The median number of treatment cycles was four. This treatment showed 25.6% responses and median overall survival of 11.1 months. In a study conducted by Pflugfelder et al. (2011) [149], patients received intravenous paclitaxel 225 mg/m^2 plus intravenous carboplatin AUC 6 on day one of a 21 day cycle, with a dose reduction after the fourth cycle to carboplatin AUC five and paclitaxel 175 mg/m^2. This study showed median progression-free survival of 10 weeks and median overall survival of 31 weeks. Response, progression-free, and overall survival were equivalent in first and second line patients. Sixty patients out of 61 died after a median follow-up of seven months. This treatment showed, in all studies, severe toxicities including neutropenia, thrombocytopenia, neurosensory problems, fatigue, nausea and vomiting [68,127,129].

The development of targeted therapies has provided new options for the management of patients with advanced melanoma. There has been particular interest in agents that target the mitogen-activated protein kinase pathway, which controls tumor growth and survival, and promotes angiogenesis. Recently, sorafenib, an oral multikinase inhibitor has been tested in combination with carboplatin and paclitaxel. A phase I trial conducted with 38 patients, who received either 100, 200, or 400 mg of sorafenib twice daily on days 2 to 19 of a 21-day cycle with carboplatin at AUC 6 and paclitaxel at 225 mg/m^2 administered on day one [130]. The overall response was 10 out of 24 treated patients with one complete response. Another study, however, showed that the treatment of 270 patients with paclitaxel at 225 mg/m^2 and carboplatin at AUC 6 once every three weeks with or without sorafenib at 400 mg twice daily on days two to 19. There was no difference in progression-free survival, which was the primary endpoint, or in response rate [131]. The control group (no sorafenib) showed a response rate of 11% with a median progression-free survival of 17.4 weeks; the median overall survival was 42 weeks. The cohort receiving sorafenib had essentially identical outcomes. The conclusion was that the addition of sorafenib to carboplatin/paclitaxel did not improve the response rate in contrast to the original observations in the phase I trial [130].

Recently, patients were randomly assigned in a two-to-one ratio to carboplatin (AUC, 5) plus paclitaxel (175 mg/m^2) and bevacizumab (15 mg/kg) administered intravenously once every three weeks. This study showed an overall response rate of 25.5%. The study did not meet the primary objective of statistically significant improvement in median survival with the addition of bevacizumab to carboplatin plus paclitaxel. A larger phase III study will be necessary to determine whether there is any benefit to the addition of bevacizumab to carboplatin plus paclitaxel in this disease setting [132].

Schmittel et al. (2006) [133] compared the combination of gemcitabine plus treosulfan with treosulfan alone in patients with metastatic melanoma; the patients received 1000 mg/m^2 of gemcitabine plus 3500 mg/m^2 of treosulfan or 3500 mg/m^2 of treosulfan on days one and eight, and in both groups the cycle was repeated on day 29. Median progression-free survival was three months and two months for patients undergoing the treatment with gemcitabine plus treosulfan and treosulfan, respectively. In a phase II clinical trial, gemcitabine plus treosulfan were tested in patients with metastatic melanoma. The patients received 1000 mg/m^2 of gemcitabine and treosulfan at a dose of 2500 or 3000 mg/m^2 in group one, and 3500 or 4000 mg/m^2 in group two on days one and eight every four weeks. In the group of patients that were treated with treosulfan in a dose less or equal to 3000 mg/m^{2,} the response rate was not observed. Among the patients treated with a dose equal to or more than 3500 mg/m^{2,} a 5% partial remission was observed, with median survival time of nine months [134]. Another study by Schmittel et al. (2005) [154] combined gemcitabine plus treosulfan and cisplatin, in which the patients received 30 or 40 mg/m^2 of cisplatin, 1000 mg/m^2 of gemcitabine and 3000 mg/m^2 of treosulfan on days one and eight repeated on day 29; the median overall survival was 7.7 months, associated with excessive haematological toxicity.

Dacarbazine 250 mg/m^2/day was combined with epirubicin 90 mg/m^2 on day one every three weeks. Partial response of 21.1% was observed [135].

Another phase III study of ipilimumab was carried out in patients with previously untreated metastatic melanoma. In this case, ipilimumab in combination with dacarbazine was compared with dacarbazine plus placebo, showing improved overall survival with the antibody therapy. Responses with the combined therapies seemed to be higher than the therapies with a single agent (17% compared to 5%) [105]. Data from preclinical and clinical studies have shown that ipilimumab can cause tumor regression in patients with metastatic melanoma with response rates of 5.8-22%. Phase III trials have demonstrated a benefit to median overall survival in the first-line setting in combination with dacarbazine versus dacarbazine alone (11.2 versus 9.1 months), and in the second-line setting in combination with glycoprotein 100 peptide vaccine (gp100) vs. gp100 alone (10.1 versus 6.4 months). The main toxicities of ipilimumab are immune related, most commonly skin and gastrointestinal troubles. Bowel perforation and treatment-related deaths have occurred, although prompt use of steroids and other immunosuppressive agents can minimize these risks [136].

In phase II study patients with metastatic melanoma received ipilimumab at three mg/kg every four weeks for four doses, either alone or with up to six-five-day courses of dacarbazine 250 mg/m^2/day. The response rate was 14.3% with ipilimumab plus dacarbazine and median overall survival was 14.3 months [137].

4. News strategies for treatment of metastatic melanoma

4.1. Signalling molecules targeted therapy

One of the most common signalling pathways affected by mutations in melanoma is the RAF/MEK/ERK pathway, a highly conserved group of proteins that regulate cell growth, division and death. In melanoma, the most common mutations are in proteins like BRAF, NRAS, HRAS, and KIT and lead to constitutive activation of the RAF/MEK/ERK pathway, which stimulates pro-proliferative genes. BRAF, the serine/threonine specific protein kinase, is triggered by somatic mutations in 50–70% of melanoma cases. A substitution of glutamic acid for valine at codon 600 (V600E) is the most common BRAF mutation known [138]. Recently, genotype-selected metastatic melanoma patients with positive BRAF mutation have been submitted to clinical trials with drabafenib (accelerated dose titration with 12 mg initial dose), an inhibitor of BRAF kinase, selective for mutations in BRAF. High response rates were achieved in patients with melanoma brain metastases leading to nine out of ten patients with a size reduction of brain lesions [139]. A phase III trial comparing drabafenib (150 mg twice daily, orally) with dacarbazine (1000 mg/m^2 intravenously every 3 weeks), higher median progression-free survival was observed in the drabafenib group than those for dacarbazine. However, dose reduction of drabafenib was needed in 28% of patients due to adverse effects including nausea, vomiting, fatigue and neutropenia. Dose reduction was also necessary in patients receiving dacarbazine (17%) [131].

Despite these front line studies that validated BRAF inhibition and genotyping analysis of BRAF mutational status as a feasible tool in patients undergoing clinical trials with signalling molecules targeted therapy, side effects remain the most important concern during therapy. In this field, another BRAF inhibitor, vemurafenib, was compared to dacarbazine, and studies demonstrated that vemurafenib-treated patients had higher overall survival rate and final analysis for progression-free survival than those who received dacarbazine. Also, the vemurafenib-treated group had relative reduction of 63% in the risk of death and of 74% in the risk of either death or disease progression, as compared to dacarbazine. Regarding adverse effects, 18% of patients treated with vemurafenib presented cutaneous squamous-cell carcinoma, keratoacanthoma, or both [10].

However, after genetic status assessment, Falchook et al. (2012) [140] demonstrated that trametinib, a reversible selective allosteric inhibitor of MEK1 and MEK2, had a good clinical activity in patients with melanoma, suggesting that MEK could be a valid therapeutic target in BRAF-mutant melanoma. Interestingly, patients were free of proliferative skin lesions such as squamous-cell carcinoma, a common adverse effect associated with BRAF inhibitors, representing an advantage of trametinib in treating early-stage diseases [140].

With regard to drug resistance, antiapoptotic proteins of the Bcl-2 family are closely involved in this process. This group of proteins regulates apoptosis by blocking the release of cytochrome *c* and the overexpression of Bcl-2, which has been partially associated with drug resistance phenomena (Soengas et al., 2003). In this field, antisense Bcl-2 therapy may be an alternative coadjutant therapy in melanoma clinical trials. In the past, in vitro experimental transfection of Bcl-2 was performed in both haematological and solid tumor cells, leading to multidrug resistant phenotype [141] and recently, oblimersen sodium was combined with dacarbazine in a clinical trial involving 771 patients with advanced melanoma [13]. This new drug decreased the expression of Bcl-2 protein by increasing the cleavage of Bcl-2 mRNA by RNase H [142,143].

Another mechanism of tumor resistance is related to the repair process of damaged DNA. The poly (ADP-ribose) polymerase-1 (PARP) is the nuclear key enzyme of this process and mediates the recruitment and activation of repair factors in the DNA break leading to base excision repair [144]. The first phase I clinical trial with inhibitor of PARP was conducted with AG014699, a prodrug of AG014447, a potent inhibitor of PARP, combined with temozolomide in patients with solid tumors and metastatic melanoma. In this clinical trial, AG014699 was well tolerated and proved to be highly and selectively toxic to cells that underwent DNA repair [145].

Finally, one of the most studied signalling molecules is NF-κB, a pathway that melanoma cells use to increase survival, proliferation and resistance to apoptosis, leading to progression of tumor and metastasis appearance [146,147]. One of the first NF-κB inhibitors used in clinical trials was bortezomib. Combined with temozolomide, a phase I clinical trial was conducted in order to establish a schedule use of these drugs, define phase II doses and assess the NF-κB activity in blood. Results demonstrated that bortezomib failed to inhibit NF-κB, and toxicities including neurotoxicity, fatigue, diarrhoea and rash were reported [18]. Furthermore, two years later another phase I trial with patients with advanced solid tumors was conducted in order to establish new maximum tolerated doses for the combination of bortezomib and temozolomide with inconclusive results [148]. In addition, both groups of authors suggested that new studies with strong preclinical rationale have to be conducted in order to cover all the changes undergone at tumor sites [18,148].

4.2. Electrochemotherapy

After years of experience in delivering genes, DNA and drugs into mammalian cells using electroporation [149,150], a local tumor ablation modality, the electrochemotherapy (ECT) has been used effectively in the treatment of various solid tumors, particularly melanoma. ECT combines chemotherapy and electroporation to increase drug uptake into cancer cells [151]. The European Standard Operating Procedures of Electrochemotherapy (ESOPE) was the largest study reported so far in patients with melanoma [152]. In this huge clinical trial, the efficacy and safety of ECT were evaluated according to the drug used, route of administration and types of electrodes for electroporation. The ESOPE project consisted of the administration of bleomycin (ineffective for systemic conventional therapy), both intravenously (15000 IU/m^2) and intratumorally (1000 IU/cm^3), followed by eletroportation. Cisplatin was also administered in some patients (only intratumorally), because previous reports had not substantiated the high efficacy of electrochemotherapy using intravenous injection of cisplatin [153]. Almost 74% of patients had complete response rate achieved on the electrochemotherapy treated tumor nodules. Furthermore, side effects were minor and acceptable by patients and showed great advantages regarding cost and effectiveness.

Recently, another approach using ECT, based on the ESOPE study, has been conducted in patients with cutaneous and subcutaneous melanoma metastases. Bleomycin was also used as a drug of choice for most cases, and ECT was conducted after intravenous administration of bleomycin (15 mg/m^2). Results demonstrated that 62% of patients had an objective response rate for all treated metastases. The authors also observed that 23% of patients had complete response of metastatic nodules and only 8% of patients showed disease progression. Because ECT was achieved using low doses of bleomycin, no systemic side effects were observed [154].

Regarding disseminated superficial metastasis, Campana et al. (2012) [175] demonstrated that several ECT cycles on metastases, unsuitable for resection or unresponsive to conventional chemotherapy, were effective only in patients with few and small metastases on the lower limb. Besides the restricted response, ECT was well tolerated and side effects were limited.

4.3. Transarterial chemoembolization

In an attempt to manage metastatic melanoma, especially liver metastases, new approaches have been tested using the dual blood vessels supply of the liver in combination with anti-cancer drugs such as irinotecan and cisplatin. This new approach, the so-called transarterial chemoembolization (TACE), takes therapeutic advantage of the hepatic artery and branches of the portal vein. By infusing chemotherapeutic agents directly into vessels followed by infusion of embolic microspheres, localized therapy and the concentration of the drug in tumor are achieved. In this field, Venturini et al. (2012) [155] enrolled five chemotherapy-naive patients with liver metastasis of uveal melanoma in an irinotecan-eluting chemoembolization trial. TACE was successfully achieved and well-tolerated in all five patients. In addition, a response rate of 80% was achieved in relation to lesion size and remission. Apart from local pain and one isolated case of cholecystitis, no further side effects were observed.

In a more complex study design including cisplatin, carboplatin, fotemustine or melphalan infusion followed by polyvinyl alcohol particles for embolization, 11 patients were monitored for five to 58 months, and 57% of them presented partial response compared to 29% with stable disease, and 14% presented new lesions detected during the follow up period. Median survival of all patients was 11.5 months after metastasis diagnosis [156]. In addition, abdominal and local pain seems to be the most common effect after TACE procedures. Huppert et al. (2010) [177] reported that pain began 1-4h after embolization and lasted around one to three days, and that morphine was necessary in some cases.

Transarterial chemoembolization has the advantages of reducing systemic toxicity of drugs and increasing intratumor effects leading to better results. However, Schusser et al. (2010) [178] also reported serious side effects after TACE protocol using fotemustin (100 mg/m^2) as a first choice, followed by cisplatin (50 mg), including splenic infarction, thrombocytopenia and gastric ulcer; all events required conservative treatment and prolonged hospitalization.

4.4. Adoptive T cells therapy

Immunotherapy has been widely reported as a promising alternative for a variety of malignancies including melanoma [157]. To divert the majority of the immune cells to react against tumor has been a huge challenge among physicians. Particularly, adoptive T cells (ATC) optimally expanded ex-vivo, in theory, could enhance anti-tumor immune response and form memory protection against recurrence. A well-established expansion of tumor-infiltrating lymphocytes (TIL) has been carefully used in clinical trials, especially in metastatic melanoma patients [79,158-160]. Recently, 93 patients with metastatic melanoma were treated with the ATC transfer of autologous TIL and IL-2 with a median follow-up of 62 months. 22% of patients showed complete regression and durable complete responses were seen in patients who had a median of three different organ sites of metastases including lung, liver, adrenal, muscle, lymphonodes, and skin [161]. However, some limitation was observed in ATC therapy. Joseph et al. (2011) [184] reported a negative influence in initial TIL outgrowth in samples obtained from patients who received systemic therapy 30 days before tumor harvest. This data suggested that parameters like prior systemic chemotherapy should be considered as important criteria for patients undergoing ATC therapy. The success of autologous TIL derived from metastatic tumor tissue is dependent on the TIL initial outgrowth and the tumor characteristics, rate of TIL and parallel systemic chemotherapy, because the latter determines the rate of TIL harvested [162].

In an attempt to make up for some limitations of ATC therapy, especially those related to TIL harvested outgrowth and based on the observation that melanoma-reactive TIL could be generated from only 50% of harvested samples [163], autologous T cells transduction with T-cell receptors (TCR) against the antigen NY-ESO-1 was carried out. A retroviral vector encoding a TCR, which recognizes the peptide NY-ESO-1, an antigen highly expressed in almost 50% of melanoma metastases, was transfected into T-cells of patients, cultured ex-vivo and transferred to patients together with HD IL-2, as a complementary therapy. Results from this vanguard clinical trial showed that five of the 11 patients with metastatic melanoma experienced an objective response including two complete responses during the follow-up period (20 months), and 2 patients demonstrated complete regressions that persisted after one year.

5. Insights in side effects prevention

It is clear that the cure for malignant melanoma is still a challenge. One can conceive of many strategies to combat the disease: i) prevention ii) several kinds of therapies, iii) amelioration of side effects caused by the therapies. In this regard, there is evidence that natural or semi-synthetic compounds can feasibly allow for a wide variety of potential drugs to be employed in a multitarget approach alone and/or in combined therapies.

Syed and Muktar (2011) [164] summarized some options in a review article about several plant products for the prevention and treatment of different kinds of cancer, including melanoma. Among the compounds they mentioned: genistein, epigallocatechin gallate, resveratrol, curcumin, fisetin, silymarin lupeol, which are able to stop the growth of tumor cells through their own multitarget drug properties [164]. In the same context, several research groups, including ours, have studied gallic acid and its ester derivatives [165-168]. It has been shown that gallic acid and gallates differing only in the number of carbon atoms in the lateral chain present antitumor properties, whose mechanism of action is also by a multitarget way, including cell growth and metastasis inhibition, action against the drug efflux, helping to avoid the development of resistance as well as a selective cytotoxicity

6. Conclusion

Significant advancements have been made in the last few years about melanoma treatment, including important information on the molecular mechanism of action of the drugs and the signalling pathways related to the disease. However, the treatment of patients with advanced melanoma remains unsatisfactory. Single agent or combinations of chemotherapies including new agents or biologic response modifiers have not resulted in response rates of durable remissions high enough to affect median survival. The approval by the FDA of ipilimumab in 2011 brought some optimism among the clinicians who treat patients with metastatic melanoma, but this therapy also has its limitations.

Promising sources of alternative molecules for cancer seem to be plants. In general, natural or semi-synthetic compounds have shown effectiveness not only in the prevention of the disease and the development of resistance, but also in important antitumoral activities in vitro and in pre-clinical assays.

Author details

Claudriana Locatelli[1], Fabíola Branco Filippin-Monteiro[2] and Tânia Beatriz Creczynski-Pasa[2]

1 Biology and Health Sciences, Universidade do Oeste de Santa Catarina,UNOESC, Videira, Brazil

2 Pharmaceutical Sciences Departament, Universidade Federal de Santa Catarina, UFSC, Florianópolis, Brazil

References

[1] de Vries E, Bray FI, Coebergh JW, Parkin DM. Changing epidemiology of malignant cutaneous melanoma in Europe 1953-1997: rising trends in incidence and mortality

but recent stabilizations in western Europe and decreases in Scandinavia. Int J Cancer 2003;107:119-126.

[2] Whiteman DC, Whiteman CA, Green AC. Childhood sun exposure as a risk factor for melanoma: a systematic review of epidemiologic studies. Cancer Causes Control 2001;12:69-82.

[3] Bressac-de-Paillerets B, Avril MF, Chompret A, Demenais F. Genetic and environmental factors in cutaneous malignant melanoma. Biochimie 2002;84:67-74.

[4] Balch CM, Buzaid AC, Soong SJ, Atkins MB, Cascinelli N, Coit DG, et al. Final version of the American Joint Committee on Cancer staging system for cutaneous melanoma. Journal of Clinical Oncology 2001;19.

[5] Monzon JG, Dancey J. Targeted agents for the treatment of metastatic melanoma. Oncotargets and Therapy 2012;5.

[6] Jemal A, Siegel R, Ward E, Hao Y, Xu J, Murray T, et al. Cancer statistics, 2008. CA Cancer J Clin 2008;58:71-96.

[7] Mouawad R, Sebert M, Michels J, Bloch J, Spano JP, Khayat D. Treatment for metastatic malignant melanoma: old drugs and new strategies. Crit Rev Oncol Hematol 2010;74:27-39.

[8] Bhatia S, Tykodi SS, Thompson JA. Treatment of metastatic melanoma: an overview. Oncology (Williston Park) 2009;23:488-496.

[9] Nashan D, Müller ML, Grabbe S, Wustlich S, Enk A. Systemic therapy of disseminated malignant melanoma: an evidence-based overview of the state-of-the-art in daily routine. J Eur Acad Dermatol Venereol 2007;21:1305-1318.

[10] Chapman PB, Hauschild A, Robert C, Haanen JB, Ascierto P, Larkin J, et al. Improved survival with vemurafenib in melanoma with BRAF V600E mutation. N Engl J Med 2011;364:2507-2516.

[11] Strumberg D, Clark JW, Awada A, Moore MJ, Richly H, Hendlisz A, et al. Safety, pharmacokinetics, and preliminary antitumor activity of sorafenib: a review of four phase I trials in patients with advanced refractory solid tumors. Oncologist 2007;12:426-437.

[12] Bartlett JB, Michael A, Clarke IA, Dredge K, Nicholson S, Kristeleit H, et al. Phase I study to determine the safety, tolerability and immunostimulatory activity of thalidomide analogue CC-5013 in patients with metastatic malignant melanoma and other advanced cancers. Br J Cancer 2004;90:955-961.

[13] Bedikian AY, Millward M, Pehamberger H, Conry R, Gore M, Trefzer U, et al. Bcl-2 antisense (oblimersen sodium) plus dacarbazine in patients with advanced melanoma: the Oblimersen Melanoma Study Group. J Clin Oncol 2006;24:4738-4745.

[14] Tarhini AA, Kirkwood JM. Oblimersen in the treatment of metastatic melanoma. Future Oncol 2007;3:263-271.

[15] Atkins M, Lee S, Flaherty L, Sosman J, Sondak V, Kirkwood J. A prospective randomized phase III trial of concurrent biochemotherapy (BCT) with cisplatin, vinblastine, dacarbazine (CVD), IL-2 and interferon alpha-2b (IFN) versus CVD alone in patients with metastatic melanoma (E3695): An ECOG-coordinated intergroup trial. Proc Am Soc Clin Oncol, 2003.

[16] Burke JR, Pattoli MA, Gregor KR, Brassil PJ, MacMaster JF, McIntyre KW, et al. BMS-345541 is a highly selective inhibitor of I kappa B kinase that binds at an allosteric site of the enzyme and blocks NF-kappa B-dependent transcription in mice. Journal of Biological Chemistry 2003;278.

[17] Liu J, Suresh Kumar KG, Yu D, Molton SA, McMahon M, Herlyn M, et al. Oncogenic BRAF regulates beta-Trcp expression and NF-kappaB activity in human melanoma cells. Oncogene 2007;26:1954-1958.

[18] Su Y, Amiri KI, Horton LW, Yu Y, Ayers GD, Koehler E, et al. A phase I trial of bortezomib with temozolomide in patients with advanced melanoma: toxicities, antitumor effects, and modulation of therapeutic targets. Clin Cancer Res 2010;16:348-357.

[19] Pisano M, Pagnan G, Dettori MA, Cossu S, Caffa I, Sassu I, et al. Enhanced anti-tumor activity of a new curcumin-related compound against melanoma and neuroblastoma cells. Mol Cancer 2010;9:137.

[20] Yang AS, Chapman PB. The history and future of chemotherapy for melanoma. Hematol Oncol Clin North Am 2009;23:583-597, x.

[21] Garbe C, Radny P, Linse R, Dummer R, Gutzmer R, Ulrich J, et al. Adjuvant low-dose interferon {alpha}2a with or without dacarbazine compared with surgery alone: a prospective-randomized phase III DeCOG trial in melanoma patients with regional lymph node metastasis. Ann Oncol 2008;19:1195-1201.

[22] Meer L, Janzer RC, Kleihues P, Kolar GF. In vivo metabolism and reaction with DNA of the cytostatic agent, 5-(3,3-dimethyl-1-triazeno)imidazole-4-carboxamide (DTIC). Biochem Pharmacol 1986;35:3243-3247.

[23] Luce JK, Thurman WG, Isaacs BL, Talley RW. Clinical trials with the antitumor agent 5-(3,3-dimethyl-1-triazeno)imidazole-4-carboxamide(NSC-45388). Cancer Chemother Rep 1970;54:119-124.

[24] Costanza ME, Nathanson L, Lenhard R, Wolter J, Colsky J, Oberfield RA, et al. Therapy of malignant melanoma with an imidazole carboxamide and bis-chloroethyl nitrosourea. Cancer 1972;30:1457-1461.

[25] Nathanson L, Wolter J, Horton J, Colsky J, Shnider BI, Schilling A. Characteristics of prognosis and response to an imidazole carboxamide in malignant melanoma. Clin Pharmacol Ther 1971;12:955-962.

[26] Middleton MR, Grob JJ, Aaronson N, Fierlbeck G, Tilgen W, Seiter S, et al. Randomized phase III study of temozolomide versus dacarbazine in the treatment of patients with advanced metastatic malignant melanoma. J Clin Oncol 2000;18:158-166.

[27] Howe HL, Wingo PA, Thun MJ, Ries LA, Rosenberg HM, Feigal EG, et al. Annual report to the nation on the status of cancer (1973 through 1998), featuring cancers with recent increasing trends. J Natl Cancer Inst 2001;93:824-842.

[28] Eggermont AM, Kirkwood JM. Re-evaluating the role of dacarbazine in metastatic melanoma: what have we learned in 30 years? Eur J Cancer 2004;40:1825-1836.

[29] Propper DJ, Braybrooke JP, Levitt NC, O'Byrne K, Christodoulos K, Han C, et al. Phase II study of second-line therapy with DTIC, BCNU, cisplatin and tamoxifen (Dartmouth regimen) chemotherapy in patients with malignant melanoma previously treated with dacarbazine. Br J Cancer 2000;82:1759-1763.

[30] Newlands ES, Blackledge GR, Slack JA, Rustin GJ, Smith DB, Stuart NS, et al. Phase I trial of temozolomide (CCRG 81045: M&B 39831: NSC 362856). Br J Cancer 1992;65:287-291.

[31] Agarwala SS, Kirkwood JM. Temozolomide, a novel alkylating agent with activity in the central nervous system, may improve the treatment of advanced metastatic melanoma. Oncologist 2000;5:144-151.

[32] Friedman HS, Kerby T, Calvert H. Temozolomide and treatment of malignant glioma. Clin Cancer Res 2000;6:2585-2597.

[33] Bleehen NM, Newlands ES, Lee SM, Thatcher N, Selby P, Calvert AH, et al. Cancer Research Campaign phase II trial of temozolomide in metastatic melanoma. J Clin Oncol 1995;13:910-913.

[34] Robertson GP. Functional and therapeutic significance of Akt deregulation in malignant melanoma. Cancer Metastasis Rev 2005;24:273-285.

[35] VanBrocklin MW, Verhaegen M, Soengas MS, Holmen SL. Mitogen-activated protein kinase inhibition induces translocation of Bmf to promote apoptosis in melanoma. Cancer Res 2009;69:1985-1994.

[36] Biswas G, Bhagwat R, Khurana R, Menon H, Prasad N, Parikh PM. Brain metastasis--evidence based management. J Cancer Res Ther 2006;2:5-13.

[37] Chang JE, Robins HI, Mehta MP. Therapeutic advances in the treatment of brain metastases. Clin Adv Hematol Oncol 2007;5:54-64.

[38] Platta CS, Khuntia D, Mehta MP, Suh JH. Current treatment strategies for brain metastasis and complications from therapeutic techniques: a review of current literature. Am J Clin Oncol 2010;33:398-407.

[39] Mehta MP, Paleologos NA, Mikkelsen T, Robinson PD, Ammirati M, Andrews DW, et al. The role of chemotherapy in the management of newly diagnosed brain meta-

stases: a systematic review and evidence-based clinical practice guideline. J Neurooncol 2010;96:71-83.

[40] Margolin K, Atkins MB, Thompson JA, Ernstoff MS, Weber J, Flaherty L, et al. Temozolomide and whole brain irradiation in melanoma metastatic to the brain: a phase II trial of the Cytokine Working Group. Journal of Cancer Research and Clinical Oncology 2002;128.

[41] Atkins MB, Gollob JA, Sosman JA, McDermott DF, Tutin L, Sorokin P, et al. A phase II pilot trial of concurrent biochemotherapy with cisplatin, vinblastine, temozolomide, interleukin 2, and IFN-alpha 2B in patients with metastatic melanoma. Clinical Cancer Research 2002;8.

[42] Paul MJ, Summers Y, Calvert AH, Rustin G, Brampton MH, Thatcher N, et al. Effect of temozolomide on central nervous system relapse in patients with advanced melanoma. Melanoma Res 2002;12:175-178.

[43] Rietschel P, Wolchok JD, Krown S, Gerst S, Jungbluth AA, Busam K, et al. Phase II study of extended-dose temozolomide in patients with melanoma. J Clin Oncol 2008;26:2299-2304.

[44] D'Atri S, Tentori L, Lacal PM, Graziani G, Pagani E, Benincasa E, et al. Involvement of the mismatch repair system in temozolomide-induced apoptosis. Mol Pharmacol 1998;54:334-341.

[45] Tang L, Tron VA, Reed JC, Mah KJ, Krajewska M, Li G, et al. Expression of apoptosis regulators in cutaneous malignant melanoma. Clin Cancer Res 1998;4:1865-1871.

[46] Soengas MS, Capodieci P, Polsky D, Mora J, Esteller M, Opitz-Araya X, et al. Inactivation of the apoptosis effector Apaf-1 in malignant melanoma. Nature 2001;409:207-211.

[47] Panka DJ, Atkins MB, Mier JW. Targeting the mitogen-activated protein kinase pathway in the treatment of malignant melanoma. Clinical Cancer Research 2006;12.

[48] Wang CY, Cusack JC, Liu R, Baldwin AS. Control of inducible chemoresistance: enhanced anti-tumor therapy through increased apoptosis by inhibition of NF-kappaB. Nat Med 1999;5:412-417.

[49] Lev DC, Ruiz M, Mills L, McGary EC, Price JE, Bar-Eli M. Dacarbazine causes transcriptional up-regulation of interleukin 8 and vascular endothelial growth factor in melanoma cells: a possible escape mechanism from chemotherapy. Mol Cancer Ther 2003;2:753-763.

[50] Ranson M, Hersey P, Thompson D, Beith J, McArthur GA, Haydon A, et al. Randomized trial of the combination of lomeguatrib and temozolomide compared with temozolomide alone in chemotherapy naive patients with metastatic cutaneous melanoma. J Clin Oncol 2007;25:2540-2545.

[51] Quéreux G, Dréno B. Fotemustine for the treatment of melanoma. Expert Opin Pharmacother 2011;12:2891-2904.

[52] Avril MF, Aamdal S, Grob JJ, Hauschild A, Mohr P, Bonerandi JJ, et al. Fotemustine compared with dacarbazine in patients with disseminated malignant melanoma: a phase III study. J Clin Oncol 2004;22:1118-1125.

[53] Jacquillat C, Khayat D, Banzet P, Weil M, Fumoleau P, Avril MF, et al. FINAL Report of The French Multicenter Phase-II study of the nitrosourea fotemustine in 153 evaluable patients with disseminated malignant-melanoma including patients with cerebral metastases. Cancer 1990;66.

[54] Khayat D, Avril MF, Gerard B, Bertrand P, Bizzari JP, Cour V. Fotemustine - an overview of its clinical activity in disseminated malignant-melanoma. Melanoma Research 1992;2.

[55] Falkson CI, Falkson G, Falkson HC. Phase II trial of fotemustine in patients with metastatic malignant melanoma. Invest New Drugs 1994;12:251-254.

[56] Petit T, Janser JC, Petit JC. Complete remission seven years after treatment for metastatic malignant melanoma. Cancer 1996;78:571.

[57] Chang J, Atkinson H, A'Hern R, Lorentzos A, Gore ME. A phase II study of the sequential administration of dacarbazine and fotemustine in the treatment of cerebral metastases from malignant melanoma. Eur J Cancer 1994;30A:2093-2095.

[58] Turrisi G, Sozzi P, Marinozzi C, Clerico MA. Persistent thrombocytopenia during melanoma treatment with fotemustine. Melanoma Res 2006;16:543-544.

[59] Feun LG, Lee YY, Plager C, Papadopoulos N, Savaraj N, Charnsangavej C, et al. Intracarotid cisplatin-based chemotherapy in patients with malignant melanoma and central nervous system (CNS) metastases. Am J Clin Oncol 1990;13:448-451.

[60] Evans LM, Casper ES, Rosenbluth R. Phase II trial of carboplatin in advanced malignant melanoma. Cancer Treat Rep 1987;71:171-172.

[61] Mohammed MQ, Retsas S. Oxaliplatin is active in vitro against human melanoma cell lines: comparison with cisplatin and carboplatin. Anticancer Drugs 2000;11:859-863.

[62] Soulié P, Raymond E, Brienza S, Cvitkovic E. [Oxaliplatin: the first DACH platinum in clinical practice]. Bull Cancer 1997;84:665-673.

[63] Lutzky J, Nunez Y, Graham P. A phase II trial of oxaliplatin in patients with advanced melanoma. ASCO Annual Meeting Proceedings, 2006.

[64] Whitehead RP, Moon J, McCachren SS, Hersh EM, Samlowski WE, Beck JT, et al. A phase II trial of vinorelbine tartrate in patients with disseminated malignant melanoma and one prior systemic therapy - A Southwest Oncology Group Study. Cancer 2004;100.

[65] Jimeno A, Hitt R, Quintela-Fandino M, Cortes-Funes H. Phase II trial of vinorelbine tartrate in patients with treatment-naive metastatic melanoma. Anti-Cancer Drugs 2005;16.

[66] Dancey J, Steward WP. The role of vindesine in oncology--recommendations after 10 years' experience. Anticancer Drugs 1995;6:625-636.

[67] Emmert S, Zutt M, Haenssle H, Neumann C, Kretschmer L. Inefficacy of vindesine monotherapy in advanced stage IV malignant melanoma patients previously treated with other chemotherapeutic agents. Melanoma Res 2003;13:299-302.

[68] Retsas S, Newton KA, Westbury G. Vindesine as a single agent in the treatment of advanced malignant melanoma. Cancer Chemother Pharmacol 1979;2:257-260.

[69] Einzig AI, Schuchter LM, Recio A, Coatsworth S, Rodriquez R, Wiernik PH. Phase II trial of docetaxel (Taxotere) in patients with metastatic melanoma previously untreated with cytotoxic chemotherapy. Med Oncol 1996;13:111-117.

[70] Wiernik PH, Einzig AI. Taxol in malignant melanoma. J Natl Cancer Inst Monogr 1993:185-187.

[71] Gogas H, Bafaloukos D, Bedikian AY. The role of taxanes in the treatment of metastatic melanoma. Melanoma Res 2004;14:415-420.

[72] Zimpfer-Rechner C, Hofmann U, Figl R, Becker JC, Trefzer U, Keller I, et al. Randomized phase II study of weekly paclitaxel versus paclitaxel and carboplatin as second-line therapy in disseminated melanoma: a multicentre trial of the Dermatologic Co-operative Oncology Group (DeCOG). Melanoma Res 2003;13:531-536.

[73] Wiernik PH, Schwartz EL, Einzig A, Strauman JJ, Lipton RB, Dutcher JP. Phase I trial of taxol given as a 24-hour infusion every 21 days: responses observed in metastatic melanoma. J Clin Oncol 1987;5:1232-1239.

[74] Legha SS, Ring S, Papadopoulos N, Raber M, Benjamin RS. A PHASE-II TRIAL OF TAXOL IN METASTATIC MELANOMA. Cancer 1990;65.

[75] Einzig AI, Hochster H, Wiernik PH, Trump DL, Dutcher JP, Garowski E, et al. A phase II study of taxol in patients with malignant melanoma. Invest New Drugs 1991;9:59-64.

[76] Walker L, Schalch H, King DM, Dietrich L, Eastman M, Kwak M, et al. Phase II trial of weekly paclitaxel in patients with advanced melanoma. Melanoma Res 2005;15:453-459.

[77] Bedikian AY, Plager C, Papadopoulos N, Eton O, Ellerhorst J, Smith T. Phase II evaluation of paclitaxel by short intravenous infusion in metastatic melanoma. Melanoma Research 2004;14.

[78] Aamdal S, Wolff I, Kaplan S, Paridaens R, Kerger J, Schachter J, et al. Docetaxel (taxotere) in advanced malignant-melanoma - a phase-ii study of the eortc early clinical-trials group. European Journal of Cancer 1994;30A.

[79] Rusthoven JJ. The evidence for tamoxifen and chemotherapy as treatment for metastatic melanoma. European Journal of Cancer 1998;34.

[80] Lens MB, Reiman T, Husain AF. Use of tamoxifen in the treatment of malignant melanoma. Cancer 2003;98:1355-1361.

[81] Karakousis CP, Lopez RE, Bhakoo HS, Rosen F, Moore R, Carlson M. Estrogen and progesterone receptors and tamoxifen in malignant melanoma. Cancer Treat Rep 1980;64:819-827.

[82] Creagan ET, Ahmann DL, Schutt AJ, Green SJ. Phase II study of mitolactol and semustine combination chemotherapy for advanced malignant melanoma. Cancer Treat Rep 1982;66:1425-1426.

[83] McCarty KS, Wortman J, Stowers S, Lubahn DB, Seigler HF. Sex steroid receptor analysis in human melanoma. Cancer 1980;46:1463-1470.

[84] Rosenberg SA, Dudley ME. Cancer regression in patients with metastatic melanoma after the transfer of autologous antitumor lymphocytes. Proc Natl Acad Sci U S A 2004;101 Suppl 2:14639-14645.

[85] Traynor K. Ipilimumab approved for metastatic melanoma. Am J Health Syst Pharm 2011;68:768.

[86] Verschraegen C. The monoclonal antibody to cytotoxic T lymphocyte antigen 4, ipilimumab, in the treatment of melanoma. Cancer Manag Res 2012;4:1-8.

[87] Ridolfi R, Chiarion-Sileni V, Guida M, Romanini A, Labianca R, Freschi A, et al. Cisplatin, dacarbazine with or without subcutaneous interleukin-2, and interferon alpha-2b in advanced melanoma outpatients: results from an Italian multicenter phase III randomized clinical trial. J Clin Oncol 2002;20:1600-1607.

[88] Bajetta E, Del Vecchio M, Nova P, Fusi A, Daponte A, Sertoli MR, et al. Multicenter phase III randomized trial of polychemotherapy (CVD regimen) versus the same chemotherapy (CT) plus subcutaneous interleukin-2 and interferon-alpha2b in metastatic melanoma. Ann Oncol 2006;17:571-577.

[89] Agarwala SS, Kirkwood JM. Temozolomide in combination with interferon alpha-2b in patients with metastatic melanoma: a phase I dose-escalation study. Cancer 2003;97:121-127.

[90] Legha SS, Ring S, Bedikian A, Plager C, Eton O, Buzaid AC, et al. Treatment of metastatic melanoma with combined chemotherapy containing cisplatin, vinblastine and dacarbazine (CVD) and biotherapy using interleukin-2 and interferon-alpha. Annals of Oncology 1996;7.

[91] Cascinelli N, Belli F, MacKie RM, Santinami M, Bufalino R, Morabito A. Effect of long-term adjuvant therapy with interferon alpha-2a in patients with regional node metastases from cutaneous melanoma: a randomised trial. Lancet 2001;358:866-869.

[92] Cameron DA, Cornbleet MC, Mackie RM, Hunter JA, Gore M, Hancock B, et al. Adjuvant interferon alpha 2b in high risk melanoma - the Scottish study. Br J Cancer 2001;84:1146-1149.

[93] Hancock BW, Wheatley K, Harris S, Ives N, Harrison G, Horsman JM, et al. Adjuvant interferon in high-risk melanoma: the AIM HIGH Study--United Kingdom Coordinating Committee on Cancer Research randomized study of adjuvant low-dose extended-duration interferon Alfa-2a in high-risk resected malignant melanoma. J Clin Oncol 2004;22:53-61.

[94] Wheatley K, Ives N, Hancock B, Gore M, Eggermont A, Suciu S. Does adjuvant interferon-alpha for high-risk melanoma provide a worthwhile benefit? A meta-analysis of the randomised trials. Cancer Treat Rev 2003;29:241-252.

[95] Håkansson A, Gustafsson B, Krysander L, Håkansson L. Effect of IFN-alpha on tumor-infiltrating mononuclear cells and regressive changes in metastatic malignant melanoma. J Interferon Cytokine Res 1998;18:33-39.

[96] Yurkovetsky ZR, Kirkwood JM, Edington HD, Marrangoni AM, Velikokhatnaya L, Winans MT, et al. Multiplex analysis of serum cytokines in melanoma patients treated with interferon-alpha2b. Clin Cancer Res 2007;13:2422-2428.

[97] Garbe C, Eigentler TK, Keilholz U, Hauschild A, Kirkwood JM. Systematic Review of Medical Treatment in Melanoma: Current Status and Future Prospects. Oncologist 2011;16.

[98] Atkins MB, Robertson MJ, Gordon M, Lotze MT, DeCoste M, DuBois JS, et al. Phase I evaluation of intravenous recombinant human interleukin 12 in patients with advanced malignancies. Clin Cancer Res 1997;3:409-417.

[99] Atkins MB, Lotze MT, Dutcher JP, Fisher RI, Weiss G, Margolin K, et al. High-dose recombinant interleukin 2 therapy for patients with metastatic melanoma: analysis of 270 patients treated between 1985 and 1993. J Clin Oncol 1999;17:2105-2116.

[100] Dillman RO, Wiemann MC, VanderMolen LA, Bury MJ, DePriest C, Church C. Hybrid high-dose bolus/continuous infusion interleukin-2 in patients with metastatic melanoma: a phase II trial of the Cancer Biotherapy Research Group (formerly the National Biotherapy Study Group). Cancer Biother Radiopharm 1997;12:249-255.

[101] Keilholz U, Punt CJ, Gore M, Kruit W, Patel P, Lienard D, et al. Dacarbazine, cisplatin, and interferon-alfa-2b with or without interleukin-2 in metastatic melanoma: a randomized phase III trial (18951) of the European Organisation for Research and Treatment of Cancer Melanoma Group. J Clin Oncol 2005;23:6747-6755.

[102] Atkins MB. Cytokine-based therapy and biochemotherapy for advanced melanoma. Clinical Cancer Research 2006;12.

[103] Balmer CM. Clinical use of biologic response modifiers in cancer treatment: an overview. Part II. Colony-stimulating factors and interleukin-2. DICP 1991;25:490-498.

[104] Bruton JK, Koeller JM. Recombinant interleukin-2. Pharmacotherapy 1994;14.

[105] Petrella T, Quirt I, Verma S, Haynes AE, Charette M, Bak K, et al. Single-agent interleukin-2 in the treatment of metastatic melanoma. Curr Oncol 2007;14:21-26.

[106] Contardi E, Palmisano GL, Tazzari PL, Martelli AM, Falà F, Fabbi M, et al. CTLA-4 is constitutively expressed on tumor cells and can trigger apoptosis upon ligand interaction. Int J Cancer 2005;117:538-550.

[107] Shah KV, Chien AJ, Yee C, Moon RT. CTLA-4 Is a Direct Target of Wnt/beta-Catenin Signaling and Is Expressed in Human Melanoma Tumors. Journal of Investigative Dermatology 2008;128.

[108] Queirolo P, Laurent S, Boitano M, Carrega P, Saverino D, Alviano F, et al. Targeting ctla-4 directly on melanoma cells: A possible novel perspective in the immunotherapy of cutaneous melanoma. Proc Am Soc Clin Oncol, 2009.

[109] Leach DR, Krummel MF, Allison JP. Enhancement of antitumor immunity by CTLA-4 blockade. Science 1996;271.

[110] Hurwitz AA, Foster BA, Kwon ED, Truong T, Choi EM, Greenberg NM, et al. Combination immunotherapy of primary prostate cancer in a transgenic mouse model using CTLA-4 blockade. Cancer Research 2000;60.

[111] Hodi FS, O'Day SJ, McDermott DF, Weber RW, Sosman JA, Haanen JB, et al. Improved survival with ipilimumab in patients with metastatic melanoma. N Engl J Med 2010;363:711-723.

[112] Robert C, Thomas L, Bondarenko I, O'Day S, M D JW, Garbe C, et al. Ipilimumab plus dacarbazine for previously untreated metastatic melanoma. N Engl J Med 2011;364:2517-2526.

[113] Sapoznik S, Hammer O, Ortenberg R, Besser MJ, Ben-Moshe T, Schachter J, et al. Novel anti-melanoma immunotherapies: disarming tumor escape mechanisms. Clin Dev Immunol 2012;2012:818214.

[114] Patel V, Gandhi H, Upaganlawar A. Ipilimumab: Melanoma and beyond. J Pharm Bioallied Sci 2011;3:546.

[115] Mansh M. Ipilimumab and cancer immunotherapy: a new hope for advanced stage melanoma. Yale J Biol Med 2011;84:381-389.

[116] Tarhini AA, Iqbal F. CTLA-4 blockade: therapeutic potential in cancer treatments. Onco Targets Ther 2010;3:15-25.

[117] Thumar JR, Kluger HM. Ipilimumab: a promising immunotherapy for melanoma. Oncology (Williston Park) 2010;24:1280-1288.

[118] Maker AV, Yang JC, Sherry RM, Topalian SL, Kammula US, Royal RE, et al. Intrapatient dose escalation of anti-CTLA-4 antibody in patients with metastatic melanoma. J Immunother 2006;29:455-463.

[119] Serrone L, Zeuli M, Sega FM, Cognetti F. Dacarbazine-based chemotherapy for metastatic melanoma: thirty-year experience overview. J Exp Clin Cancer Res 2000;19:21-34.

[120] Del Prete SA, Maurer LH, O'Donnell J, Forcier RJ, LeMarbre P. Combination chemotherapy with cisplatin, carmustine, dacarbazine, and tamoxifen in metastatic melanoma. Cancer Treat Rep 1984;68:1403-1405.

[121] Lattanzi SC, Tosteson T, Chertoff J, Maurer LH, O'Donnell J, LeMarbre PJ, et al. Dacarbazine, cisplatin and carmustine, with or without tamoxifen, for metastatic melanoma: 5-year follow-up. Melanoma Res 1995;5:365-369.

[122] Chapman PB, Einhorn LH, Meyers ML, Saxman S, Destro AN, Panageas KS, et al. Phase III multicenter randomized trial of the Dartmouth regimen versus dacarbazine in patients with metastatic melanoma. J Clin Oncol 1999;17:2745-2751.

[123] Chiarion Sileni V, Nortilli R, Aversa SM, Paccagnella A, Medici M, Corti L, et al. Phase II randomized study of dacarbazine, carmustine, cisplatin and tamoxifen versus dacarbazine alone in advanced melanoma patients. Melanoma Res 2001;11:189-196.

[124] Su PJ, Chen JS, Liaw CC, Chang HK, Wang HM, Yang TS, et al. Biochemotherapy with carmustine, cisplatin, dacarbazine, tamoxifen and low-dose interleukin-2 for patients with metastatic malignant melanoma. Chang Gung Med J 2011;34:478-486.

[125] Atzpodien J, Neuber K, Kamanabrou D, Fluck M, Bröcker EB, Neumann C, et al. Combination chemotherapy with or without s.c. IL-2 and IFN-alpha: results of a prospectively randomized trial of the Cooperative Advanced Malignant Melanoma Chemoimmunotherapy Group (ACIMM). Br J Cancer 2002;86:179-184.

[126] Creagan ET, Suman VJ, Dalton RJ, Pitot HC, Long HJ, Veeder MH, et al. Phase III clinical trial of the combination of cisplatin, dacarbazine, and carmustine with or without tamoxifen in patients with advanced malignant melanoma. J Clin Oncol 1999;17:1884-1890.

[127] E B, MG Z, F N, N Z. Tamoxifen does not improve response when added to chemotherapy in metastatic melanoma. Proc Am Soc Clin Oncol, 1993: 393.

[128] McClay EF, McClay ME, Jones JA, Winski PJ, Christen RD, Howell SB, et al. A phase I and pharmacokinetic study of high dose tamoxifen and weekly cisplatin in patients with metastatic melanoma. Cancer 1997;79:1037-1043.

[129] Antoine EC, Rixe O, Vuillemin E, Benhammouda A, Borel C, Ghironzi GC, et al. A phase II study of tamoxifen combined with cisplatin-interleukin 2 and alpha-interferon in metastatic melanoma. Am J Clin Oncol 1995;18:421-424.

[130] Rixe O, Benhammouda A, Antoine E. Final results of a prospective multicentric study on 91 metastatic malignant melanoma patients treated by chemo-imunotherapy with cisplatin, interleukin-2 and interferon-a. Proc Am Soc Clin Oncol, 1994: 399.

[131] Fierro MT, Bertero M, Novelli M, Appino A, Doveil GC, Colonna S, et al. Therapy for metastatic melanoma: effective combination of dacarbazine, carmustine, cisplatin and tamoxifen. Melanoma Res 1993;3:127-131.

[132] Johnson DH, Presant C, Einhorn L, Bartolucci AA, Greco FA. Cisplatin, vinblastine, and bleomycin in the treatment of metastatic melanoma - a phase-ii study of the southeastern-cancer-study-group. Cancer Treatment Reports 1985;69.

[133] Bajetta E, Rovej R, Buzzoni R, Vaglini M, Bonadonna G. Treatment of advanced malignant melanoma with vinblastine, bleomycin, and cisplatin. Cancer Treat Rep 1982;66:1299-1302.

[134] Nathanson L, Kaufman SD, Carey RW. Vinblastine, infusion, bleomycin, and cis-dichlorodiammine-platinum chemotherapy in metastatic melanoma. Cancer 1981;48:1290-1294.

[135] Seigler HF, Lucas VS, Pickett NJ, Huang AT. DTIC, CCNU, bleomycin and vincristine (BOLD) in metastatic melanoma. Cancer 1980;46:2346-2348.

[136] Vuoristo MS, Hahka-Kemppinen M, Parvinen LM, Pyrhonen S, Seppa H, Korpela M, et al. Randomized trial of dacarbazine versus bleomycin, vincristine, lomustine and dacarbazine (BOLD) chemotherapy combined with natural or recombinant interferon-alpha in patients with advanced melanoma. Melanoma Research 2005;15.

[137] Pyrhönen S, Hahka-Kemppinen M, Muhonen T, Nikkanen V, Eskelin S, Summanen P, et al. Chemoimmunotherapy with bleomycin, vincristine, lomustine, dacarbazine (BOLD), and human leukocyte interferon for metastatic uveal melanoma. Cancer 2002;95:2366-2372.

[138] Kivelä T, Suciu S, Hansson J, Kruit WH, Vuoristo MS, Kloke O, et al. Bleomycin, vincristine, lomustine and dacarbazine (BOLD) in combination with recombinant interferon alpha-2b for metastatic uveal melanoma. Eur J Cancer 2003;39:1115-1120.

[139] Young DW, Lever RS, English JS, MacKie RM. The use of BELD combination chemotherapy in advanced malignant melanoma. Cancer 1985;55:1879-1881.

[140] Stables GI, Doherty VR, MacKie RM. Nine years' experience of BELD combination chemotherapy (bleomycin, vindesine, CCNU and DTIC) for metastatic melanoma. Br J Dermatol 1992;127:505-508.

[141] Legha SS, Ring S, Papadopoulos N, Plager C, Chawla S, Benjamin R. A prospective evaluation of a triple-drug regimen containing cisplatin, vinblastine, and dacarbazine (CVD) for metastatic melanoma. Cancer 1989;64:2024-2029.

[142] Eton O, Legha SS, Bedikian AY, Lee JJ, Buzaid AC, Hodges C, et al. Sequential biochemotherapy versus chemotherapy for metastatic melanoma: results from a phase III randomized trial. J Clin Oncol 2002;20:2045-2052.

[143] Kim KB, Eton O, East MJ, Hodges C, Papadopoulos NE, Grimm EA, et al. Pilot study of high-dose, concurrent biochemotherapy for advanced melanoma. Cancer 2004;101:596-603.

[144] Jungnelius U, Ringborg U, Aamdal S, Mattsson J, Stierner U, Ingvar C, et al. Dacarbazine-vindesine versus dacarbazine-vindesine-cisplatin in disseminated malignant melanoma. A randomised phase III trial. European Journal of Cancer 1998;34.

[145] Ringborg U, Jungnelius U, Hansson J, Strander H. Dacarbazine-vindesine-cisplatin in disseminated malignant melanoma. A phase I-II trial. Am J Clin Oncol 1990;13:214-217.

[146] Hodi FS, Soiffer RJ, Clark J, Finkelstein DM, Haluska FG. Phase II study of paclitaxel and carboplatin for malignant melanoma. Am J Clin Oncol 2002;25:283-286.

[147] Rao RD, Holtan SG, Ingle JN, Croghan GA, Kottschade LA, Creagan ET, et al. Combination of paclitaxel and carboplatin as second-line therapy for patients with metastatic melanoma. Cancer 2006;106:375-382.

[148] Kottschade LA, Suman VJ, Amatruda T, McWilliams RR, Mattar BI, Nikcevich DA, et al. A phase II trial of nab-paclitaxel (ABI-007) and carboplatin in patients with unresectable stage IV melanoma : a North Central Cancer Treatment Group Study, N057E(1). Cancer 2011;117:1704-1710.

[149] Pflugfelder A, Eigentler TK, Keim U, Weide B, Leiter U, Ikenberg K, et al. Effectiveness of carboplatin and paclitaxel as first- and second-line treatment in 61 patients with metastatic melanoma. PLoS One 2011;6:e16882.

[150] Flaherty KT, Schiller J, Schuchter LM, Liu G, Tuveson DA, Redlinger M, et al. A phase I trial of the oral, multikinase inhibitor sorafenib in combination with carboplatin and paclitaxel. Clin Cancer Res 2008;14:4836-4842.

[151] Hauschild A, Grob JJ, Demidov LV, Jouary T, Gutzmer R, Millward M, et al. Dabrafenib in BRAF-mutated metastatic melanoma: a multicentre, open-label, phase 3 randomised controlled trial. Lancet 2012;380:358-365.

[152] Kim KB, Sosman JA, Fruehauf JP, Linette GP, Markovic SN, McDermott DF, et al. BEAM: a randomized phase II study evaluating the activity of bevacizumab in combination with carboplatin plus paclitaxel in patients with previously untreated melanoma. J Clin Oncol 2012;30:34-41.

[153] Schmittel A, Schmidt-Hieber M, Martus P, Bechrakis NE, Schuster R, Siehl JM, et al. A randomized phase II trial of gemcitabine plus treosulfan versus treosulfan alone in patients with metastatic uveal melanoma. Ann Oncol 2006;17:1826-1829.

[154] Schmittel A, Schuster R, Bechrakis NE, Siehl JM, Foerster MH, Thiel E, et al. A two-cohort phase II clinical trial of gemcitabine plus treosulfan in patients with metastatic uveal melanoma. Melanoma Res 2005;15:447-451.

[155] Lopez M, Perno CF, Di Lauro L, Papaldo P, Ganzina F, Barduagni A. Controlled study of DTIC versus DTIC plus epirubicin in metastatic malignant melanoma. Invest New Drugs 1984;2:319-322.

[156] Minchom A, Young K, Larkin J. Ipilimumab: showing survival benefit in metastatic melanoma. Future Oncol 2011;7:1255-1264.

[157] Hersh EM, O'Day SJ, Powderly J, Khan KD, Pavlick AC, Cranmer LD, et al. A phase II multicenter study of ipilimumab with or without dacarbazine in chemotherapy-naïve patients with advanced melanoma. Invest New Drugs 2011;29:489-498.

[158] Davies H, Bignell GR, Cox C, Stephens P, Edkins S, Clegg S, et al. Mutations of the BRAF gene in human cancer. Nature 2002;417:949-954.

[159] Falchook GS, Long GV, Kurzrock R, Kim KB, Arkenau TH, Brown MP, et al. Dabrafenib in patients with melanoma, untreated brain metastases, and other solid tumors: a phase 1 dose-escalation trial. Lancet 2012;379:1893-1901.

[160] Falchook GS, Lewis KD, Infante JR, Gordon MS, Vogelzang NJ, Demarini DJ, et al. Activity of the oral MEK inhibitor trametinib in patients with advanced melanoma: a phase 1 dose-escalation trial. Lancet Oncol 2012;13:782-789.

[161] Schmitt CA, Rosenthal CT, Lowe SW. Genetic analysis of chemoresistance in primary murine lymphomas. Nat Med 2000;6:1029-1035.

[162] Jansen B, Schlagbauer-Wadl H, Brown BD, Bryan RN, van Elsas A, Müller M, et al. bcl-2 antisense therapy chemosensitizes human melanoma in SCID mice. Nat Med 1998;4:232-234.

[163] Klasa RJ, Gillum AM, Klem RE, Frankel SR. Oblimersen Bcl-2 antisense: facilitating apoptosis in anticancer treatment. Antisense Nucleic Acid Drug Dev 2002;12:193-213.

[164] de Murcia G, Ménissier de Murcia J. Poly(ADP-ribose) polymerase: a molecular nick-sensor. Trends Biochem Sci 1994;19:172-176.

[165] Plummer R, Jones C, Middleton M, Wilson R, Evans J, Olsen A, et al. Phase I study of the poly(ADP-ribose) polymerase inhibitor, AG014699, in combination with temozolomide in patients with advanced solid tumors. Clin Cancer Res 2008;14:7917-7923.

[166] Kashani-Sabet M, Shaikh L, Miller JR, Nosrati M, Ferreira CM, Debs RJ, et al. NF-kappa B in the vascular progression of melanoma. J Clin Oncol 2004;22:617-623.

http://dx.doi.org/10.5772/55192

[167] Ascierto PA, Streicher HZ, Sznol M. Melanoma: a model for testing new agents in combination therapies. J Transl Med 2010;8:38.

[168] Portnow J, Frankel P, Koehler S, Twardowski P, Shibata S, Martel C, et al. A phase I study of bortezomib and temozolomide in patients with advanced solid tumors. Cancer Chemother Pharmacol 2012;69:505-514.

[169] Neumann E, Schaefer-Ridder M, Wang Y, Hofschneider PH. Gene transfer into mouse lyoma cells by electroporation in high electric fields. EMBO J 1982;1:841-845.

[170] Hargrave B, Downey H, Strange R, Murray L, Cinnamond C, Lundberg C, et al. Electroporation-mediated gene transfer directly to the swine heart. Gene Ther 2012.

[171] Mir LM. Therapeutic perspectives of in vivo cell electropermeabilization. Bioelectrochemistry 2001;53:1-10.

[172] Marty M, Sersa G, Garbay JR, Gehl J, Collins CG, Snoj M, et al. Electrochemotherapy - An easy, highly effective and safe treatment of cutaneous and subcutaneous metastases: Results of ESOPE study. Ejc Supplements 2006;4.

[173] Sersa G, Stabuc B, Cemazar M, Miklavcic D, Rudolf Z. Electrochemotherapy with cisplatin: the systemic antitumor effectiveness of cisplatin can be potentiated locally by the application of electric pulses in the treatment of malignant melanoma skin metastases. Melanoma Res 2000;10:381-385.

[174] Kis E, Oláh J, Ócsai H, Baltas E, Gyulai R, Kemény L, et al. Electrochemotherapy of cutaneous metastases of melanoma--a case series study and systematic review of the evidence. Dermatol Surg 2011;37:816-824.

[175] Campana LG, Valpione S, Mocellin S, Sundararajan R, Granziera E, Sartore L, et al. Electrochemotherapy for disseminated superficial metastases from malignant melanoma. Br J Surg 2012;99:821-830.

[176] Venturini M, Pilla L, Agostini G, Cappio S, Losio C, Orsi M, et al. Transarterial Chemoembolization with Drug-eluting Beads Preloaded with Irinotecan as a First-Line Approach in Uveal Melanoma Liver Metastases: Tumor Response and Predictive Value of Diffusion-weighted MR Imaging in Five Patients. Journal of Vascular and Interventional Radiology 2012;23.

[177] Huppert PE, Fierlbeck G, Pereira P, Schanz S, Duda SH, Wietholtz H, et al. Transarterial chemoembolization of liver metastases in patients with uveal melanoma. Eur J Radiol 2010;74:38-44.

[178] Schuster R, Lindner M, Wacker F, Krössin M, Bechrakis N, Foerster MH, et al. Transarterial chemoembolization of liver metastases from uveal melanoma after failure of systemic therapy: toxicity and outcome. Melanoma Res 2010;20:191-196.

[179] Rosenberg SA, Restifo NP, Yang JC, Morgan RA, Dudley ME. Adoptive cell transfer: a clinical path to effective cancer immunotherapy. Nat Rev Cancer 2008;8:299-308.

[180] Dudley ME, Wunderlich JR, Shelton TE, Even J, Rosenberg SA. Generation of tumor-infiltrating lymphocyte cultures for use in adoptive transfer therapy for melanoma patients. J Immunother 2003;26:332-342.

[181] Dudley ME, Wunderlich JR, Yang JC, Sherry RM, Topalian SL, Restifo NP, et al. Adoptive cell transfer therapy following non-myeloablative but lymphodepleting chemotherapy for the treatment of patients with refractory metastatic melanoma. J Clin Oncol 2005;23:2346-2357.

[182] Dudley ME, Yang JC, Sherry R, Hughes MS, Royal R, Kammula U, et al. Adoptive cell therapy for patients with metastatic melanoma: evaluation of intensive myeloablative chemoradiation preparative regimens. J Clin Oncol 2008;26:5233-5239.

[183] Rosenberg SA, Yang JC, Sherry RM, Kammula US, Hughes MS, Phan GQ, et al. Durable complete responses in heavily pretreated patients with metastatic melanoma using T-cell transfer immunotherapy. Clin Cancer Res 2011;17:4550-4557.

[184] Joseph RW, Peddareddigari VR, Liu P, Miller PW, Overwijk WW, Bekele NB, et al. Impact of clinical and pathologic features on tumor-infiltrating lymphocyte expansion from surgically excised melanoma metastases for adoptive T-cell therapy. Clin Cancer Res 2011;17:4882-4891.

[185] Tran KQ, Zhou J, Durflinger KH, Langhan MM, Shelton TE, Wunderlich JR, et al. Minimally cultured tumor-infiltrating lymphocytes display optimal characteristics for adoptive cell therapy. J Immunother 2008;31:742-751.

[186] Syed DN, Mukhtar H. Botanicals for the prevention and treatment of cutaneous melanoma. Pigment Cell Melanoma Res 2011;24:688-702.

[187] Locatelli C, Rosso R, Santos-Silva MC, de Souza CA, Licinio MA, Leal P, et al. Ester derivatives of gallic acid with potential toxicity toward L1210 leukemia cells. Bioorganic & Medicinal Chemistry 2008;16:3791-3799.

[188] Locatelli C, Leal PC, Yunes RA, Nunes RJ, Creczynski-Pasa TB. Gallic acid ester derivatives induce apoptosis and cell adhesion inhibition in melanoma cells: The relationship between free radical generation, glutathione depletion and cell death. Chem Biol Interact 2009;181:175-184.

[189] de Cordova CAS, Locatelli C, Assuncao LS, Mattei B, Mascarello A, Winter E, et al. Octyl and dodecyl gallates induce oxidative stress and apoptosis in a melanoma cell line. Toxicology in Vitro 2011;25:2025-2034.

[190] Locatelli C, Carvalho DR, Mascarello A, de Cordova CA, Yunes RA, Nunes RJ, et al. Antimetastatic activity and low systemic toxicity of tetradecyl gallate in a preclinical melanoma mouse model. Invest New Drugs 2011.

Chapter 10

Targeted Agents for the Treatment of Melanoma: An Overview

Hsiang-Wen Tseng, Wen-Tai Li+ and
Jung-Feng Hsieh+

Additional information is available at the end of the chapter

http://dx.doi.org/10.5772/54938

1. Introduction

Malignant melanoma is an important healthcare issue. The incidence of melanoma has increased dramatically during the last few decades and melanoma is now one of the most common forms of cancer. This aggressive form of skin cancer is characterized by its high capacity for invasion and metastasis. Patients with advanced stages of the disease have universally poor prognoses with a median survival of 3–11 months, depending on various prognostic factors. Primary cutaneous melanomas are divided into four groups on the basis of histopathology: superficial spreading melanoma, nodular melanoma, lentigo maligna melanoma, and acral lentiginous melanoma. Superficial spreading melanoma is the most common form. In the early growth phase, tumor cells spread laterally into the epidermis, forming an irregular pattern with an uneven color on the skin. Nodular melanoma occurs most often on the chest or back where it has a tendency to grow vertically into the skin, penetrating deeply if not removed. Nodular melanoma lesions are often characterized by a darkly pigmented lump on the skin surface. Lentigo maligna melanoma most commonly occurs on the facial areas of elderly people. It grows slowly and may take several years to develop. Acral lentiginous melanoma is usually found on the palms of the hands, the soles of the feet, or around the toenails. Melanoma is usually curable in its early stages; however, the disease may be fatal if it spreads to other parts of the body. Malignant melanoma usually develops via the transformation and proliferation of melanocytes that reside in the basal cell layer of the epidermis. Melanoma can also develop when melanocytes no longer respond to normal cellular growth control mechanisms, which allows the tumor cells to metastasize into nearby tissues or other organs, where they invade and compromise organ function. Thus, the development of alternative treatment for melanoma is critically important. Recent advances in oncology have led to novel therapeutics that is capable of targeting known oncogenes and immunotherapeutic antibodies. Clinical trials of these agents have demonstrated measurable benefits to patients with metastatic melanoma. In this chapter, we review clinical studies of recently developed targeted agents and summarize their current effectiveness in melanoma treatment.

2. Immune modulators for melanoma treatment

Melanoma is characterized as one of the most immunogenic tumors because of the presence of tumor-infiltrating lymphocytes in resected melanoma, occasional spontaneous regression, and clinical responses to immune stimulation. The immunogenicity of melanoma has led investigators to study novel immune strategies for overcoming immune system evasion by tumors. Therapies targeted at the immune checkpoints (e.g., cytotoxic T lymphocyte-associated antigen 4, CTLA-4) have transformed the treatment of advanced melanoma in recent years. T cells self-regulate their activation through CTLA-4 expression. CTLA-4 functions as a negative co-stimulatory molecule for the T cell; therefore, therapies that antagonize CTLA-4 remove the brakes from T cells leading to a net effect of T cell hyper-responsiveness [1]. At present, clinical trials of anti-CTLA-4 monoclonal antibody treatment are being conducted for melanoma. Several human monoclonal antibodies, i.e., tremelimumab (CP-675,206; Pfizer Pharmaceuticals, New York), ipilimumab (MDX-010; Bristol-Myers Squibb, Medarex, Princeton, NJ) and urelumab (BMS-663513), are under investigation. These antibodies have been demonstrated to induce tumor regression and may prolong time to disease progression [2-3]. As shown in Table 1, three such antibodies, i.e., tremelimumab, ipilimumab, and urelumab, are in clinical development.

Drug Name	Mechanisms
Tremelimumab (CP-675,206)	Anti-CTLA-4
Ipilimumab (MDX-010)	Anti-CTLA-4
Urelumab (BMS-663513)	Anti-CD137

Table 1. Clinical trials of selected monoclonal antibodies for melanoma treatment

2.1. Tremelimumab

Melanoma is an immunogenic tumor, which suggests that manipulation of the immune system using monoclonal antibody treatment to suppress the CTLA-4 inhibitory function could produce a favorable clinical result. Tremelimumab is a fully human IgG2 antibody, which is directed against human CTLA-4. CTLA-4 plays a pivotal role in this interaction by dampening immune responses to self-antigens. CTLA-4 is a cell surface receptor expressed on activated T cells. In mice, the T cell-mediated killing of tumors is enhanced by blocking CTLA4 binding to its natural ligands, such as CD80 and CD86, which are expressed on antigen-presenting cells. Blocking antibodies to CTLA-4 were shown to induce tumor regression in selected mouse models [4]. When translated to the clinic, the administration of blocking antibodies to CTLA-4 produced objective tumor responses in a subset of patients with metastatic melanoma [5]. Tremelimumab is a fully human IgG2 monoclonal antibody tested in patients with cancer, the majority of whom have had metastatic melanoma. Pfizer previously developed tremelimumab for the potential intravenous (i.v.) treatment of cancers. They were also developing tremelimumab as a potential treatment for melanoma. Clinical trials using tremelimumab demonstrated that this antibody could induce long-lasting tumor regressions in 7%–10% of patients with metastatic melanoma. These tumor responses are mediated by the intratumoral infiltration of cytotoxic T cells, as demonstrated in patient-derived tumor biopsies. Grade 3 or 4 toxicities in the range of 20% to 25% are mainly inflammatory or autoimmune in nature, which are on-target effects after inhibiting CTLA-4-mediated self-tolerance. The lack of any survival advantage during the early analysis of a phase III clinical trial comparing tremelimumab with standard chemotreatment for metastatic melanoma highlights the importance of gaining a better understanding of how this antibody modulates the human immune system and how to better select patients for this mode of treatment [6].

Tremelimumab is being developed by Pfizer for the treatment of various cancers. It is currently in worldwide phase III development for malignant melanoma. Tremelimumab at 15 mg/kg every 3 months was compared with standard chemotreatment during a pivotal phase III clinical trial in patients with previously untreated metastatic melanoma without brain metastasis and a baseline lactate dehydrogenase level below double the upper normal limit. The Data Safety Monitoring Board (DSMB) determined that the second interim analysis crossed the prospectively defined futility boundaries for improvement in overall survival (OS). The trial had a very short follow-up, with most patients only followed for 6–11 months after the initial dose. During that period, the survival curve of the tremelimumab group was ahead of the curve of the chemotreatment arm by 1 month [7]. The interim results of this trial have been updated recently; however, insignificant improvements in survival were observed with tremelimumab. A subset analysis suggested that patients with a low baseline C-reactive protein (CRP) had a markedly improved outcome when treated with tremelimumab compared with chemotreatment. CRP may be an indicator of the tumor microenviroment because this acute reactive protein is produced in the liver in response to peripheral inflammation [8]. Furthermore, Pfizer and the Debiopharm Group entered into a co-development agreement to conduct a phase III trial of tremelimumab for the treatment of patients with unresectable, stage IV melanoma. A biomarker will be used to select patients considered likely to respond to tremelimumab. Under the terms of the agreement, Debiopharm will assume responsibility for conducting the phase III trial of tremelimumab, while Pfizer will retain responsibility for the worldwide commercialization of the compound. The financial terms of the agreement were not disclosed [9]. In addition, tremelimumab had been discontinued for melanoma. Therefore, the clinical development of tremelimumab has provided evidence of long-lasting responses in a small subset of patients with metastatic melanoma.

2.2. Ipilimumab

Ipilimumab is a fully human monoclonal IgG1κ antibody against CTLA-4, an immune inhibitory molecule expressed in activated T cells and suppressor T regulatory cells. Activation of the cellular immune response involves the interaction of T cell receptors with major histocompatibility complex molecules on antigen-presenting cells (APCs). This requires co-stimulation where ligand B7 on APC binds to CD28 on T cells, which triggers T cell proliferation. A negative co-stimulation signal is transduced by CTLA-4, which is present in T cells, and interaction of CTLA-4 with the same B7 ligand inhibits T cell activation and proliferation [10]. Ipilimumab is a human MAB against CTLA-4 that enhances the co-stimulation of cytotoxic T cells, resulting in their proliferation and an antitumor response. It is licensed for the treatment of unresectable or metastatic malignant melanoma, and multiple clinical trials using this medication for the treatment of other malignancies are ongoing. As the clinical response to ipilimumab is derived from immunostimulation, predictably it also generates autoimmunity, leading to immune-related adverse events in the majority of patients [11]. Ipilimumab was approved by the Food and Drug Administration (FDA) in February 2011 and by the European Medicines Agency in July 2011 for use in the treatment of advanced malignant melanoma in patients not responding to chemotreatment, with or without previous exposure to immunotreatment [12]. Two significant phase III clinical trials of ipilimumab in patients with unresectable/metastatic malignant melanoma have been conducted. In the first trial, ipilimumab at 3 mg/kg significantly improved OS from 6.4 to 10 months [13]. In the second trial, ipilimumab at 10 mg/kg in combination with dacarbazine significantly improved the 3-year survival rate from 12.8 to 20.2% compared with dacarbazine alone [14]. Therefore, the dose of ipilimumab used in clinical trials ranged from 3 to 10 mg/kg.

Ipilimumab was approved by the FDA in March 2011 as a monotreatment (3 mg/kg every 3 weeks for 4 doses) for the treatment of advanced melanoma in pre-treated or chemotreatment-naive patients. Four months later, ipilimumab received rapid approval by the European Commission, after a positive opinion was expressed by the Committee for Medicinal Products for Human Use. However, the EU limits its use to previously treated patients with advanced melanoma. Phase III trials are testing ipilimumab in an adjuvant setting in patients with high-risk stage III or IV melanoma after surgical removal of the tumor. A neoadjuvant potential use of ipilimumab is currently under evaluation in patients with stage IIIB/C melanoma before lymphadenectomy. In this trial, ipilimumab is also administered after surgery as maintenance treatment. The trial aims to analyze the host immune responses in nodal metastatic melanoma and in the peripheral blood by comparing the immunological parameters at baseline and after treatment. Data on 17 patients indicated that ipilimumab induces a significant increase in the frequency of circulating regulatory T cells (Tregs), i.e., increase in the induction of tumor-infiltrating Tregs at 6 weeks [15]. Ipilimumab is the first agent that has been demonstrated to improve OS in patients with metastatic melanoma, which has a very poor prognosis, in randomized phase III clinical trials [16].

2.3. Urelumab (BMS-663513)

CD-137 is a member of the tumor necrosis factor receptor (TNFR) family and functions as a costimulatory molecule. BMS-663513 is a fully human monoclonal antibody agonist of CD-137, which is a TNFR expressed on the surfaces of activated white blood cells [17]. CD-137 stimulation enhances the immune response, specifically an antitumor immune response, via various

http://dx.doi.org/10.5772/54938

mechanisms [18]. Phase I and II trials initially focused on patients with melanoma, but they were expanded to patients with renal cell carcinoma (RCC) and ovarian cancer. Urelumab (BMS-663513) was tolerable across a wide dose range (0.3–15 mg/kg). As a single agent, urelumab has demonstrated clinical activity that justifies its further evaluation as a single agent and in combination with other treatment modalities [19].

3. c-KIT inhibitors for melanoma treatment

Targeted treatments act by selectively inhibiting molecules, usually proteins, the expression or overexpression of which have specific roles in the growth of the target neoplasm. Thus, one of the main characteristics of targeted antineoplastic treatment is that the drugs act specifically on their intended target and that those targets have specific effects on the tumor [20]. The number of possible therapeutic targets in melanoma is increasing with an improvement in our understanding of the biology of this tumor. One of these, c-KIT, has been considered a potential therapeutic target in melanoma for a long time. Indeed, c-KIT is a protein that acts as a fundamental growth factor receptor in epidermal melanocytes and has an essential role in the differentiation and migration of melanocytic cells during embryonic development [21]. c-KIT inhibitors have been used for melanoma treatment. c-KIT, which is also known as CD117, is a receptor tyrosine kinase (RTK) that is mutated in approximately 20% of acral, mucosal, and chronic sun-induced skin damage [22]. The ligand for KIT is stem cell factor (SCF) and binding of SCF to c-KIT induces the activation of downstream signaling pathways that mediate growth and survival signals within the cell, including the PI3K-AKT-mTOR and RAS-RAF-MEK-ERK pathways. KIT has been implicated in the pathogenesis of several cancers including acute myeloid leukemia (AML) and gastrointestinal stromal tumors (GIST). Unlike GIST, where c-KIT mutations tend to be deletions or insertions in exon 11, c-KIT mutations in melanoma occur at multiple sites in the gene, including the juxtamembrane domain at exons 11 and 13 and the kinase domain at exon 17. They are usually point mutations that do not correlate with the KIT copy number or CD117 expression [23]. As shown in Table 2, two c-KIT inhibitors, i.e., imatinib and dasatinib, are under evaluation for treating melanoma.

Name	Mechanisms
Imatinib	c-KIT inhibitors
Dasatinib	c-KIT inhibitors

Table 2. Clinical trials of c-KIT inhibitors for treating melanoma

3.1. Imatinib

Targeting KIT may be a therapeutic strategy for patients with CSD, acral, or mucosal melanomas that harbor an activating c-KIT mutation in exons 9, 11, or 13 [24]. Imatinib (Figure 1), an oral tyrosine kinase inhibitor (TKI) with known activity against c-KIT-activated tumors, was tested in three phase II trials in patients with melanomas that harbored c-KIT mutations. The first trial enrolled patients with metastatic melanomas that expressed at least one protein tyrosine kinase [c-KIT, platelet-derived growth factor receptors (PDGFRs), c-abl, or abl-related gene], and a response was observed in only 1 patient, i.e., in the patient who had the highest level of c-KIT expression. Of note, c-KIT mutations were not required prior to entry in this trial. In the second trial, 28 patients with c-KIT mutations and amplifications with advanced unresectable melanoma arising from acral, mucosal, and chronic sun-induced skin damage were orally administered 400 mg imatinib mesylate twice daily in 6-week cycles until disease progression or unacceptable toxicity [25].

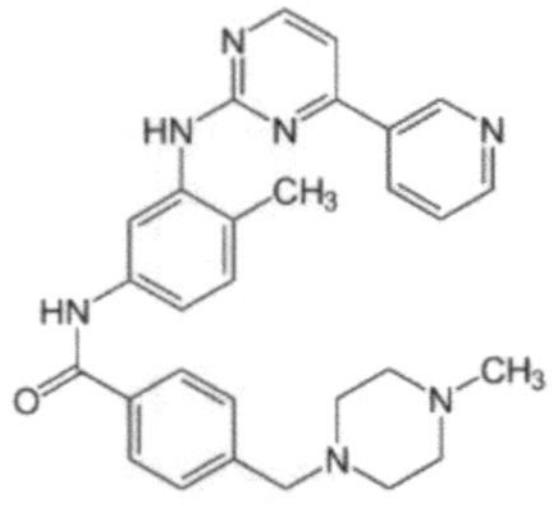

Figure 1. Chemical structure of imatinib.

Novartis developed and launched imatinib, an inhibitor of tyrosine kinases including Bcr-Abl and c-KIT. The product is indicated for the treatment of newly diagnosed Philadelphia chromosome-positive (Ph+) chronic myeloid leukemia (CML) and Ph+ CML in blast crisis during the accelerated phase or chronic phase after interferon treatment. It is also indicated for the treatment of KIT-positive GIST, including unresectable and/or metastatic disease and resected disease after surgery, in adults with newly diagnosed Ph+ acute lymphoblastic leukemia (ALL) in combination with chemotreatment, as a single agent for relapsed or refractory Ph+ ALL. It is also indicated for the treatment of adults with unresectable, recurrent, and/or metastatic dermatofibrosarcoma protuberans (DFSP); hypereosinophilic syndrome (HES); chronic eosinophilic leukemia (CEL); aggressive systemic mastocytosis (ASM); and myelodysplastic/myeloproliferative diseases (MDS/MPD) associated with PDGFR gene rearrangements.

3.2. Dasatinib

Dasatinib (Figure 2, BMS-354825; Sprycel®; Bristol-Myers Squibb Co) is a multi-targeted inhibitor of RTKs, including BCR-ABL fusion protein, stem cell factor receptor (c-KIT) and Src family kinases (SFKs). The phase II trial results were presented at the 45th ASCO meeting in 2009, showing that daily treatment with dasatinib has modest activity in patients with melanoma. Accrual is almost complete. Toxicity is frequent; therefore, alternate schedules to allow breaks in dosing might be better and should be evaluated. Combination studies may be warranted on the basis of preclinical evaluations of molecularly defined subsets of patients. Dasatinib is indicated for the treatment of newly diagnosed adults with Ph+ CML in the chronic phase and of adults with chronic, accelerated, myeloid, or lymphoid blast phase Ph+ CML with resistance or intolerance to prior treatment, including imatinib. Dasatinib is also indicated for the treatment of adults with Ph+ ALL with resistance or intolerance to prior treatment, including imatinib. Dasatinib was launched in the US in July 2006 for the second-line treatment of CML and Ph+ ALL. The drug was launched in the UK and some European countries for the second-line treatment of CML by the end of 2006. Dasatinib was launched in Japan in April 2009. In October 2010, the drug was approved in the US for the first-line treatment of Ph+ CML. By December 2010, the drug was approved in the EC for the treatment of newly diagnosed, chronic phase CML in adult patients. In June 2011, the drug was approved for the first-line treatment of CML in Japan. The company is also developing the drug for other cancer indications, including breast, prostate, and pancreatic cancers, and non-small-cell lung cancer (NSCLC). By October 2008, phase III trials began for castration-resistant prostate cancer. Therefore, an application for this indication was expected in 2012 or 2013. In December 2006, phase II trials were initiated for breast cancer. By December 2006, a phase II trial for systemic mastocytosis was also initiated. In May 2007, a phase II trial for sarcoma began in the US. A phase II trial for NSCLC was initiated in November 2007. In December 2007, Bristol-Myers Squibb were also investigating dasatinib for multiple myeloma (MM) and other hematological malignancies, and a phase I/II trial was also underway for melanoma. By May 2009, a phase II trial was ongoing for head and neck cancer. By October 2009, a phase II trial was completed for polycythemia vera. By June 2010, a phase II trial began for colorectal cancer. In June 2011, a phase II trial began in the US for locally advanced pancreatic cancer, while phase II trials also began in Europe for pancreatic cancer by September 2011.

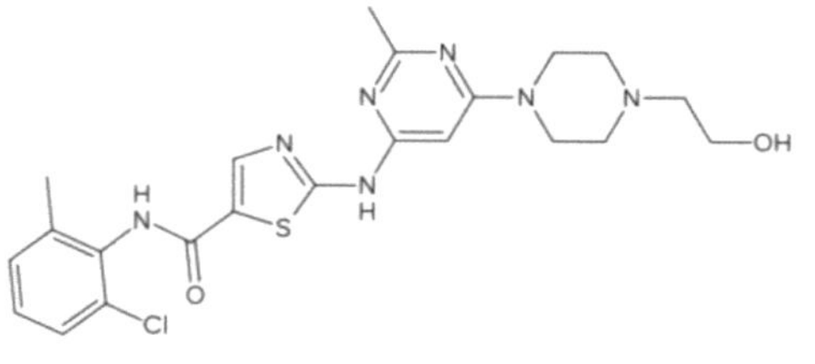

Figure 2. Chemical structure of dasatinib.

4. BRAF/MEK inhibitors for melanoma treatment

The mitogen-activated protein kinase (MAPK) pathway relays extracellular signals from the plasma membrane of the cell to the nucleus via an ordered series of phosphorylation events. MAPKs regulate diverse cellular programs including embryogenesis, proliferation, differentiation, and apoptosis via the cell surface sensing the metabolic state and environment of the cell [26]. The RAS/RAF/MEK/ERK pathway plays a role in normal organogenesis; however, it can lead to malignant cellular proliferation, inhibition of apoptosis, and invasion when aberrantly activated. In melanoma, the most commonly mutated gene is BRAF, with a frequency of 50%–70%. More than 90% of these mutations result in a substitution of valine for glutamic acid at position 600 (V600E). BRAF V600E leads to ERK activation, which results in the proliferation and survival advantage of melanoma cells [27-28]. BRAF phosphorylates regulatory serine residues on MEK1/2, and BRAF mutation results in the activation of the RAS/RAF/MEK/ERK pathway, leading to cellular proliferation and a series of antiapoptotic and potentially immunoregulatory events that culminate in tumor progression. Advanced melanomas harboring BRAF mutations appear to be associated with truncal primaries and an earlier age at onset; however, chronic UV-induced skin damage may be absent. Clinically, the disease associated with BRAF mutation has been shown to follow a more aggressive clinical course with a shorter OS for patients not treated with BRAF inhibitors [29]. As shown in Table 3, five BRAF inhibitors are under evaluation for melanoma.

Name	Mechanisms
Sorafenib	Multi-target BRAF inhibitors
RAF265	Multi-target BRAF inhibitors
Dabrafenib	Selective BRAF inhibitors
Vemurafenib	BRAF V600E inhibitor
Selumetinib	MEK inhibitor

Table 3. Clinical trials of BRAF inhibitors for treating melanoma

4.1. Sorafenib

Sorafenib (Figure 3, Nexavar, BAY-43-9006; Bayer) is a small molecule and a multikinase inhibitor (including the vascular endothelial growth factor receptors VEGFR-1, VEGFR-2, and VEGFR-3, PDGFR, as well as FLT3, C-KIT, and BRAF). It yielded negative results in metastatic melanoma trials when tested as a single agent and in combination with other chemotherapeutic agents, despite its success in treating metastatic renal, hepatocellular carcinomas (HCCs) [30], and thyroid cancer. In first-line treatment, a phase III, randomized, double-blind, placebo-controlled trial using chemotreatment-naive patients with unresectable stage III or IV melanoma was initiated for sorafenib treatment in 2005. The objective was to compare improvements in OS in patients receiving sorafenib or placebo in combination with both carboplatin and paclitaxel. In 2010, the results were presented at the 46th ASCO meeting, showing that the addition of sorafenib to carboplatin and paclitaxel did not improve OS, i.e., no significant differences were observed between the treatment groups in terms of OS, PFS, or RR. The median OS for the sorafenib combination group was 11.1 months compared with 11.3 months for the carboplatin plus paclitaxel group. The median PFS was 4.9 months versus 4.1 months, respectively. Grade 3 or 4 adverse events occurred in 78% patients in the sorafenib group (versus 84%). As a second-line treatment, a total of 270 patients received placebo plus carboplatin and paclitaxel (median PFS, 17.9 weeks) or sorafenib plus carboplatin and paclitaxel (median PFS, 17.4 weeks). The addition of sorafenib to carboplatin and paclitaxel did not improve any of the endpoints compared with that of placebo to carboplatin and paclitaxel. Therefore, it cannot be recommended in a second-line setting for patients with advanced melanoma [31]. In the first phase II trial, which included 39 patients and used sorafenib as mono-treatment, one complete response and seven partial responses were achieved. In a second phase I/II trial with 35 patients, where the drug was combined with carboplatin and paclitaxel, the number of partial responses increased to 11, while 19 minor responses were observed. Subsequently, a two-armed phase II trial was undertaken. In this trial, an increase in the disease-free interval was observed in the group that received sorafenib, although there was no improvement in OS. Since then, other phase III trials have been undertaken in which sorafenib has been combined with other cytostatic agents, such as temozolomide, carboplatin, or paclitaxel. However, no improvements were observed in the outcomes. In these trials, the response was not correlated with the presence of BRAF V600E mutation. It is believed that sorafenib actually targets VEGFR-2 or PDGFR-β more strongly than BRAF in these patients. At present, its main indications are for the treatment of clear cell renal carcinoma and unresectable HCC, where angiogenesis seems to play a more important role [32]. Some preclinical studies suggest that sorafenib would be more effective in the small group of melanomas with BRAF mutations, rather than in melanomas with V600E mutation [33].

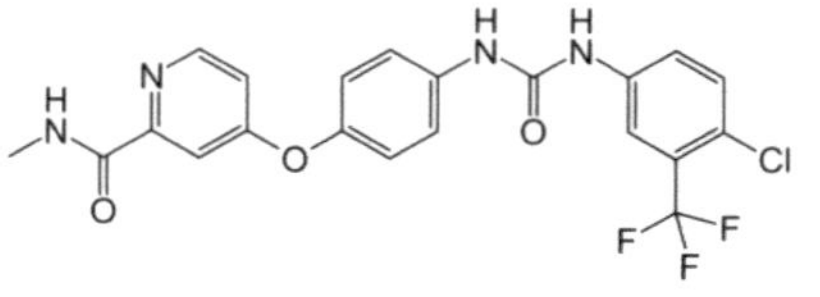

Figure 3. Chemical structure of sorafenib.

4.2. RAF265

RAF265 (Figure 4) is an orally bioavailable small molecule with preclinical antitumor activity that is currently being tested in phase I clinical trials for locally advanced or metastatic melanoma. RAF265 is a novel, orally dosed, small-molecule BRAF kinase and VEGFR-2 inhibitor with potent preclinical antitumor activity in mutant BRAF tumor models. The preclinical effectiveness of RAF265 for the treatment of melanoma has been evaluated. Advanced metastatic melanoma tumors from 34 patients were orthotopically implanted into nude mice. The tumors that grew in mice (17 of 34) were evaluated to determine their response to RAF265 (40 mg/kg/daily) for 30 days. Nine of the 17 successfully implanted (53%) tumors had mutant BRAF, whereas 8 (47%) tumors had wild-type BRAF. Tumor implants from 7 of 17 patients (41%) responded to RAF265 treatment with a >50% reduction in tumor growth [34]. In 2011, the clinical data of this first human study were presented at the 47th ASCO meeting. The first in human study, and RAF-265 was shown to be effective in patients with mutated and wild-type BRAF melanomas. The observed 11-day mean half-life of RAF-265 indicated that an intermittent dosing schedule should be investigated. At the 42nd ACSO meeting, the MTD of oral RAF-265 was reported as 48 mg with a continuous daily dosing schedule. Dose-limiting hematological toxicities following qd dosing (67 mg) highlighted the need to explore intermittent dosing. RAF265 is also a multitargeted small molecule inhibitor of the BRAF V600E mutant and VEGFR. A phase I trial that treated advanced melanoma patients with RAF265 demonstrated an overall response rate of 16% for patients with BRAF mutation-positive melanoma and 13% for patients with wild-type BRAF or unknown status of BRAF mutation [35].

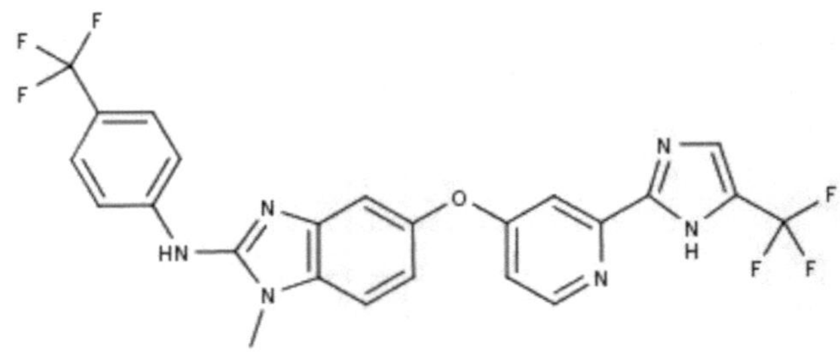

Figure 4. Chemical structure of RAF265.

4.3. Dabrafenib

Dabrafenib (Figure 5, GlaxoSmithKline PLC), a 4-(3-aminosulfonylphenyl)-5-(pyrimidin-3-yl) thiazole, is a highly selective and potent adenosine triphosphate-competitive BRAF inhibitor with >100-fold selectivity for mutant BRAF over wild-type BRAF in cell lines. In addition, dabrafenib leads to dose-dependent inhibition of MEK and ERK phosphorylation in BRAF mutant cell lines, and it induces tumor regression in melanoma xenografts. Dabrafenib was first clinically tested in study BRF112680, which was the first phase I human dose escalation study designed to evaluate its clinical efficacy, safety, and pharmacokinetics. Preliminary analysis of the initial phase I trial and an extended phase II cohort indicated that dabrafenib was active in the treatment of intracerebral melanoma metastases, with commensurate extracranial activity. In 21 of 34 subjects with BRAF V600E mutant melanoma, the clinical activity at dosages of 150 mg twice daily was determined on the basis of the objective tumor responses, judged using RECIST criteria, observed as soon as 8 weeks after treatment initiation, although the corresponding response rate in melanomas harboring V600K mutation was considerably lower at 19% [36]. In August 2012, GSK applied for the US and EU approval of dabrafenib for unresectable or metastatic melanoma with BRAF V600 mutations.

4.4. Vemurafenib

Recently, the highly specific and potent BRAF V600E inhibitor, designated as vemurafenib (Figure 6, RO5185426, RG7204, PLX4032; Plexxikon Inc.), has delivered highly promising results. It was launched in the US after FDA approval for BRAF V600E mutation-positive unresectable or metastatic melanoma in 2011 and in the UK in 2012. In a phase III randomized, controlled trial, patients with metastatic melanoma and BRAF mutation received first-line

http://dx.doi.org/10.5772/54938

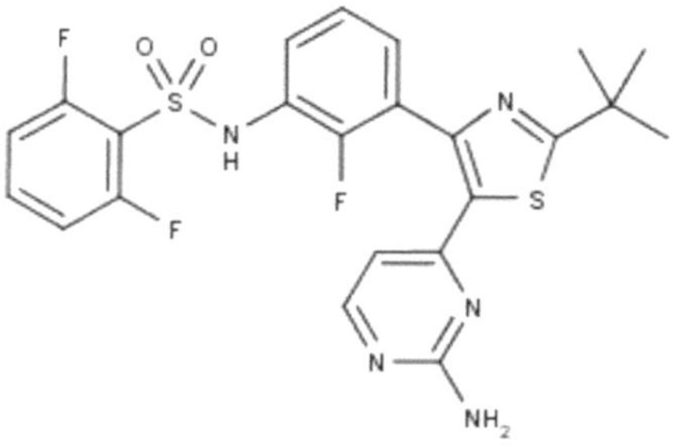

Figure 5. Chemical structure of dabrafenib.

treatment with vemurafenib or dacarbazine, and the primary endpoint was OS. These results showed that in addition to improved OS, vemurafenib significantly reduced the risks of death and disease progression by 63% and 74%, respectively, compared with dacarbazine. The response rate in patients who received vemurafenib was 48.4%, which was almost 9 times higher than that in patients who received chemotreatment (5.5%). Furthermore, 84% of the patients who received vemurafenib were alive after 6 months compared with 64% who received chemotreatment, i.e., the median OS with vemurafenib (10.5 months) was longer than that with dacarbazine [37]. Vemurafenib produced improved OS and PFS rates in patients. Thus, it offers a novel, first-line, personalized treatment for patients with mutated BRAF [38].

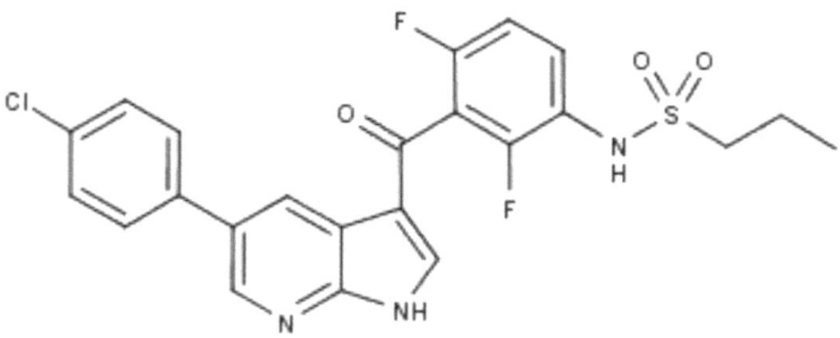

Figure 6. Chemical structure of vemurafenib.

4.5. Selumetinib

MEK is a protein that belongs to the MAPK pathway downstream of BRAF. Selumetinib (Figure 7, AZD6244; AstraZeneca), an orally available selective inhibitor of MEK1/2, was developed for the potential treatment of patients with cancers, such as NSCLC, pancreatic cancer, colorectal cancer, biliary cancer, and thyroid carcinoma, in phase II trials [39]. By 2006, a phase II trial was underway to compare selumetinib with temozolomide for unresectable late-stage malignant melanoma. However, disappointing data were reported in December 2007, and Astra Zeneca reported that it did not plan to advance selumetinib as a monotreatment for melanoma and would investigate other options. In March 2010, the enrollment of 91 patients was completed in a phase II trial of selumetinib in combination with dacarbazine compared with dacarbazine alone for the first-line treatment of melanoma with BRAF mutation. In January 2012, the top-line data were expected in the first half of 2012. By November 2010, AstraZeneca had begun a phase II trial of the drug plus temozolomide in patients with metastatic melanoma of the eye. The trial was ongoing in January 2011. In May 2008, a phase II trial of selumetinib plus chemotreatment for melanoma was planned to start in the second half of 2008. By June 2006, selumetinib had entered a phase II trial for malignant melanoma. The randomized, open-label, multicenter trial compared the drug with temozolomide in 180 patients with unresectable stage III/IV disease. Astra Zeneca began dosing patients in the trial in September 2006. The top-line data reported in December 2007 showed that the drug had failed to improve PFS. At that time, Astra Zeneca did not plan to conduct a phase III trial for this indication and was considering other options. Additional data were presented at the 44th ASCO annual meeting; however, no significant difference was observed in the primary endpoint of PFS in the overall group or mutation subgroup between the two treatment arms. Similar data were also reported in the interim analysis of OS. In February 2010, additional data were presented at the Biomarkers Fifth Annual Congress in Manchester, UK. Patients harboring bRaf gene mutations showed some signs of better clinical responses. In June 2010, similar data were presented at the 46th ASCO meeting in Chicago, IL. A 12% response rate was observed in patients with bRaf mutations. Further results were expected. By November 2010, enrollment was completed.

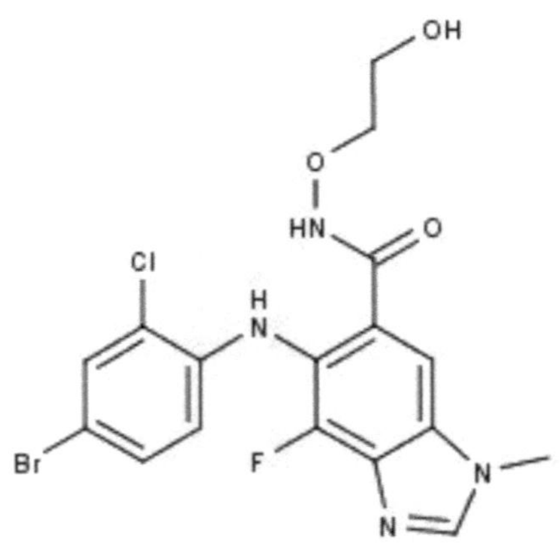

Figure 7. Chemical structure of selumetinib.

5. AKT inhibitors for melanoma treatment

The phosphoinositide 3-kinase (PI3K) pathway is an important driver of cell proliferation and survival, particularly in cells that respond to growth factor receptor engagement. The

http://dx.doi.org/10.5772/54938

PI3K/AKT/mTOR pathway is another signaling transduction pathway that is aberrantly activated in several cancers, including melanoma [40]. As shown in Table 4, AKT inhibitor such as perifosine is under evaluation for melanoma.

Name	Mechanisms
Perifosine	AKT inhibitor

Table 4. Clinical trials of AKT inhibitors for treating melanoma

Aeterna Zentaris is developing perifosine (Figure 8), an oral alkylphosphocholine signal transduction modulator that inhibits Akt activation in the PI3K pathway, for the potential treatment of various cancers, but primarily MM, neuroblastoma, and RCC. In December 2009, a phase III trial began for MM. In May 2012, Aeterna Zentaris stated that it was continuing phase III MM trials in North America. In August 2011, a phase I trial for recurrent pediatric solid tumors was ongoing. In June 2012, data from the phase I/Ib study were presented. Later that month, the results of two RCC phase II trials were reported. The licensees, Handok Pharmaceuticals, Yakult Honsha, and Hikma, are developing the drug for various cancers, including colorectal cancer. In January 2012, Yakult Honsha initiated a phase I/II trial in patients with refractory advanced colorectal cancer in Japan. In June 2012, Yakult Honsha initiated a phase I combination trial for MM in Japan. Keryx previously collaborated with Aeterna Zentaris for producing drugs to treat various cancers. In December 2009, Keryx began a phase III trial for MM. In December 2011, it was reported that the trial was actively recruiting patients in the US and Canada. In April 2012, Keryx and Aeterna Zentaris planned to evaluate whether the phase III trials for MM would continue as planned. In January 2012, the potential launch of the drug was anticipated by the end of the year, with the completion of the phase III MM trial at the beginning of 2013. In July 2009, Keryx initiated a phase I trial in pediatric patients with solid tumors. In June 2010, the data from the trial were reported. By June 2009, Keryx was developing the drug for colorectal cancer. In April 2010, a phase III trial was initiated. In April 2012, the results showed that the trial had failed to meet its primary endpoint. Later that month, the indication was no longer listed in Keryx's future projects, while in June 2012, it was no longer listed in Aeterna Zentaris's future projects. In July 2007, a phase II trial was initiated for RCC. In May 2009, the clinical data were presented. In June 2007, phase II data were reported for macroglobulinemia. In January 2010, additional data were reported. In February 2007, a phase I trial for ovarian cancer was initiated. In October 2011, the trial was ongoing. In December 2006, Keryx started a phase II trial for rare sarcomas. In November 2007, the preliminary results were reported. In October 2011, the trial was completed. In August 2006, a phase II trial was initiated for GIST. The trial was completed in October 2011. In March 2006, Keryx initiated phase II trials for refractory and relapsed leukemia. In October 2009, another phase II trial was initiated, and the data were reported in December 2010. Aeterna Zentaris had previously been developing the drug for NSCLC. In September 2005, a radio-treatment combination trial began for NSCLC. In June 2009, negative data were reported from the trial and the company planned to concentrate on MM and metastatic colon cancer. Aeterna

Zentaris was advised not to pursue trials in pancreatic cancer or head and neck cancer. Trials have also been conducted in prostate cancer, liver cancer, breast cancer, melanoma, and glioma.

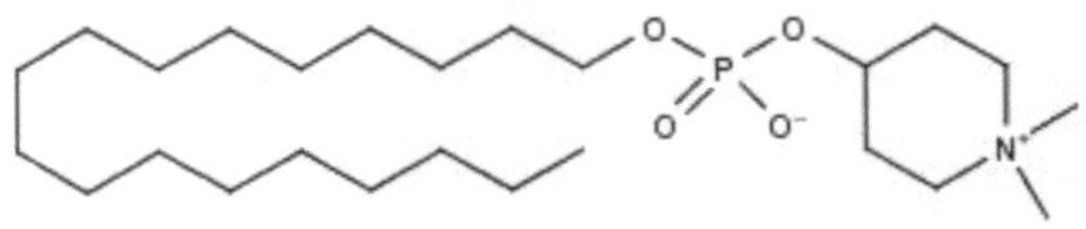

Figure 8. Chemical structure of perifosine.

6. mTOR inhibitors for melanoma treatment

Everolimus (RAD001, Afinitor) is an orally active inhibitor of Mammalian Target of Rapamycin complex 1 (mTORC1), a multifunctional signal transducing protein implicated in cancer [41]. Everolimus possesses antitumor and antiangiogenic/antivascular activities [42]. Previously, it was shown that the antiangiogenic/antivascular activities produced by mTORC1 inhibition using everolimus were partially overlapping, but they were also distinct from those following VEGFR inhibition by the TKI PTK/ZK (PTK787/ZK 222584; vatalanib) [43]. As shown in Table 5, everolimus is under evaluation for melanoma.

Name	Mechanisms
Everolimus	mTOR inhibitor

Table 5. Clinical trials of mTOR inhibitors for treating melanoma

Novartis has developed and launched everolimus (Figure 9), an oral analog of the mTOR inhibitor sirolimus, as an immunosuppressant to inhibit growth factor-induced cell proliferation and angiogenesis. The product is indicated in Europe and Japan under the trade name Certican for the prophylaxis of organ rejection in adults at low-to-moderate immunological risk of receiving an allogeneic renal or cardiac transplant. This product is also indicated under the trade name Zortress in the US to prevent organ rejection in adult kidney transplant recipients. Under the name Afinitor, everolimus is indicated for the second-line treatment of advanced RCC in Japan, after the failure of treatment with sunitinib or sorafenib in the US, or after the failure of treatment with VEGF-targeted treatment in the EU. It is also indicated for the treatment of patients with subependymal giant cell astrocytomas (SEGA) associated with tuberous sclerosis complex (TSC) who require therapeutic intervention but are not candidates for curative surgical resection, for the treatment of advanced neuroendocrine tumors (NET) of pancreatic origin, for the treatment of non-cancerous renal angiomyolipoma tumors that do not require immediate surgery in adult patients with TSC (in the US), and for use in combination with exemestane for the treatment of postmenopausal women with advanced hormone-

http://dx.doi.org/10.5772/54938

receptor positive, HER2-negative breast cancer after the failure of treatment with non-steroidal aromatase inhibitors, including letrozole or anastrozole. In April 2004, everolimus was launched as Certican in Germany for the prevention of heart and kidney transplant rejection and then in EU in 2005. In April 2010, everolimus was launched as Zortress in the US for the prevention of kidney transplant rejection in adults. In March 2007, everolimus was launched for heart transplant rejection in Japan. It was approved for renal transplant rejection in Japan in December 2011. In March 2009, everolimus was launched as Afinitor in the US for the second-line treatment of advanced RCC. In August 2009, the EC approved Afinitor for the second-line treatment of advanced RCC. In April 2010, Afinitor was launched in Japan for RCC. By June 2010, a phase II trial was underway for treatment-naive papillary RCC. In October 2010, Afinitor was approved in the US for the treatment of patients with SEGA associated with TS, while EU approval was granted in September 2011 under the trade name Votubia. In February 2012, a application was submitted in Japan for TS, while an additional dispersible tablet formulation for pediatric use was also applied for at the same time. In May 2011, everolimus was approved by the FDA for pancreatic NET. In September 2011, everolimus was approved in the EU for pancreatic NET. In December 2011, approval was granted in Japan for pancreatic NET. In July 2012, the FDA approved everolimus for use in combination with exemestane for the treatment of postmenopausal women with ER+/HER2− breast cancer after the failure of treatment with letrozole or anastrozole. In July 2012, the EC approved the drug for the treatment of ER+/HER2− advanced breast cancer in postmenopausal women without symptomatic visceral disease after recurrence or progression following treatment with a non-steroidal aromatase inhibitor. In April 2012, everolimus was approved in the US for the treatment of non-cancerous renal angiomyolipoma tumors that do not require immediate surgery in adult patients with TSC. An EU application for angiomyolipoma tumors not requiring immediate surgery in adult patients with TSC was filed in January 2012. The drug is also being developed for other solid tumor indications. By September 2008, phase III trials were underway investigating the use of the drug plus octreotide in the treatment of carcinoid tumors. In February 2009, applications for carcinoid cancer were planned for 2H09. A phase II trial for bladder cancer began in December 2008. In May 2010, a phase III trial began for advanced HCC. In January 2011, an application for HCC was expected in 2013. In June 2010, a phase III program for advanced ER+ and HER2+ breast cancer was ongoing in first- and second-line settings. In July 2009, phase II trials began for head and neck cancer. A phase I trial for colorectal cancer began in June 2010. In October 2010, a phase I trial was planned for cervical cancer. In June 2012, a phase I/II trial for glioma was planned to start in November 2012. A phase II trial for neurofibromas associated with neurofibromatosis was planned for December 2011. A phase I trial for esophageal cancer was planned for January 2012. Drugs are being developed for hematological tumors. A phase I trial for non-Hodgkin's lymphoma (NHL) began in March 2008, while development for NHL was ongoing in January 2012. In June 2009, phase III trials were initiated for diffuse large B-cell lymphoma. In January 2011, Novartis did not expect an application for this indication before 2015. In January 2010, a phase II trial was initiated for Hodgkin's lymphoma. The data were reported in December 2011. In June 2010, the data were reported from a phase I/II trial for multiple myeloma. In February 2008, a phase I trial began using patients with AML. In December 2011, a phase II extension study was planned. In December 2008, phase II data were presented for Waldenström's macroglobulinemia. Label extension during transplants was also ongoing. In March 2005, a phase III trial was initiated for lung transplantation. In September 2011, a second phase III trial began for lung transplant rejection. In January 2008, phase III trials for the prevention of liver transplant rejection were ongoing. In October 2011, a US regulatory application for liver transplant rejection was expected later in that year. Development for non-cancer indications was also ongoing. In December 2006, a phase III trial began for autosomal dominant polycystic kidney disease, and the results were published in August 2010. In February 2009, a phase II trial of everolimus in combination with ranibizumab for the potential treatment of age-related macular degeneration began. The drug was previously developed for the treatment of RA, inflammatory bowel disease, and genetic disorders. However, no development has been reported for these indications. In terms of cancer indications, everolimus was also previously developed for Kaposi's sarcoma, although this indication was discontinued by June 2011 because of lack of efficacy in phase II trials. Phase II development was underway by May 2005 for GIST, for hormone-refractory prostate cancer by August 2005, for small cell lung cancer by February 2006, and for NSCLC by June 2007. Phase II data for melanoma were also reported in June 2009.

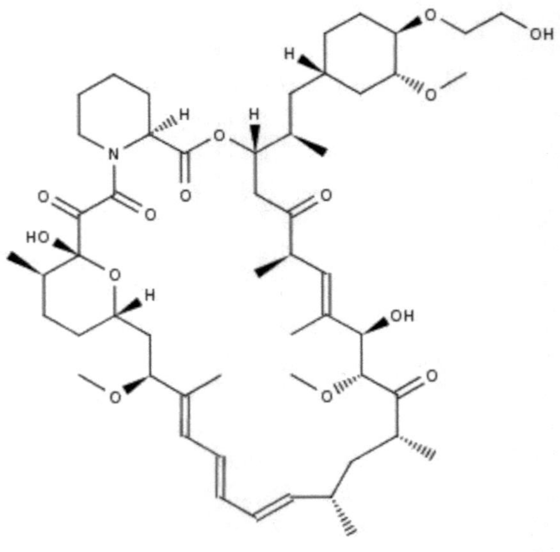

Figure 9. Chemical structure of everolimus.

7. Conclusions

This report reviews the clinical studies of recently developed targeted agents, including immune modulators, c-KIT inhibitors, BRAF/MEK inhibitors, AKT inhibitors, and mTOR

http://dx.doi.org/10.5772/54938

inhibitors, for the treatment of melanoma. Current research is focused on understanding the intrinsic mechanisms of these drugs. This will lead to rationally designed combinations of first- and second-line therapies, which will hopefully improve the efficacy and tolerability in selected groups of patients with melanoma. Understanding the molecular basis of melanoma and translating this knowledge into targeted treatment that improve the survival of patients with advanced melanoma is very important. Immune modulatory antibodies such as tremelimumab, ipilimumab, and BMS-663513 may have a crucial role in initiating and maintaining a melanoma-specific immune response.

Acknowledgements

We thank the National Science Council in Taiwan for grant support (NSC 99-2313-B-030-001-MY3).

Author details

Hsiang-Wen Tseng[1], Wen-Tai Li[+2] and Jung-Feng Hsieh[+3*]

*Address all correspondence to: 075101@mail.fju.edu.tw

1 Industrial Technology Research Institute, Biomedical Thechnology and Device Research Laboratories, Taiwan

2 National Research Institute of Chinese Medicine, Taiwan

3 Department of Food Science, Fu Jen Catholic University, Taiwan

[+]Wen-Tai Li and Jung-Feng Hsieh contributed equally to this work.

References

[1] Melero, I, Hervas-stubbs, S, Glennie, M, Pardoll, D. M, & Chen, L. (2007). Immunostimulatory monoclonal antibodies for cancer therapy. Nature reviews Cancer, , 7, 95-106.

[2] Phan, G. Q, Yang, J. C, Sherry, R. M, Hwu, P, Topalian, S. L, Schwartzentruber, D. J, Restifo, N. P, Haworth, L. R, Seipp, C. A, Freezer, L. J, Morton, K. E, Mavroukakis, S. A, Duray, P. H, Steinberg, S. M, Allison, J. P, Davis, T. A, & Rosenberg, S. A. (2003). Cancer regression and autoimmunity induced by cytotoxic T lymphocyte-associated

antigen 4 blockade in patients with metastatic melanoma. Proc. Natl. Acad. Sci. USA., 100, 8372-8377.

[3] Ribas, A, Camacho, L. H, Lopez-berestein, G, Pavlov, D, Bulanhagui, C. A, Millham, R, Comin-anduix, B, Reuben, J. M, Seja, E, Parker, C. A, Sharma, A, Glaspy, J. A, & Gomez-navarro, J. (2005). Antitumor activity in melanoma and anti-self responses in a phase I trial with the anti-cytotoxic T lymphocyte-associated antigen 4 monoclonal antibody CP-675,206. J. Clin. Oncol., 23, 8968-8977.

[4] Leach, D. R, Krummel, M. F, & Allison, J. P. (1996). Enhancement of antitumor immunity by CTLA-4 blockade. Science,, 271, 1734-1736.

[5] Korman, A. J, Peggs, K. S, & Allison, J. P. (2006). Checkpoint blockade in cancer immunotherapy. Adv. Immunol., 90, 297-339.

[6] Ribas, A. (2010). Clinical development of the anti-CTLA-4 antibody tremelimumab. Semin. Oncol., 37, 450-454.

[7] Ribas, A, Hauschild, A, Kefford, R, Punt, C. A, Haanen, J. B, Marmol, M, Garbe, C, Gomez-navarro, J, Pavlov, D, & Marshall, M. (2008). Phase III, open-Label, randomized, comparative study of tremelimumab (CP-675,206) and chemotherapy (temozolomide or dacarbazine) in patients with advanced melanoma. J. Clin. Oncol. 26, abstr 9011.

[8] Marshall, M, Ribas, A, & Huang, B. (2010). Evaluation of baseline serum C-reactive protein and benefit from tremelimumab compared to chemotherapy in first-line melanoma. J Clin Oncol. 28, abstr 2609.

[9] Pfizer IncDebiopharm Group. (2010). Pfizer and Debiopharm collaborate to co-develop investigational compound tremelimumab (CP-675,206) in advanced melanoma. www.debiopharm.com.

[10] Chambers, C. A, Kuhns, M. S, Egen, J. G, & Allison, J. P. (2001). CTLA-4-mediated inhibition in regulation of T cell responses: mechanisms and manipulation in tumor immunotherapy. Annu. Rev. Immunol., 19, 565-594.

[11] Juszczak, A, Gupta, A, Karavitaki, N, Middleton, M. R, & Grossman, A. B. (2012). Ipilimumab: a novel immunomodulating therapy causing autoimmune hypophysitis: a case report and review. Eur. J. Endocrinol., 167, 1-5.

[12] Hanaizi, Z, Van Zwieten-boot, B, Calvo, G, Lopez, A. S, Van Dartel, M, Camarero, J, Abadie, E, & Pignatti, F. (2012). The European Medicines Agency review of ipilimumab (Yervoy) for the treatment of advanced (unresectable or metastatic) melanoma in adults who have received prior therapy: summary of the scientific assessment of the Committee for Medicinal Products for Human Use. Eur. J. Cancer., 48, 237-242.

[13] Robert, C, Thomas, L, Bondarenko, I, O'Day, S, M D, J. W, Garbe, C, Lebbe, C, Baurain, J. F, Testori, A, Grob, J. J, Davidson, N, Richards, J, Maio, M, Hauschild, A, Miller, W. H. Jr, Gascon, P, Lotem, M, Harmankaya, K, Ibrahim, R, Francis, S, Chen, T. T,

Humphrey, R, Hoos, A, & Wolchok, J. D.(2011). Ipilimumab plus dacarbazine for previously untreated metastatic melanoma. N. Engl. J. Med. , 364, 2517-2526.

[14] Vaubel, J. M, Linette, G. P, Hogg, D, Ottensmeier, C. H, Lebbé, C, Peschel, C, Quirt, I, Clark, J. I, Wolchok, J. D, Weber, J. S, Tian, J, Yellin, M. J, Nichol, G. M, Hoos, A, & Urba, W. J.(2010). Improved survival with ipilimumab in patients with metastatic melanoma. N. Engl. J. Med. , 363, 711-723.

[15] Tarhini, A. A, Edington, H, Butterfield, L. H, Sinha, M, Moschos, S. J, Tawbi, H, & Shuai, Y. (2011). Neoadjuvant ipilimumab in patients with stage IIIB/C melanoma: immunogenicity and biomarker analysis. J. Clin. Oncol. 29, abstr 8536.

[16] Graziani, G, Tentori, L, & Navarra, P. (2012). Ipilimumab: a novel immunostimulatory monoclonal antibody for the treatment of cancer. Pharmacol. Res. , 65, 9-22.

[17] Molckovsky, A, & Siu, L. L. (2008). First-in-class, first-in-human phase I results of targeted agents: highlights of the 2008 American society of clinical oncology meeting. J. Hematol. Oncol. , 29, 1-20.

[18] Melero, I, Murillo, O, Dubrot, J, Hervás-stubbs, S, & Perez-gracia, J. L. (2008). Multilayered action mechanisms of CD137 (4-1BB)-targeted immunotherapies. Trends. Pharmacol. Sci. , 29, 383-390.

[19] Sznol, M, Hodi, F. S, Margolin, K, Mcdermott, D. F, Ernstoff, M. S, Kirkwood, J. M, Wojtaszek, C, Feltquate, D, & Logan, T. (2008). Phase I study of BMS-663513 a fully human anti-CD137 agonist monoclonal antibody, in patients (pts) with advanced cancer (CA). J. Clin. Oncol. 26, abstr 3007.

[20] Martí, R. M, Sorolla, A, & Yeramian, A. (2012). New therapeutic targets in melanoma. Actas. Dermosifiliogr. , 103, 579-590.

[21] Yoshida, H, Kunisada, T, Grimm, T, Nishimura, E. K, Nishioka, E, & Nishikawa, S. I. (2001). Review: melanocyte migration and survival controlled by SCF/c-kit expression. J. Investig. Dermatol. Symp. Proc. , 6, 1-5.

[22] Curtin, J. A, Busam, K, Pinkel, D, & Bastian, B. C. (2006). Somatic activation of KIT in distinct subtypes of melanoma. J. Clin. Oncol. , 24, 4340-4346.

[23] Finn, L, Markovic, S. N, & Joseph, R. W. (2012). Therapy for metastatic melanoma: the past, present, and future. BMC Med. 10, 23.

[24] Spagnolo, F, & Queirolo, P. (2012). Upcoming strategies for the treatment of metastatic melanoma. Arch. Dermatol. Res. , 304, 177-184.

[25] Carvajal, R. D, Antonescu, C. R, Wolchok, J. D, Chapman, P. B, Roman, R. A, Teitcher, J, Panageas, K. S, Busam, K. J, Chmielowski, B, Lutzky, J, Pavlick, A. C, Fusco, A, Cane, L, Takebe, N, Vemula, S, Bouvier, N, Bastian, B. C, & Schwartz, G. K. (2011). KIT as a therapeutic target in metastatic melanoma. JAMA. , 305, 2327-2334.

[26] Raman, M, Chen, W, & Cobb, M. H. (2007). Differential regulation and properties of MAPKs. Oncogene. , 26, 3100-3112.

[27] Davies, H, Bignell, G. R, Cox, C, Stephens, P, Edkins, S, Clegg, S, Teague, J, Woffendin, H, Garnett, M. J, Bottomley, W, Davis, N, Dicks, E, Ewing, R, Floyd, Y, Gray, K, Hall, S, Hawes, R, Hughes, J, Kosmidou, V, Menzies, A, Mould, C, Parker, A, Stevens, C, Watt, S, Hooper, S, Wilson, R, Jayatilake, H, Gusterson, B. A, Cooper, C, Shipley, J, Hargrave, D, Pritchard-jones, K, Maitland, N, Chenevix-trench, G, Riggins, G. J, Bigner, D. D, Palmieri, G, Cossu, A, Flanagan, A, Nicholson, A, Ho, J. W, Leung, S. Y, Yuen, S. T, Weber, B. L, Seigler, H. F, Darrow, T. L, Paterson, H, Marais, R, Marshall, C. J, Wooster, R, Stratton, M. R, & Futreal, P. A. (2002). Mutations of the BRAF gene in human cancer. Nature. , 417, 949-954.

[28] Davar, D, & Kirkwood, J. M. (2012). New therapies in the treatment of melanoma. Expert. Opin. Investig. Drugs. 21, 1643-1659.

[29] Long, G. V, Menzies, A. M, Nagrial, A. M, Haydu, L. E, Hamilton, A. L, Mann, G. J, Hughes, T. M, Thompson, J. F, Scolyer, R. A, & Kefford, R. F. (2011). Prognostic and clinicopathologic associations of oncogenic BRAF in metastatic melanoma. J. Clin. Oncol. , 29, 1239-1246.

[30] Mangana, J, Levesque, M. P, Karpova, M. B, & Dummer, R. Sorafenib in melanoma. (2012). Expert. Opin. Investig. Drugs. , 21, 557-568.

[31] Hauschild, A, Agarwala, S. S, Trefzer, U, Hogg, D, Robert, C, Hersey, P, Eggermont, A, Grabbe, S, Gonzalez, R, Gille, J, Peschel, C, Schadendorf, D, Garbe, C, Day, O, Daud, S, White, A, Xia, J. M, Patel, C, Kirkwood, K, & Keilholz, J. M. U. (2009). Results of a phase III, randomized, placebo-controlled study of sorafenib in combination with carboplatin and paclitaxel as second-line treatment in patients with unresectable stage III or stage IV melanoma. J. Clin. Oncol. , 27, 2823-2830.

[32] Wellbrock, C, & Hurlstone, A. (2010). BRAF as therapeutic target in melanoma. Biochem. Pharmacol. , 80, 561-567.

[33] Smalley, K. S, Xiao, M, Villanueva, J, Nguyen, T. K, Flaherty, K. T, Letrero, R, Van Belle, P, Elder, D. E, Wang, Y, Nathanson, K. L, & Herlyn, M. (2009). CRAF inhibition induces apoptosis in melanoma cells with non-BRAF mutations. Oncogene. 28, 85-94.

[34] Su, Y, Vilgelm, A. E, Kelley, M. C, Hawkins, O. E, Liu, Y, Boyd, K. L, Kantrow, S, Splittgerber, R. C, Short, S. P, Sobolik, T, Zaja-milatovic, S, Dahlman, K. B, Amiri, K. I, Jiang, A, Lu, P, Shyr, Y, Stuart, D. D, Levy, S, Sosman, J. A, & Richmond, A. (2012). RAF265 inhibits the growth of advanced human melanoma tumors. Clin. Cancer Res. , 18, 2184-2198.

[35] Sharfman, W. H, Hodi, F. S, & Lawrence, D. P. (2011). Results from the first-inhuman (FIH) phase I study of the oral RAF inhibitor RAF265 administered daily to patients with advanced cutaneous melanoma. ASCO Annual Meeting. 2011, 8508.

[36] Kefford, R, Arkenau, H, Brown, M. P, Millward, M, Infante, J. R, Long, G. V, Ouellet, D, Curtis, M, Lebowitz, P. F, & Falchook, G. S. (2010). Phase I/II study of GSK2118436, a selective inhibitor of oncogenic mutant BRAF kinase, in patients with metastatic melanoma and other solid tumors. J. Clin. Oncol. 28, 15s.

[37] Chapman, P. B, Hauschild, A, Robert, C, Haanen, J. B, Ascierto, P, Larkin, J, Dummer, R, Garbe, C, Testori, A, Maio, M, Hogg, D, Lorigan, P, Lebbe, C, Jouary, T, Schadendorf, D, Ribas, A, Day, O, Sosman, S. J, Kirkwood, J. A, Eggermont, J. M, Dreno, A. M, Nolop, B, Li, K, Nelson, J, Hou, B, Lee, J, Flaherty, R. J, Mcarthur, K. T, & Brim-3, G. A. Study Group. (2011). Improved survival with vemurafenib in melanoma with BRAF mutation. N. Engl. J. Med. 364, 2507-2516., 600E

[38] Heakal, Y, Kester, M, & Savage, S. (2011). Vemurafenib (PLX4032): an orally available inhibitor of mutated BRAF for the treatment of metastatic melanoma. Ann. Pharmacother. , 45, 1399-1405.

[39] Troiani, T, Vecchione, L, Martinelli, E, Capasso, A, Costantino, S, Ciuffreda, L. P, Morgillo, F, Vitagliano, D, Aiuto, D, De Palma, E, Tejpar, R, Van Cutsem, S, De Lorenzi, E, Caraglia, M, Berrino, M, & Ciardiello, L. F. (2012). Intrinsic resistance to selumetinib, a selective inhibitor of MEK1/2, by cAMP-dependent protein kinase A activation in human lung and colorectal cancer cells. Br. J. Cancer. , 106, 1648-1659.

[40] Cully, M, You, H, Levine, A. J, & Mak, T. W. (2006). Beyond PTEN mutations: the PI3K pathway as an integrator of multiple inputs during tumorigenesis. Nat. Rev. Cancer. , 6, 184-192.

[41] O'Reilly, T, Lane, H. A, Wood, J. M, Schnell, C, Littlewood-Evans, A, Brueggen, J, & McSheehy, P. M. (2011) Everolimus and PTK/ZK show synergistic growth inhibition in the orthotopic BL16/BL6 murine melanoma model. Cancer Chemother Pharmacol., 67, 193-200.

[42] Lane, H. A, Wood, J. M, Mcsheehy, P. M, Allegrini, P. R, Boulay, A, Brueggen, J, Littlewood-evans, A, Maira, S. M, Martiny-baron, G, & Schnell, C. R. Sini, P. & O'Reilly, T. (2009). mTOR inhibitor RAD001 (everolimus) has antiangiogenic/vascular properties distinct from a VEGFR tyrosine kinase inhibitor. Clin. Cancer Res. , 15, 1612-1622.

[43] Wood, J. M, Bold, G, Buchdunger, E, Cozens, R, Ferrari, S, Frei, J, Hofmann, F, Mestan, J, Mett, H, O'Reilly, T, Persohn, E, Rösel, J, Schnell, C, Stover, D, Theuer, A, Towbin, H, Wenger, F, Woods-Cook, K, Menrad, A, Siemeister, G, Schirner, M, Thierauch, K. H, Schneider, M. R, Drevs, J, Martiny-Baron, G, & Totzke, F. (2000). PTK787/ZK 222584, a novel and potent inhibitor of vascular endothelial growth factor receptor tyrosine kinases, impairs vascular endothelial growth factor-induced responses and tumor growth after oral administration. Cancer Res., 60, 2178-2189.

Chapter 11

Porphyrin and Phthalocyanine Photosensitizers as PDT Agents: A New Modality for the Treatment of Melanoma

Shawn Swavey and Matthew Tran

Additional information is available at the end of the chapter

http://dx.doi.org/10.5772/54940

1. Introduction

1.1. Melanoma — Background

In the United States, skin cancer is the most common type of cancer, which is further divided into three types of cancer: basal cell, squamous cell and melanoma. Basal cell and squamous cell cancers are the most common types of skin cancer, but they are less deadly and more readily treated than melanoma. While it is the least common of the skin cancers, more than 68,000 Americans are diagnosed with melanoma each year, and an additional 48,000 are diagnosed with early forms of cancer that involve the top layer of the skin. [1] It is the leading cause of death from skin cancer, due to its metastatic behavior. The frequency of melanoma has more than doubled in the past thirty years, especially in Western industrialized societies. [2]

Melanoma is a malignant tumor that originates in the melanocytes. Melanocytes are found randomly throughout the basal cells and are found in the deepest portions of the epidermis. They are responsible for making the pigments (melanin) found in the skin. The level of pigment released by melanocytes is directly related to skin color. It has been found that exposure to ultraviolet radiation triggers the melanocytes to create more pigments, which leads to what we observe as tanned skin. Studies show that melanoma has different, common locations of occurrence in men and women. [1] Men have been found to commonly develop melanoma on the skin of the head, neck, between the shoulders and the hips, whereas women often develop melanoma on the skin of the lower legs or between the shoulders or hips. Melanoma can occur on any skin surface, but it is more prone to develop on preexisting moles. There are five stages of melanoma [1]; Stage 0; Melanoma is only located in the top layer of the skin and the basil lamina is intact. This is referred to as *melanoma in situ*, Stage I; the melanoma lies in the epidermis. The tumor is no more than 1 mm thick and has penetrated the basil lamina and extended into the papillary dermis, Stage II; The tumor is between 1 and 2 mm thick and extends into the papillary-reticular dermis interface, Stage III; The tumor extends into the reticular dermis and the melanoma cells have spread into at least one lymph node or to nearby tissues, and Stage IV; The cancer cells have metastasized to the lungs or other organs, skin areas, or lymph nodes far from the original growth. The tumor has also extended into the subcutaneous fat. Detecting melanoma early is crucial to the survival rate of the patient.

2. Risk factors for melanoma

There are several risk factors attributed to the development of melanoma in individuals. Exposure to ultraviolet radiation has been shown to be a major risk factor in the development of melanoma. Severe sunburns increase the likelihood of developing melanoma later in one's life. Although tanning decreases the likelihood of sunburns, it is not a method of counteracting cancer, for it increases the duration of sun exposure. In addition, individuals with fair skin or who are prone to severe, blistering sunburns are at a high risk of developing melanoma. Melanoma is far less common in dark skinned individuals. In addition, the duration of sun exposure over one's life is a factor in the risk of radiation induced melanoma. A person who has lived most of his/her life in an area of high sun exposure is more likely to develop melanoma. Similarly, people who live in higher altitudes, where the sun is stronger, are at a greater risk for developing melanoma than those who live at lower altitudes. Another risk factor is personal history of melanoma. An individual who has been diagnosed with melanoma before is likely to contract another form of melanoma. In addition, someone who has been diagnosed with basal cell or squamous cell skin cancer is at a high risk of developing another form of skin cancer, including melanoma. Family history of the disease is also a contributing factor. Individuals who have ancestral cases of melanoma are at a high risk of developing the disease themselves. The risk of developing melanoma is increased when the family incidences are in one's immediate family. Approximately 8-12% of cases of cutaneous melanoma are inherited. [3]

3. Current treatment regimens for melanoma

There are several existing treatments for melanoma, including surgery, chemotherapy [4], radiation therapy [5], biological therapy [6], and to a lesser extent, photodynamic therapy. These treatments can be used in any combination to varying degrees of success. Since melanoma is typically a more invasive form of skin cancer, many of these treatments act as deterrents rather than cures. However, if the melanoma is diagnosed and treated early enough, it can be cured with a high degree of success.

The primary treatment for melanoma is surgery. In the surgical process, the tumor is excised along with some of the surrounding healthy tissue so that there is a minimal chance of leaving cancer cells in the area. Chemotherapy is another fairly common procedure for treating melanoma. Chemotherapy is a type of cancer treatment that relies on drugs in order to stop or slow the growth of cancer cells. However, chemotherapy indiscriminately harms healthy cells that also grow rapidly, such as those located in the mouth, intestines, and hair. The effectiveness of chemotherapy relies on the type and severity of the cancer in question, and depending on the aforementioned factors, it can cure, control, or ease cancer. Chemotherapy can be administered alone, but it is typically used in conjunction with other cancer treatments, such as biological therapy, radiation therapy, or surgery. The treatment can be administered in a variety of ways: injection, intra-arterial, intraperitoneal, intravenous, topical, or oral. The therapy sessions are spread out so that there is a recovery period in between treatments.

Radiation therapy is another type of therapy used in the treatment of melanoma. Like chemotherapy, radiation therapy can cure, stop, or slow cancer growth depending on the type and severity of the disease. Also similar to chemotherapy, radiation therapy is indiscriminate in its treatment, affecting nearby healthy cells in addition to the afflicted cells. Radiation therapy employs radiation to kill cancer cells, and this radiation can be administered either internally or externally. Because internal radiation therapy places the radiation source inside the body, it allows for a more precise treatment of the cancer in question than external beam treatment. Radiation therapy also possesses serious side effects, many of which can be more severe if chemotherapy is received in addition to radiation therapy. The most common side effects include fatigue and skin changes such as dryness, itching, peeling, or blistering. Biological therapy is also used as a cancer treatment. Biological therapy, like chemotherapy, relies on drugs in order to combat cancer. However, biological therapy differs from chemotherapy because it aids the immune system in fighting cancer. Like many of the other treatments, biological therapy can be used to stop or slow growth, and it makes it easier for the immune system to destroy cancer cells.

Although it has been around for over three decades and has been successfully used to treat other forms of skin cancer, photodynamic therapy (PDT) has not received as much attention especially in the United States as a treatment option for melanoma. The major reason for this lack of attention stems from the fact that PDT requires visible light of specific wavelengths to be effective; however, the pigments found particularly in melanoma block this light making PDT less effective. As will be described in this chapter, researchers are looking at innovative ways to develop PDT into a useful treatment option for melanoma.

4. Photodynamic Therapy (PDT)

4.1. Discovery and applications

Photodynamic therapy (PDT), the therapeutic use of light, was first discovered by Raab [7] when he reported that the combination of acridine orange and light could destroy living organisms. In the 1920's it was noted by Policard [8] that the effects of fluorescence were inherently more for tumor tissue than the healthy tissue. A great deal of research has been done on PDT, which represents an interesting treatment modality for numerous health related conditions, especially but not limited to cancer treatment. It is now believed that PDT also treats immunological effects (new antibiotics) [9], inflammation [10] and bacterial infections. [11]

Traditional cancer treatment includes radiation, surgery and/or chemotherapy, all of which have deleterious side effects. As an alternative to these treatments PDT offers a more targeted and less invasive treatment regimen. Until now, photodynamic therapy has been used for treatment of bladder cancers, brain cancers, breast metastases, skin cancers, gynecological malignancies, colorectal cancers, thoracic malignancies, and oral, head and neck cancers. [12]

Although it is not completely understood, researchers have reported that PDT activates and suppresses the immune system, [13] by a combination of effects that begins after the light treatment, the curative properties arise from the death of the irradiated cancer cells. The damage to the plasma membrane and membrane of the cellular organelles by singlet oxygen can trigger other events with far reaching consequences. The mechanism by which PDT induces specific immune responses has been suggested by Korbelik. [14] Summarizing, PDT-treated tissue release large quantities of cell debris, and inflammatory signals, cytokines and chemo-tactic agents which trigger the tissue to secrete immunosuppressive factors. The work of Musser [15] showed that PDT-induced immune suppression was also a function of the photosensitizer used.

Another PDT-induced effect is inflammation. It is reported that vascular destruction, observed after PDT is similar to the inflammatory response after tissue injury or bacterial infection. [16] This process is characterized by the release of a wide range of potent mediators including vasoactive substances, components of clotting cascades, proteinases, peroxidases, radicals, leucocytes, chemoattractants, cytokines, growth factors, and other immunoregulators.

5. Mechanisms of action for PDT

PDT typically utilizes a photosensitizer, molecular oxygen and light to destroy cancer cells. Two mechanisms [17] of the actions for PDT are recognized, Fig 1. In anoxic environments, the light induced excitation of the photosensitizer can promote an electron to a higher energy state. At this point a variety of reactions can take place. For example, this excited photosensitizer can react directly with organic substrates by electron exchange, filling the hole vacated by the excited electron, producing an oxidized substrate and reduced photosensitizer. Guanine, the most susceptible base to oxidation, is the presumed target leading to the formation of various oxo-guanine complexes and ultimately the decomposition of cellular DNA. [18] The reduced photosensitizer can react with oxygen to produce superoxide anions (O_2-) which can then form the highly reactive hydroxyl radical ($OH^{\bullet}$). The excited photosensitizer can also react with superoxide radicals ($O_2^{\bullet}$) to produce superoxide anions (O_2-) which can then create the highly reactive hydroxyl radical ($OH^{\bullet}$). Collectively these reactions are classified as Type-I photoreactions and are characterized by a dependence on the target-substrate concentration, Fig 2.

http://dx.doi.org/10.5772/54940

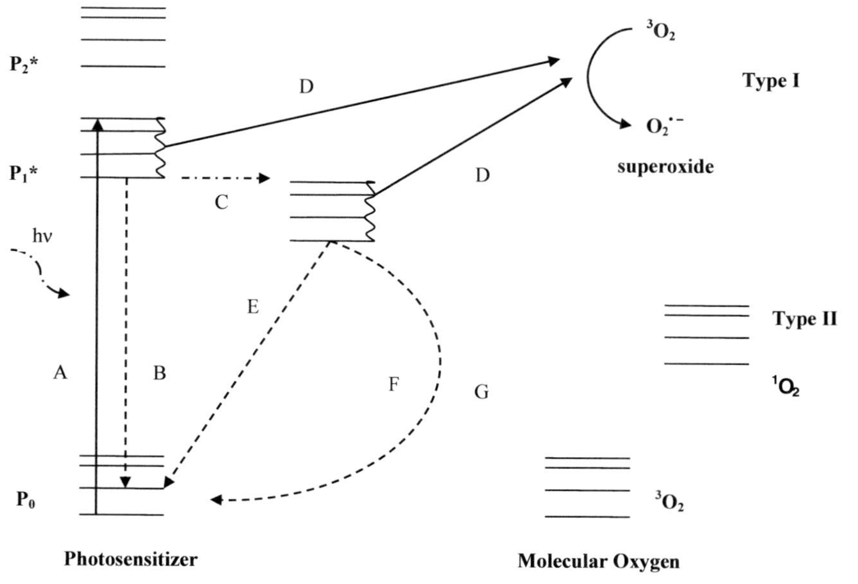

Figure 1. A diagram shows the various energy and electron transfer during PDT: (A) excitation; (B) fluorescence; (C) intersystem crossing; (D) electron transfer; (E) phosphorescence; (F) internal conversion; (G) non-radiated transfer of energy to singlet oxygen. P_0 is the ground state of photosensitizer, P_1* and P_2* are the excited state of photosensitizer, $^3O_2$ is the triplet ground state oxygen, $^1O_2$ is the singlet excited state oxygen

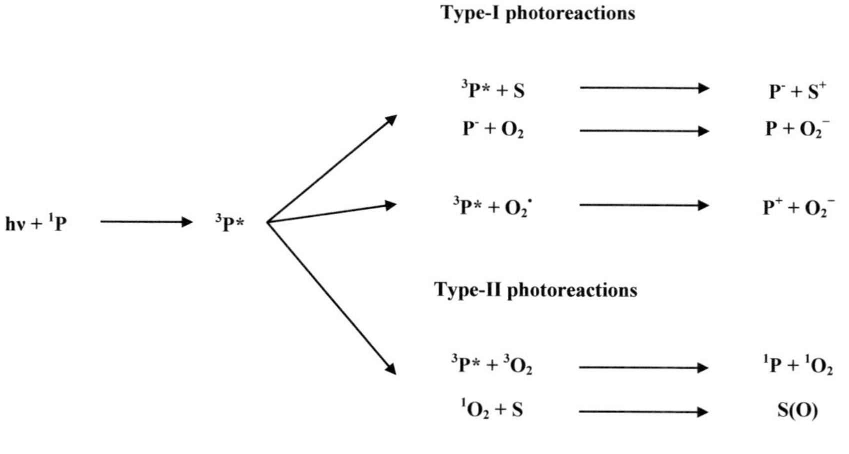

Figure 2. Type-I and type-II photoreactions, where ^1P is a photosensitizer in a singlet ground state, $^3P^*$ is a photosensitizer in a triplet excited state, S is a substrate molecule, P- is reduced photosensitizer molecule, S^+ is an oxidized substrate molecule, O_2 is molecule oxygen (triplet ground state), O_2- is the superoxide anion, $^3O_2$ is triplet ground-state oxygen, $^1O_2$ is singlet excited state, and S(O) is an oxygen adduct of a substrate.

The second mechanism also involves excitation of the photosensitizer with light but in this mechanism energy is transferred to the ground state of molecular oxygen resulting in excited singlet oxygen which goes on to destroy cellular function. [19] It was first identified that the cyto-toxic product of the photochemical reaction for PDT to be singlet oxygen by Weishaupt *et al.* in 1976. [20] The photosensitizer and oxygen interact through the triplet states because oxygen has a unique, triplet-ground state and low-lying excited states. The energy required for the triplet to singlet transition in oxygen is 22 kcal mol^{-1} which corresponds to the energy of a wavelength of 1274 nm (infrared light). [21] The energy needed to produce singlet oxygen is relatively low. Photochemical reactions of this type are known as Type-II photoreactions and are characterized by a dependence on oxygen concentration, Fig 2. [22] It is believed that the Type-II mechanism dominates during PDT. [23]

6. Photosensitizers

6.1. Development of photosensitizers and photofrin

Numerous attempts were made to treat tumor tissue with photosensitizing agents since the potential of photo treatment was discovered. Before the 1960s, scientists applied natural macrocycles to patients and tumor-bearing animals in an attempt to more accurately detect tumor tissue by florescence. [24-27] During the 1960s, Schwartz isolated a tumor localizing impurity from hematoporphyrin preparations that was later named hematoporphyrin derivative (HpD), Fig 3. Meanwhile, Lipson was investigating how to detect tumor tissue by fluorescence of hematoporphyrin. Unable to obtain reproducible results with hematoporphyrin, Lipson began experimenting with Schwartz's HpD. He used it as a tumor detection agent, [28] and first recognized that it could work as a photosensitizer to destroy tumor tissue. [29] In the 1970s, Dougherty's group discovered that fluorescein diacetate could photodynamically destroy TA-3 cells in vitro [30] and found that it could be used as a photosensitizer. [31] Following that, the group of Weishaupt identified that the cytotoxic product of photodynamic reaction to be singlet oxygen. [13] However, fluorescein has a low singlet oxygen quantum yield and a long wavelength absorption in the green portion of the electromagnetic spectrum that does not penetrate deeply into tissue. Macrocyclic photosensitizers were then examined as photosensitizers because they are efficient singlet oxygen generators and have absorption maxima in the red portion of the electromagnetic spectrum.

Eventually, Schwartz's Hpd was rediscovered by Dougherty, which by then was known to have a high singlet oxygen quantum yield, an absorption maximum in the red, and is selectively retained in tumor tissues. [30] After several years spent isolating and identifying the active fractions of HpD, a purified version named Photofrin®, was approved for use in the United States against early- and late-stage lung cancers and esophageal cancers and dysplasia with other indications pending. [30] This drug upon photoexcitation in the visible region (red) of the spectrum generates singlet oxygen from triplet oxygen through energy transfer (type II mechanism) resulting in cell death. [31]

http://dx.doi.org/10.5772/54940

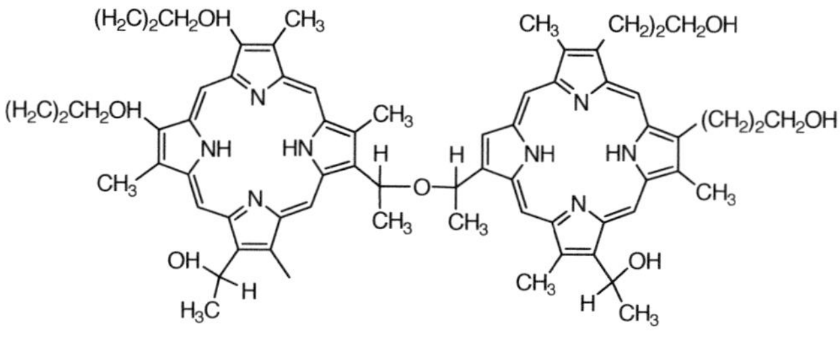

Marycin

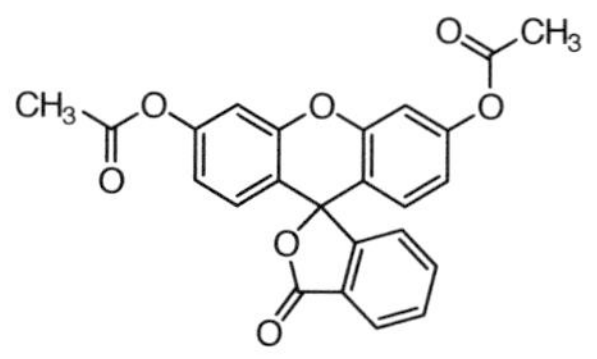

Fluorescein Diacetate

Figure 3. Marycin, an HpD isolated [28] in 1988 and Fluorescein diacetate

This chapter will focus on macrocycles (porphyrins and phthalocyanines) as potential photosensitizers for the treatment of melanoma by photodynamic therapy. There are a number of reviews of porphyrin and phthalocyanine photosensitizers and their use as PDT agents for a variety of cancers. [32-41]

7. Porphyrin Photosensitizers

7.1. Porphyrin background

Porphyrins have been extensively studied as potential photosensitizers in photodynamic therapy (PDT). [42]- [45] Their planar aromatic structure coupled with their photophysical properties and synthetic versatility has made them attractive components for PDT. [46] Although synthetic routes toward porphyrins leads to relatively low yields, their starting materials are typically inexpensive and their synthesis is generally straightforward, as illustrated for the porphyrin synthesis of *meso*-tetrapyridylporphyrin, Fig. 4. The synthesis typically requires reaction of pyrrole with the aldehyde of choice to give the appropriate substitution at the *meso*-positions. The *meso*-positions are indicated in Fig. 4 by the numbers 5, 10, 15, 20. Purification by column chromatography gives the desired porphyrin. As illustrated in the electronic spectra of Fig. 4 porphyrins display a very intense Soret band at approximately 410 nm and four lower energy Q-bands. The lowest energy Q-band, with absorptivities in the tens of thousands, at approximately 650 nm is the transition of interest for PDT. In addition, porphyrins have been associated with high affinity for tumor sites and efficient formation of ROS. [47] Specifically, cationic porphyrins have been studied primarily for their water solubility and their strong electrostatic interactions with negatively charged phosphate oxygen atoms of the DNA backbone. [48] This section will focus on studies, performed in the past decade, involving porphyrins as photosensitizers for the treatment of melanoma.

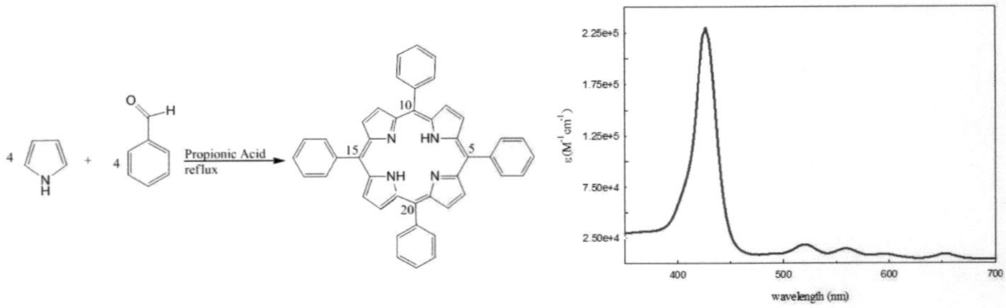

Figure 4. Synthesis and electronic spectra of *meso*-tetrapyridylporphyrin (H_2TPP).

8. Porphyrins, PDT and melanoma

In 1999 Busetti, Soncin and coworkers studied the effects of PDT on melanoma tumors in mice. [49] The inefficiency of Photofrin to treat highly pigmented melanoma has been related to the absorption of the wavelengths of light necessary to activate Photofrin by the melanin in the tumors. For this reason Busetti and coworkers chose a benzoporphyrin derivative monoacid ring A (BPD-MA), verteporfin, trade name visudyne, Fig. 5. Verteporfin has been used to eliminate abnormal blood vessels in the eye associated with macular degeneration.

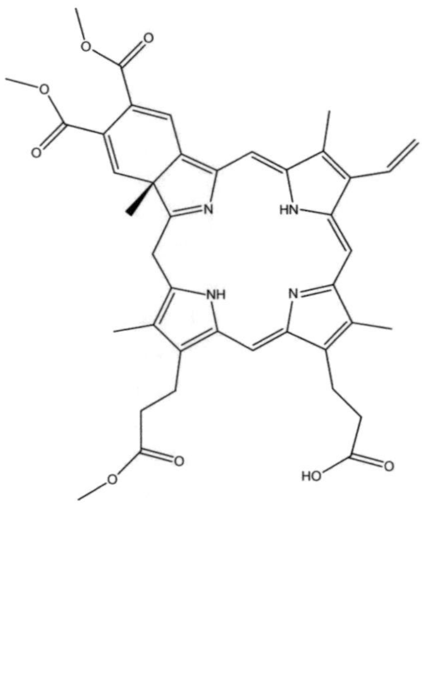

Figure 5. Structure of verteporfin.

The studies were conducted on C57/BL6 mice implanted with heavily pigmented melanoma B16. Injection of the photosensitizer, 5.5 μmol/kg body weight, was allowed 3 h for a maximum concentration to be reached in the cells. The researchers noted limited selectivity of BPD-MA toward tumor cells and adjacent tissue. The majority of the BPD-MA was cleared through the bile-gut pathway within 24 h of injection, with small amounts found in the liver. Irradiation of the tumors involved an argon-pump dye laser at 690 nm, within the photodynamic window of 600-800 nm. Three hours after injection of the photosensitizer the tumors were irradiated with energy of 520 mJ cm^{-2}. Large necrotic areas of the tumor were observed at this time as well as reduction in tumor growth. The researchers noted that mice implanted with B16 tumors and irradiated after injection of the photosensitizer were tumor free for up to two weeks after treatment. The phototoxicity observed for BPD-MA treated mice was not observed in tumors irradiated in the absence of the photosensitizer.

In a subsequent study researchers investigated a porphyrin dimer as a potential PDT agent for the treatment of melanoma. The dimer, 10, 15, 20-tritolylporphyrin-5-(4-amidophenyl)-[5-(4-phenyl)-10, 15, 20-tritolyporphyrin] (T-D), Fig. 6, was synthesized by the Adler method of refluxing mixed aromatic aldehydes with pyrrole in propionic acid. [50] The dimer (T-D) was synthesized from the monomeric porphyrin units by a known literature method.

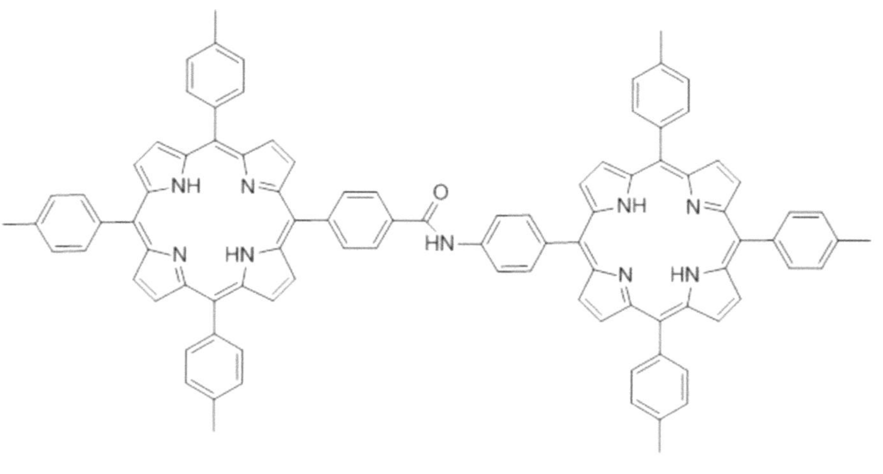

Figure 6. Structure of 10, 15, 20-tritolylporphyrin-5-(4-amidophenyl)-[5-(4-phenyl)-10, 15, 20-tritolyporphyrin] (T-D)

The electronic spectra of the dimer displayed an intense Soret band at 423 nm with less intense Q-bands at 517, 552, 592, and 649 nm in organic solvents. Photoexcitation for PDT treatment focused on the 649 band, although its molar absorptivity was relatively low (7550 M^{-1} cm^{-1}). Singlet oxygen generation for the excited dimer gave a very high quantum yield of 0.8. Due to the complexes insolubility in aqueous buffer solutions the dimer was dissolved in dimethyl sulfoxide (DMSO) and diluted to 10^{-8} to 10^{-5} M concentrations in aqueous phosphate buffer for the cell studies.

Photodynamic experiments were performed on human (SKMEL 188) melanoma cells and mouse (S91) melanoma cells. The melanoma cells were incubated with various concentrations of the T-D solutions for 24 h before irradiation. Melanoma cells incubated with 10^{-7} M T-D phosphate buffer solutions were irradiated with an LH313K lamp filtered to cut off wavelengths below 630 nm. Energy doses between 13.5 and 82 J cm^{-2} were used with irradiation times of 30 min. Cells were incubated for 36 h after irradiation before determining cell death. Both human and mouse melanoma cells showed a 3-fold decrease in size compared to cells irradiated without T-D at 81 J cm^{-2}. Although the dimer is insoluble in aqueous solutions and requires high energy irradiation for phototoxicity the authors point out that this complex has some distinct advantages over Photofrin for the treatment of pigmented melanoma, namely, chemical homogeneity, low aggregation (which can lead to excited state quenching), and good solubility in hydrophobic base with relatively long-lived triplet excited states, leading to significant singlet oxygen production.

9. Halogenated porphyrins

Synthetically enhancing porphyrins as PDT agents has been achieved through incorporation of halogens into the porphyrin structure. [51-54] Halogens covalently bound to phenyl groups at the *meso*-positions promote intersystem crossing, increasing singlet oxygen production; for example, halogenated tetraaryl porphyrins combined through a diarylethyne linker (where the halogens are chloro and fluoro substituted phenyl groups), Fig 7, had significantly longer excited state lifetimes when compared to their non-halogenated analogs. [51]

In addition, PDT agents with fluorophenyl substituents have been efficiently converted to porphyrin-saccharide conjugates to enhance their uptake in cancer cells, while in a separate study water soluble fluorinated porphyrins have shown more efficient PDT activity than their non-fluorinated counterparts. [53,54]

Researchers in 2007 looked at a water soluble porphyrin incorporating chloro groups. [55] The porphyrin, 5, 10, 15, 20-tetrakis-(2-chloro-3-sulfophenyl)porphyrin ($TCPPSO_3H$), Fig. 8, was synthesized by reacting 2-chlorobenzaldeyde with pyrrole by the method of Adler and Longo, followed by sulfonation. The electronic spectrum of the complex is typical of porphyrins with an intense Soret band and four lower energy lower intensity Q-bands. The lowest energy Q-band at 633 nm displayed a molar absorptivity of 504 $M^{-1}cm^{-1}$ in aqueous pH 7 phosphate buffer. Singlet oxygen quantum yields were determined to be 0.74, significantly higher than the non-halogenated analog.

http://dx.doi.org/10.5772/54940

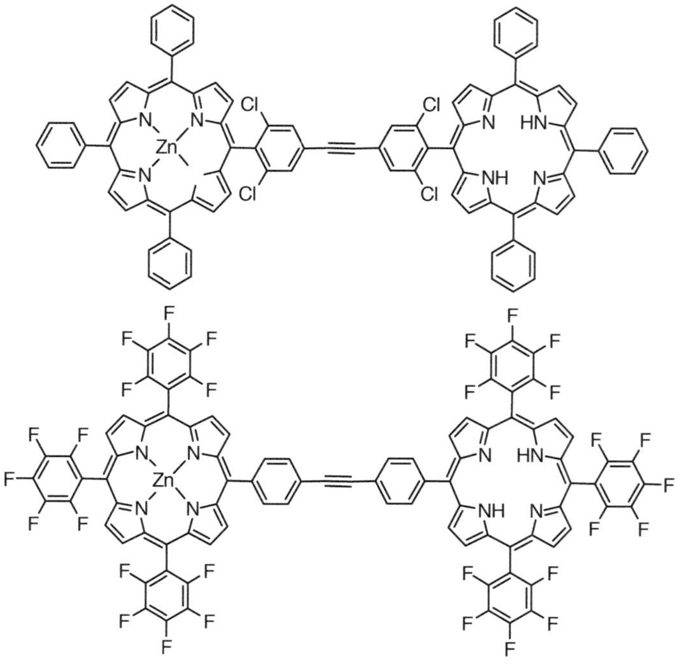

Figure 7. Structures of the halogenated tetraaryl porphyrins combined through a diarylethyne linker.

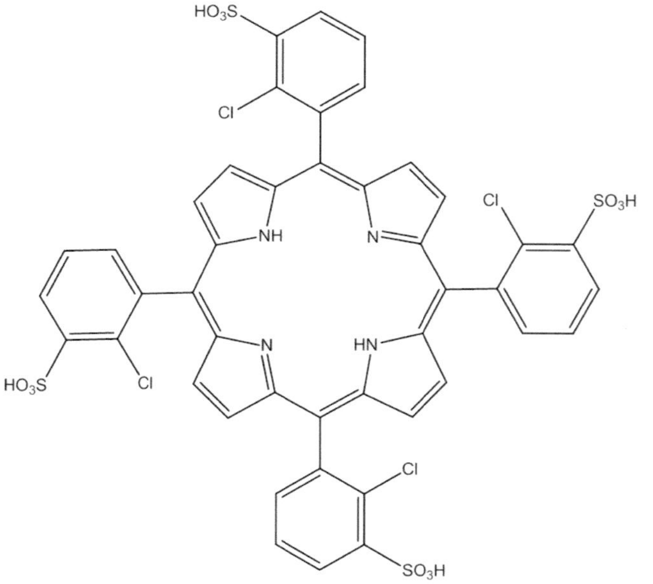

Figure 8. Structure of 5, 10, 15, 20-tetrakis-(2-chloro-3-sulfophenyl)porphyrin ($TCPPSO_3H$).

The melanoma cells studied were mouse (S91) and human (SKEML 188). At concentrations of $TCPPSO_3H$ of 2 x 10^{-4} M or greater dark toxicity in S91 melanoma cells was observed. The S91 melanoma cells were determined to be more sensitive to the photosensitizer in the dark than the human SKMEL 188 cells; therefore, concentrations of 2 x 10^{-5} M buffered solutions of $TCPPSO_3H$ were used for PDT experiments on both cell lines. Cellular uptake of $TCPPSO_3H$ buffered solutions reached a peak after two hours with the S91 cells being five times greater than the SKMEL 188 cells. Thirty minute irradiation with 4 J cm^{-2} or higher led to 90% cell toxicity for both types of cells. S91 cells were still dead 24 h post PDT treatment with 20 μM $TCPPSO_3H$ and 6.2 J cm^{-2} light doses.

In a more recent study halogenated porphyrin photosensitizers were studied as PDT agents, Fig. 9, against A375 melanoma cells. [56] It has been noted that halogenated structures can interfere with the activity of P-glycoprotein (P-gp). This can enhance drug therapy by preventing the function of the P-gp to eliminate these drugs from the cells. Complexes 2-5, Fig. 9, (the halogenated porphyrins) led to the highest quantum yields for singlet oxygen formation compared to the non-halogenated complex, 1 Fig. 9. Photobleaching after 24 h of irradiation was minimal for complexes 1-5. In addition, no dark toxicity was observed for the complexes in the presence of melanoma cells.

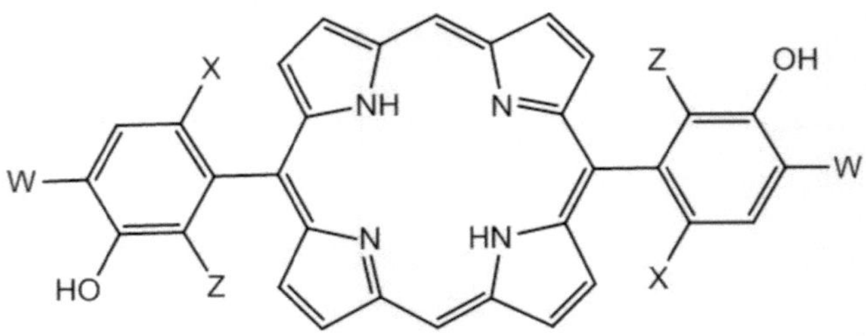

1. X = Z = W = H
2. X = Br, Z = W = H
3. X = Z = H, W = I
4. X = W = H, Z = I
5. Z = Cl, Z = W = H

Figure 9. Structure of halogenated porphyrins.

For the PDT experiments melanoma cells were incubated for 24 h with concentrations of complexes 1-5 ranging from 50 nM to 10 μM. Irradiation of the cells after incubation with the complexes, performed with 10 J cm^{-2}, was evaluated 24 h post PDT treatment. Surprisingly, all of the complexes, including the non-halogenated photosensitizer, showed thirty times the efficiency for photokilling than Photofrin against A375 melanoma cells; however, no appreciable difference was noted between the halogenated and non-halogenated complexes. Further studies are needed to determine the effect of the halogenated porphyrins on P-gp inhibition.

Apart from production of singlet oxygen another mechanism of PDT action, as stated earlier, is the formation of reactive oxygen species (ROS) within the cell. ROS, for example, hydrogen

http://dx.doi.org/10.5772/54940

peroxide, hydroxyl radicals, or superoxide anions are highly reactive leading to oxidative damage of cellular biomolecules. Cells are equipped with enzymes capable of counter acting a limited amount of ROS; however, PDT can lead to an overproduction of ROS which cellular mechanisms are unable to handle. To this end, researchers have synthesized and investigated a series of water soluble porphyrins containing Zn(II), Pd(II) metal centers, as well as, the free-base porphyrin. [57] The sulfonated porphyrin analogs of *meso*-tetrakis-(4-sulfonatophenyl)porphyrin ($TPPS_4$) are illustrated in Fig. 10. Fluorescence probes were used to determine the production of hydrogen peroxide after PDT treatment in human melanoma (G361) cells. Production of hydrogen peroxide by PDT leads, through a series of reactions, to the formation of hydroxyl radicals, the most reactive and deadly form of ROS. The photosensitizers in this study were noted to be homogeneously distributed throughout the cells, excluding the nucleus. The most effective of the photosensitizers in this study was the Zn(II)$TPPS_4$ complex, generating the highest concentration of ROS in the melanoma cells (G361) at 100 μM concentrations and light doses of 5 J cm^{-2}; however, the optimal concentration leading to photocytotoxicity was determined to be 10 μM. Cell viability was linked to light dose, photosensitizer concentration, and the type of photosensitizer.

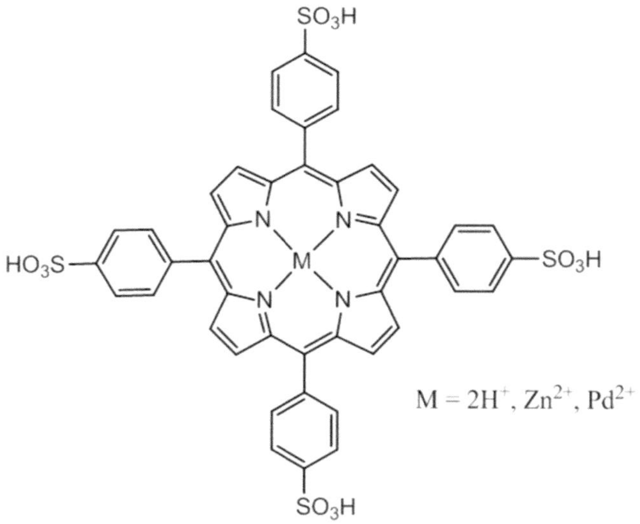

Figure 10. Structure of *meso*-tetrakis-(4-sulfonatophenyl)porphyrin ($TPPS_4$)

In a unique application, researchers have combined PDT with boron neutron capture therapy (BNCT). [58] The porphyrin photosensitizer in this study was appended with 36 boron atoms, *meso*-tetra-(4-nido-carboranylphenyl)porphyrin (H_2TCP), as illustrated in Fig. 11.

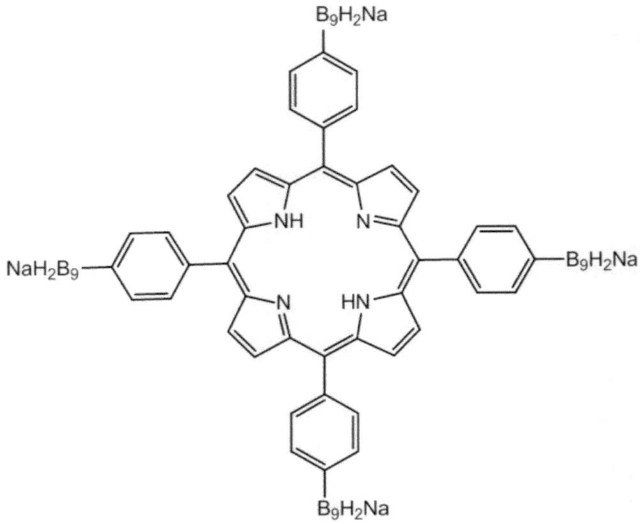

Figure 11. Structure of *meso*-tetra-(4-nido-carboranylphenyl)porphyrin (H_2TCP).

As a PDT agent H_2TCP was measured to generate singlet oxygen in aqueous solutions with a quantum yield of 0.44. Boron neutron capture therapy (BNCT) is used for cancer treatment by injection of a non-toxic radio-sensitizing agent. Irradiation of ^{10}B-enriched tumor lesions with low energy neutrons results in the release of highly toxic $^{4}He^{2+}$ and $^{7}Li^{3+}$ causing severe damage to biological molecules and eventually leading to cell death. Like PDT, BNCT is a targeted treatment modality which the authors anticipated could be used in a synergistic fashion to give maximum tumor killing with minimal collateral damage to healthy cells.

For this study pigmented melanoma (B16F1) cells were subcutaneously transplanted into mice through injection. After seven days tumors were measured at 0.6 cm in diameter, at this point treatment was initiated. The photosensitizer H_2TCP showed no photobleaching after 20 min irradiation indicating its stability under these conditions. The appropriate solution for PDT treatment was obtained when H_2TCP was dissolved in 20% dimethylsulfoxide – 30% polyethyleneglycol – 50% water. Distribution of the photosensitizer was observed in melanoma cells after 24 h incubation. Irradiation with 600-700 nm light for 10 min led to complete cell death at 20 μM concentrations of H_2TCP. There was no dark toxicity toward the melanoma cells at concentrations as high as 50 μM H_2TCP. Fluorescence experiments of the cell studies suggest that the predominant pathway to cell death was necrotic. Mouse studies indicated that injections of H_2TCP of 5 μg/kg were almost completely eliminated from the plasma within 3 h post injection. In addition, maximum tumor accumulation of the photosensitizer was achieved at 3 h post injection with little change after 24 h. Unfortunately poor tumor selectivity was also observed with equal amounts of the photosensitizer being recovered from the skin as well as the tumor tissue. Before PDT and BNCT studies are conducted the authors feel it is important to further investigate other methods of photosensitizer transport to enhance its localization in the tumor cells. This complex does offer the hope of a combined targeted therapy for the treatment of melanoma.

10. Ruthenium complexes and ruthenated porphyrins

Although Photofrin® was approved by U.S. Food and Drug Administration (FDA) for use in the United States, it suffers from dark toxicity and purification difficulties. In order to overcome these, another class of compounds which have received a great deal of attention as potential PDT agents are ruthenium complexes containing polypyridyl ligands. [59-62] For example, excitation of the Metal to Ligand Charge Transfer (MLCT) state of a Ru(II) polypyridyl complex, Fig 12, has been shown to lead to the formation of ROS resulting in efficient cleavage of supercoiled DNA. [63] The Ru(II) polypyridyl complexes have intense, overlapping MLCT transitions in the visible region of the spectrum for acceptor ligand and ligand-based $\pi \rightarrow \pi^*$ transitions in the UV region. The complexes efficiently absorb light throughout the UV and visible allowing for efficient excitation. The MLCT emissions of these Ru complexes are quenched by oxygen to produce $^1O_2$.

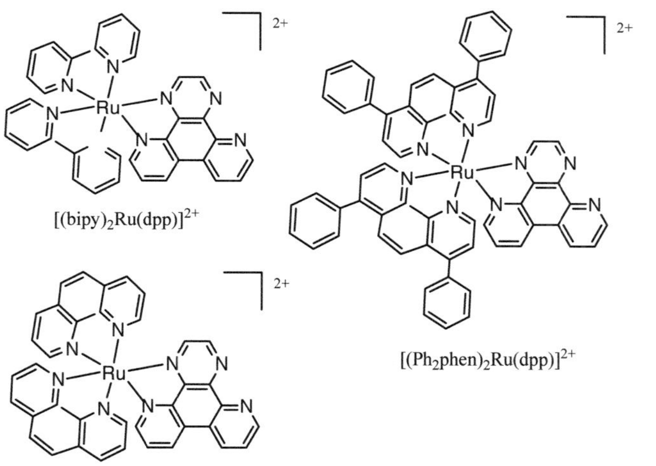

Figure 12. DNA photocleavage agents [(TL)2Ru(dpp)]Cl2 with TL = 2,20-bipyridine (bpy), 1,10-phenanthroline (phen) or 4,7-diphenyl- 1,10-phenanthroline (Ph2phen), with the polyazine bridging ligand 2,3-bis(2-pyridyl)pyrazine (dpp).

Ruthenium complexes coordinated to the periphery of porphyrin molecules have also been shown to interact with DNA. [64-71] In one study a mono-ruthenated porphyrin, Fig 13, caused single strand breaks of circular plasmid DNA when irradiated with UV light. It was suggested that the mechanism of photocleavage was related to the formation of radical cations of guanine. [66] A separate study of a tetra-ruthenated porphyrin, Fig 13, suggested electrostatic binding to DNA and photocleavage of circular plasmid DNA through formation of singlet oxygen. [69]

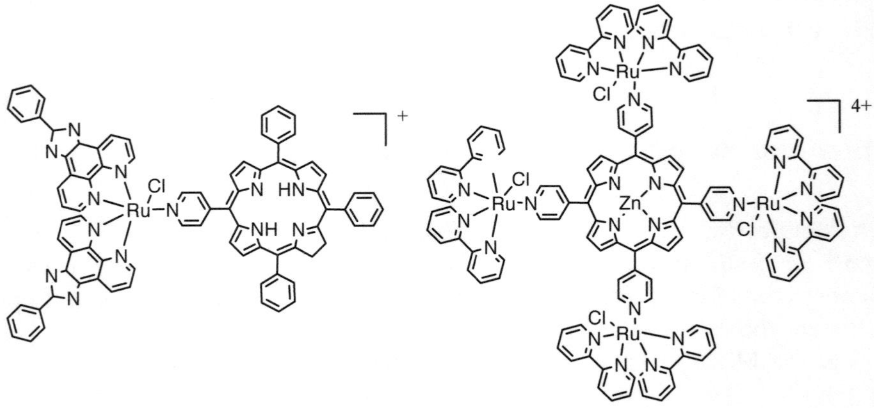

Figure 13. The structure of the mono-ruthenated porphyrin: [MPyTPPARu(pip)2Cl]$^{+}$ and the structure of tetra-ruthenated porphyrin: μ-{meso-5,10,15,20-tetra(4-pyridyl)porphyrin}- tetrakis-{bis-(bipyridine)chlororuthenium(II)}$^{4+}$.

11. Melanoma and ruthenium porphyrins

Reactions of Ru(η^6-arene)(μ-Cl) complexes with 5, 10, 15, 20-(4-pyridyl)porphyrin (TPP) in refluxing methanol gave tetranuclear ruthenium porphyrins in excellent yield, Fig. 14. [72]

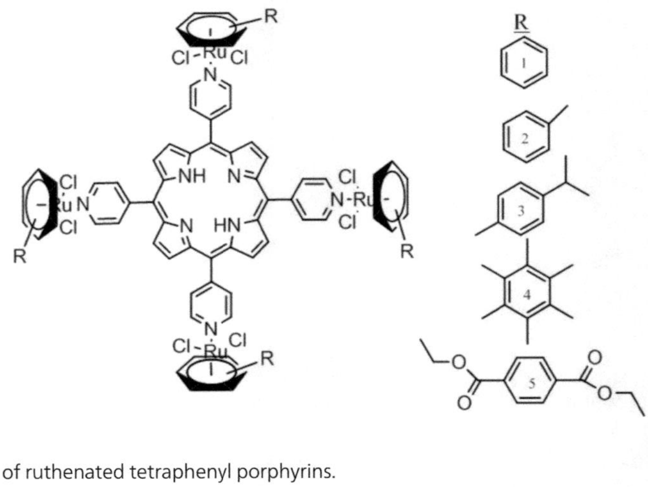

Figure 14. Structures of ruthenated tetraphenyl porphyrins.

The complexes in this study were used to investigate growth inhibition of human Me300 melanoma cells. The melanoma cells were incubated with various concentrations of complexes 1-5 over a 24 h period. Cell survival was determined by accepted protocol (MTT assay). Dark toxicity experiments revealed that complexes 3 and 4 were moderately toxic while complexes

http://dx.doi.org/10.5772/54940

1, 2, and 5 were less toxic to the cells. Localization of complex 2 in the cells cytoplasm was determined by fluorescence measurements; however, nuclear localization was not observed.

Melanoma cells incubated with 10 μM concentrations of complexes 1-5 for 24 h were irradiated using a red laser at 652 nm, with a light dosage range of 5-30 J cm^{-2}. After irradiation 24 h was allowed to lapse before cell cytotoxicity was measured. In the absence of the photosensitizers, 1-5, irradiation of the melanoma cells was determined to be ineffective at cell killing. Light doses as low as 5 J cm^{-2} in the presence of the complexes indicated 60-80% melanoma cell killing. Little difference in phototoxicity was observed for the complexes after PDT treatment under the same conditions. Therrien and coworkers have studied a variety of interesting ruthenium substituted porphyrin photosensitizers for their effects as PDT agents against pigmented melanoma. [73-75]

In an attempt to combine the tumor affinity of porphyrins with the enhanced excited state lifetimes afforded by halogens and the added benefits of coordinated ruthenium polyazine groups we have investigated the synergistic effects of these substituents as PDT agents for the treatment of melanoma. [76,77] In our most recent study we synthesized a series of ruthenated pyridyl porphyrins containing one pentafluorophenyl group at the *meso*-position combined with a series of transition metal ions, Fig. 15. [77]

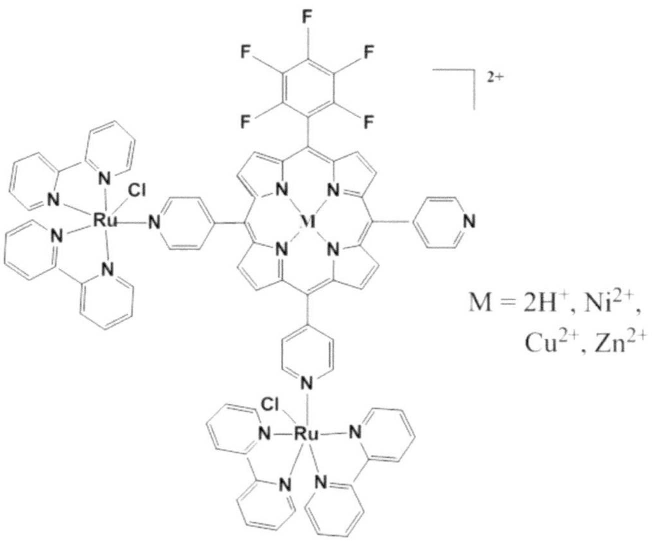

I-IV

Figure 15. Transition metal and free base ruthenium porphyrin analogs.

Early experiments of the free base porphyrin showed extraordinary ability to photocleave circular plasmid DNA when irradiated with light above 400 nm. When various transition metal ions (Ni(II), Cu(II), and Zn(II)) were inserted into the porphyrin the photocleavage ability was markedly reduced. Cell studies were performed on human dermal skin fibroblast cells and malignant melanoma cells obtained from a 53 year old male. Normal and melanoma cells were incubated for 24 h at 37 ºC in the dark with complex concentrations of 5 and 10 μM. The complexes (I-IV) did not show any dark toxicity toward either normal fibroblast or melanoma cells. PDT experiments were performed by irradiating the cultured cells (containing the photosensitizers) for either 30 or 60 min intervals with a 60 W tungsten lamp. In the case of the free base porphyrin (I) irradiation of 30 min at concentrations as low as 3 μM indicated complete cell killing of both normal fibroblast and melanoma cells. In contrast, irradiation times of 60 min at concentrations of the Ni(II) and Cu(II) complexes (II and III) of 10 μM showed no cell damage for either the normal fibroblast or melanoma cells. The Zn(II) complex (IV) showed the greatest potential as a PDT agent. Irradiation for 30 min at concentrations of the Zn(II) porphyrin of 5 and 10 μM showed minimal cell damage of the normal fibroblast cells but induced complete cell killing of the melanoma cells. Further studies are needed to determine the effect of the central metal ions on the phototoxicity of these complexes.

12. Phthalocyanine photosensitizers – Background

Phthalocyanines represent another form of macrocyle, similar in many ways to porphyrins. Synthetic routes to phthalocyanines vary; however, one common method involves reacting o-cyanobenzamide with phthalimide to give the tetrabenzoporphyrazin, more commonly named, phthalocyanince (Pc), Fig. 16.

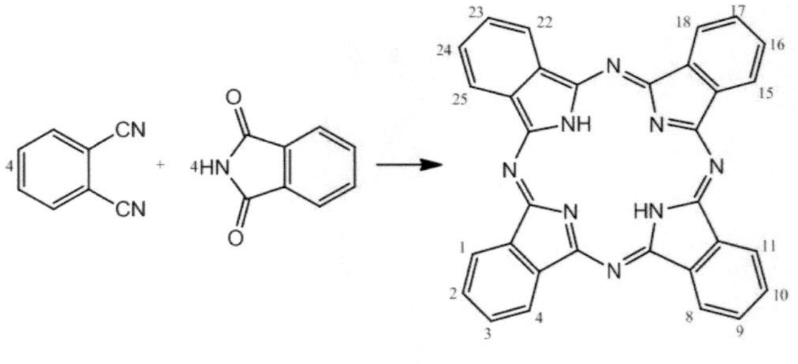

Figure 16. Synthesis of phthalocyanine.

Phthalocyanines have the ability, like porphyrins, to coordinate metal ions within their nitrogen core, they are a tetradentate ligand. This has offered numerous ways to synthetically alter their physical properties. If not at the metal center, substitutions of Pc's is typically made at the benzo-periphery (positions 1-4, 8-11, 15-18, and 22-25, Fig. 16). Two advantages Pc's seem to have over porphyrins, as potential PDT agents, is their comparatively high yields and their spectroscopic properties. Like porphyrins, Pc's have a Soret band at higher energy ca. 400 nm and Q-bands at lower energy; however, in the case of Pc's the low energy Q-bands (650-750 nm) are typically much more intense than the Soret bands, opposite of porphyrins. These intense absorptions fit very nicely within the photodynamic window needed for PDT.

http://dx.doi.org/10.5772/54940

One major drawback is that Pc's lack the specificity toward tumor cells that porphyrins possess, this has led to numerous synthetic manipulations to try and find ways to get the Pc's into the tumor.

13. Phthalocyanines, PDT and melanoma

Researchers in 1999 compared Photofrin (HpD), Zn(II) phthalocyanine (ZnPc), Zn(II) naphthalocyanine (ZnNc), and a newly synthesized tetrabenzamido-substituted Zn(II) phthalocyanine (ZnNcA) as PDT agents against B16 pigmented melanoma. Pathogen-free male C57B1/6 mice between 6 and 8 weeks of age were transplanted with 1 mm^3 pieces of melanoma tumor tissue. Six days post-transplant, tumor diameters were between 3 and 4 mm, at this point PDT treatment was initiated. [78] Tumor infected mice were injected with the photosensitizers and irradiated 24 h after injection with wavelengths between 630-780 nm. Twenty one days after PDT treatment HpD and ZnPc treated mice showed no effect on the tumors. Some tumor growth delay was observed 15 days post PDT treatment with the ZnNc photosensitizer. Higher photosensitizer concentrations and increased irradiation energy did not produce increased phototherapeutic effects for these photosensitizers. In the case of the ZnNcA photosensitizer treated mice pronounced tumor necrosis post irradiation was observed with tumor diameters held at 4 mm up to 19 days after treatment. ZnNcA shows singlet oxygen generation quantum yields of 0.33 with good accumulation in the tumor which has been linked to its success against these particular tumors.

Aggregation is a common issue with macrocyclic complexes. To address this two new silicon(IV) centered phthalocyanines have been synthesized, Fig. 17. [79]

Both of the complexes in Fig. 17 have electronic spectra displaying intense Q-bands at 668 nm. In this study M6 achromic melanoma cells were incubated with the desired photosensitizer for 1 h prior to irradiation. Irradiation experiments involved a 250 W tungsten-halogen lamp containing a filter to cut off wavelengths below 480 nm. After the cells were irradiated they were washed with PBS buffer solutions and grown in a fresh culture for 6 h. Due to low water solubility of HexSiPc, this photosensitizer was incorporated in EYL (egg yolk lecithin) lisosomes. Under these conditions the maximum concentration of Cl_2SiPc in M6 cells was 2.18 ng and 15.3 ng for HexSiPc, obtained after 90 min of incubation. No evidence of dark toxicity was observed for concentrations of Cl_2SiPc between 10^{-10} and 10^{-8} M or for concentrations of HexSiPc between 10^{-10} and 10^{-5} M. The Cl_2SiPc complex showed little M6 killing after 1 h of incubation and 20 min irradiation with a 250 W tungsten-halogen lamp. The HexSiPc photosensitizer, on the other hand, (entrapped in EYL) gave LD_{90} of 3×10^{-7} M after 20 min of irradiation and 2×10^{-9} M after 2 h of irradiation with a 250 W tungsten-halogen lamp. It was concluded that the superior photokilling observed for HexSiPc was linked to lipid peroxidation.

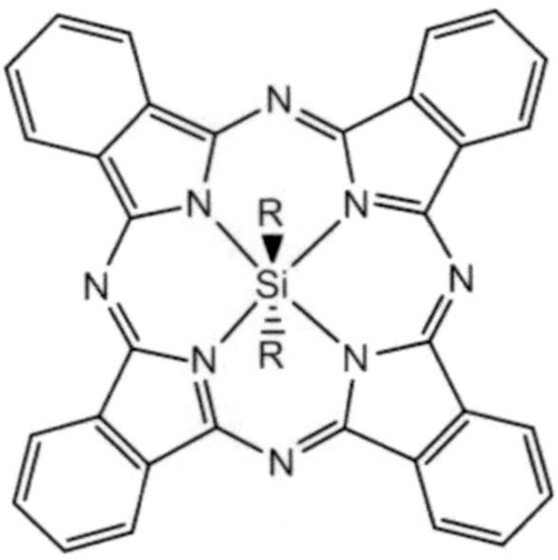

R = Cl (Cl_2SiPc)
R = O-Si(n-hex)$_3$ (HexSiPc)

Figure 17. Structure of (Cl_2SiPc) and (HexSiPc).

Another study aimed at decreasing Pc aggregation while increasing its lipophilicity included a series of SiPc complexes containing various substituents coordinated to the silicon metal center, one of which is illustrated in Fig. 18. [80]

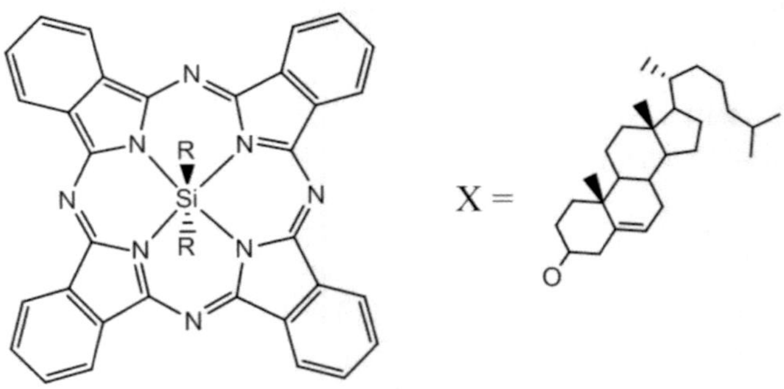

Chol-O-SiPc

Figure 18. Structure of bis(cholesteryloxy) derivative of SiPc.

This study involved human pigmented melanoma cells SKMEL-2. The photosensitizers were dissolved in tetrahydrofuran (THF) and entrapped in liposomes to increase tumor affinity. Irradiation experiments were performed using a 250 W tungsten-halogen lamp filtered to cut off wavelengths below 480 nm. The melanoma cells were incubated with the substituted SiPc liposome entrapped complexes prior to irradiation for 20 min. Of the six Si-substituted Pc's in this study the best photokilling was observed for the complex illustrated in Fig. 18. Photokilling efficacy of Chol-O-SiPc, in vitro, was seven to nine times greater than the known reference chloro-aluminum phthalocyanine with LD_{50} = 6-8 x 10^{-9} M. The mechanism of photokilling of this complex was evaluated by kinetic studies indicating that faster mitochondrial mediated apoptosis was occurring by PDT with this complex as compared to the reference Pc.

As noted earlier generation of ROS leads to cell death and blood vessel damage; crucial to tumor regression. In a study of G361 human melanoma cells with a disulfonated chloroaluminum phthalocyanine ($ClAlPcS_2$) photosensitizer, researchers were interested in looking at the generation of ROS and hydrogen peroxide after PDT treatment. The complex, $ClAlPcS_2$, was made water soluble by conversion to its ammonia salt. [81] The electronic spectra of this complex displayed an intense Q-band at 670 nm. PDT experiments were performed by irradiation with a semiconductor laser at 675 nm and energies of 10 and 20 J cm^{-2}. At lower light doses of energy (10 J cm^{-2}) and higher concentrations of Pc, 7.5 and 75 μg/mL, increased generation of ROS was observed; however, at light doses of 20 J cm^{-2} and concentrations of Pc of 0.75 μg/mL larger amounts of ROS were generated as compared to higher concentrations and higher light doses. The most ROS generated were at a concentration of 75 μg/mL and light dose of 10 J cm^{-2}. G361 melanoma cell viability studies indicated that the optimal phototoxicity could be obtained with a light dose of 25 J cm^{-2} and concentrations of photosensitizer of 5 μg/mL and 10 μg/mL.

Phthalocyanines, like porphyrins, have also been combined with boron isotopes in an attempt to obtain a synergistic treatment method involving PDT and BNCT (boron neutron capture therapy). The ZnPc coupled to boron, in this study, is illustrated in Fig. 19. [82]

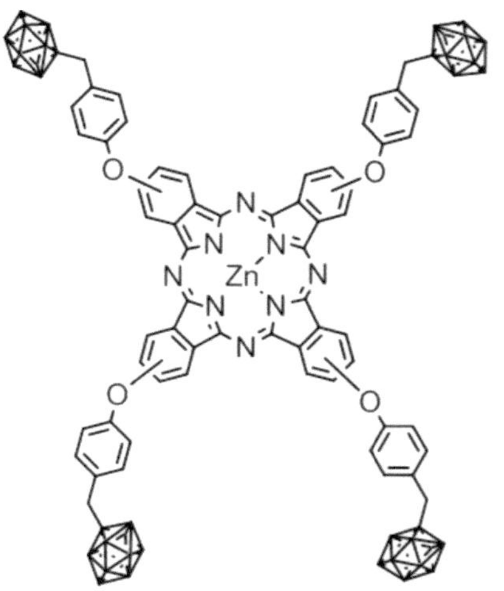

Figure 19. Structure of ZnB_4Pc.

Due to low water solubility the ZnB_4Pc complex was incorporated into liposomes. The complex was stable for one week in liposomal aqueous suspensions. The photosensitizer-liposome suspension was used to study B16F1 melanotic melanoma cells. After 18 h of incubation with the melanoma cells the peak concentration of ZnB_4Pc complex obtained was 7 μm, with no dark toxicity observed. Red light irradiation of B16F1 cells incubated for 1 h with 7 μM ZnB_4Pc-liposomes resulted in > 95% cell death. No regrowth of melanotic melanoma cells after several days post-irradiation was observed.

Pigmented melanoma cells were transplanted into C57BL/6 mice subcutaneously. The best results for PDT treatment of melanoma transplanted mice after injection of ZnB_4Pc was observed with irradiation 3 h post injection with wavelengths between 600-700 nm. PDT experiments conducted 24 and 48 h post injection were ineffective in shrinking the tumors, leading the authors to conclude that the PDT treatment was affecting the blood vessels associated with the tumor. Moreover, significant tumor growth delay was observed when BNCT treatment was conducted 24 h post injection of the ZnB_4Pc complex suggesting that this complex offers a dual pathway toward melanoma treatment.

Various synthetic routes have been taken to reduce aggregation of phthalocyanines while increasing their water solubility. A recent study looked at coordination of N-methylated piperazine substituents at the axial positions of a silicon(IV) phthalocyanine. [83] N-methylation lends a cationic charge to the complex making it water soluble while the bulky Si-coordinated substituents prevent aggregation, Fig. 20.

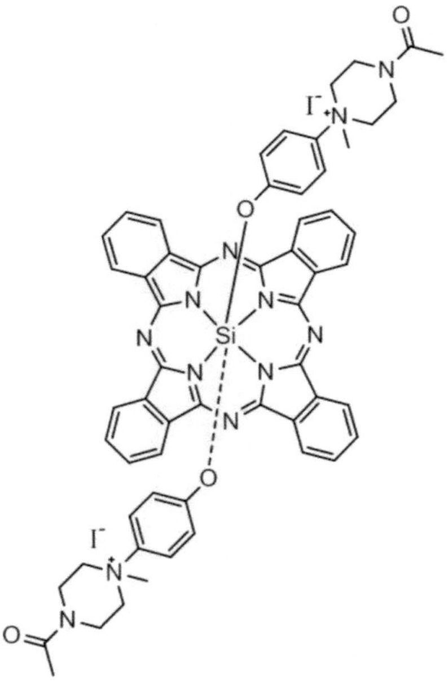

Figure 20. Structure of bis(4-(4-acetylpiperazine)phenoxy)phthalocyanoto silicon(IV) N-methyl derivative.

Suprisingly, this structurally complicated phthalocyanine was synthesized with a yield of 73%. Electronic absorption spectra of the complex reveals an intense Q-band at 685 nm in N,N-dimethylformamide (DMF). In aqueous solution the Q-band shifts to lower energy, 690 nm, while obeying the Beer-Lambert law, indicating no aggregation at the concentrations studied.

Investigations of singlet oxygen production gave a quantum yield of 0.49. To enhance biocompatibility and selectivity the phthalocyanine was complexed with bovine serum albumin (BSA), a common protein carrier for anticancer drugs. Studies were conducted on B16 melanoma cells using 0.1 μM concentrations of photosensitizer. At this concentration no dark toxicity was observed. PDT treatment was conducted with red light greater than 610 nm at 60 J cm^{-2} resulting in complete killing of the B16 melanoma cells.

There are a limited number of studies in which phthalocyanines have been combined with ruthenium complexes for the purpose of PDT. Researchers in 2009 synthesized a Tb(III) phthalocyanine capable of hydrogen bonding to a polypyridyl Ru(II) complex in aqueous solution, Fig. 21. [84] The idea was to incorporate the photosensitizing ability of the phthalocyanine to generate singlet oxygen under oxygen rich conditions, when irradiated with low energy light and photolytic release of nitric oxide from the ruthenium complex under hypoxic conditions. This would give dual capabilities for photodynamic damage since nitric oxide has been linked to antitumor activity.

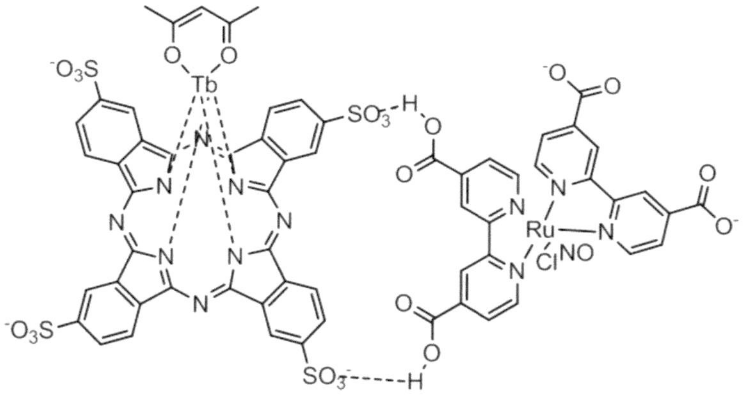

Figure 21. Structure of *cis*-[Ru(H-dcbpy-$)_2$(Cl)(NO)][Na_4(Tb(TsPc)(acac)]

Although the complex was not isolated it was assumed to form hydrogen bonds in aqueous solution. The electronic spectrum of a one to one mixture of the complexes in aqueous solution reveals two intense absorption bands at 642 nm and 682 nm. PDT studies were performed on B16F10 pigmented murine melanoma cells. When irradiated at 691 nm the quantum yield for singlet oxygen production was measured to be 0.41. Some dark toxicity was observed; however, upon irradiation, 80% of the melanoma cells had undergone photocytotoxicity. In the absence of the phthalocyanine there was reduced cell viability which was linked to the release of nitric oxide upon irradiation of the ruthenium complex.

Studies have indicated that nanoparticles enhance tumor targeting. To take advantage of this property researchers have combined phthalocyanines with gold nanoparticles dispersed in an emulsion, Fig. 22. Electronic spectra of the free C_{11}Pc and C_{11}Pc-Np display an intense Q-band at 696 nm. [85]

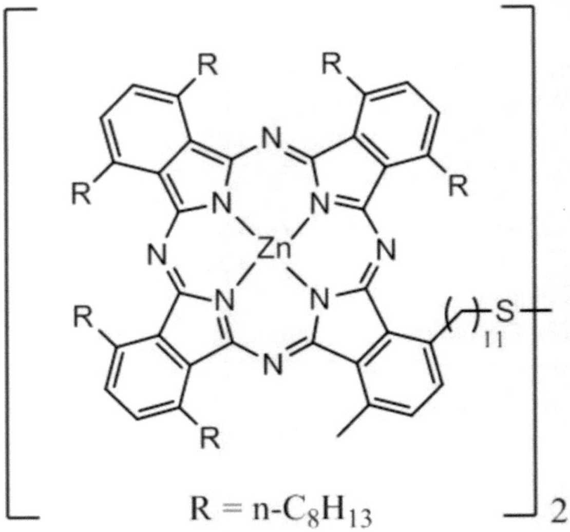

Figure 22. Structure of C_{11}Pc.

Mice (C57) transplanted with B78H1 amelonotic clone of murine melanoma were used in this study. At 10 to 15 days post melanoma transplantation (tumor external diameters of 0.4 to 0.6 cm) the C_{11}Pc and C_{11}Pc-Np emulsions were injected at a dose of 1.5 µmol/kg body weight. The highest accumulation of photosensitizer found in the tumor was observed at 24 h post injection, while at 3 h post injection significant amounts of photosensitizer was found in the serum. Irradiation studies were performed at 3 h and 24 h post injection with wavelengths of light between 600 nm and 700 nm. It was noted that untreated mice died within 3 weeks of melanoma transplant. Suprisingly, little effect on tumor growth was observed when tumors were irradiated 24 after photosensitizer injection, when the photosensitizer was at a maximum concentration within the tumor. However, irradiation 3 h post injection led to significant tumor growth delay for both C_{11}Pc and C_{11}Pc-Np. The authors indicate that the observed growth delay was most likely due to vascular damage to the tumor cells leading to low blood flow to the cells.

14. Other macrocycles for PDT of melanoma and concluding remarks

We would be remiss if we did not acknowledge the great deal of research devoted to photosensitizer macrocycles other than porphyrins and phthalocyanines for the treatment of melanoma. Although this chapter has focused primarily on porphyrins and phthalocyanines there are other similar complexes under investigation as PDT agents for melanoma. One of the more promising photosensitizers being studied is based on the macrocycle texaphyrin. The lutetium texaphyrin in this study, Fig. 23, showed water solubility and intense absorbance between 700 nm and 760 nm. [86]

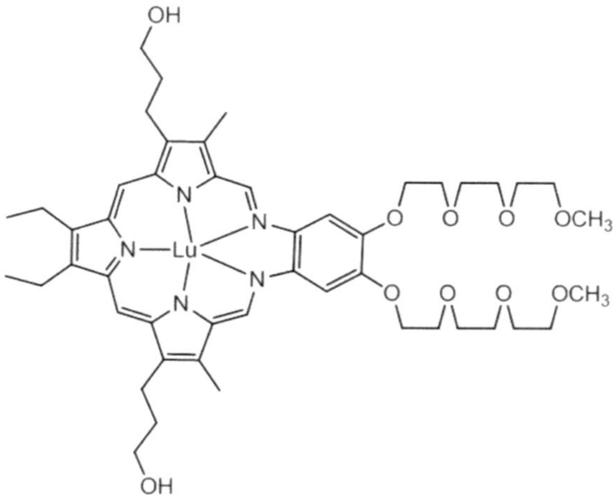

Figure 23. Structure of Lu-texaphyrin (PCI-0123).

PCI-0123 was studied in C57BL/6 mice transplanted with the pigmented murine melanoma B16F10. PDT studies of the tumor transplanted mice injected with PCI-0123 irradiated with 732 nm light showed delay in tumor growth and increased life spans. The interested reader is encouraged to review the following references for further information on other macrocycles being studied as PDT agents for the treatment of melanoma. [87-93]

It is clear that a great deal of research is ongoing toward finding new PDT agents for the treatment of melanoma. This trend will certainly increase as the incidence of melanoma continues to increase throughout the world. There are many challenges yet to be overcome; however, photosensitizers capable of treating melanoma by PDT are continually being developed. Two major hurdles which must be addressed are, first, overcoming the ability of pigmented melanoma to absorb wavelengths needed to activate the photosensitizer and second, the metastatic nature of melanoma. Great strides have been made to develop photosensitizers capable of phototoxicity in pigmented melanoma. Unfortunately, it is unlikely that PDT will be a viable option (on its own) for the treatment of advanced stage melanoma which has begun to metastasize. In combination with traditional melanoma treatments PDT is becoming a more accepted regimen for the treatment of this most deadly form of skin cancer.

Author details

Shawn Swavey and Matthew Tran

Department of Chemistry, University of Dayton, Dayton, Ohio, USA

References

[1] Steen, S, Nemunaitis, J, Fisher, T, & Kuhn, J. Proc. (Bayl. Univ. Med. Cent.), (2008).

[2] Jack, A, Boyes, C, Aydin, N, Alam, K, & Wallack, M. Surg. Oncol., (2006).

[3] Hendi, A. Atlas of Skin Cancers", Springer, New York; (2011).

[4] "Radiation Therapy and You"National Institute of Health, May (2012).

[5] "Chemotherapy and You"National Institute of Health, June (2011).

[6] "Biological Therapy"National Institute of Health, January, (2004).

[7] Raab, O, & Biol, Z. (1900).

[8] Policard, A. (1924). *Compt. Rend. Soc. Biol.,*.

[9] Andrei, V. N, Dabney, D. W, Jenna, T. S, Luigi, M. G, & Richard, C. W. Antimicrobial Agents and Chemotherapy, (2002).

[10] Mcmahon, K. S, Wieman, T. J, Moore, P. H, & Fingar, V. H. (1994). *Cancer Res.,*.

[11] Neurath, R. A, Strick, N, Cebinath, A. K, & Mol, J. Recog., (1995).

[12] (Dougherty, a) T. J, Gomer, C. J, & Henderson, B. W. et al. J. Natl. Cancer Inst. 1998, 90, 889. (b) R.K. Pandey, G. Zheng. Porphyrins as Photosensitizers in Photodynamic Therapy. Kadish, Smith, Guilard. (eds). Academic Press: San Diego., (2000). , 6

[13] Pandey, R. K, & Porph, J. (2000). *Phthalocyan.,*.

[14] Korbelik, M, & Clin, J. Laser Med. Surg. (1996).

[15] Musser, D. A, & Fiel, R. J. (1991). *Photochem. Photobiol.,*.

[16] Georgakoudi, I, & Foster, T. H. Photochem. Photobiol., (1998).

[17] Ravanant, J. -L, Douki, T, & Cadet, J. J. Photochem. Photobiol. B., (2001).

[18] Belvedere, A, Bosca, F, Catalfo, A, Cuquerella, M. C, De Guidi, G, & Miranda, M. A. Chem. Res. Toxicol., (2002).

[19] Weishaupt, K. R, Gomer, C. J, & Dougherty, T. J. (1976). *Cancer Res.,*.

[20] Turro, N. J. Modern Molecular Photochemistry. University Science Books: California, (1991). , 1991, 583-593.

[21] Foote, C. S. Mechanisms of photo-oxygenation. In Porphyrin Localization and Treatment of Tumors. Doiron DR, Gomer CJ. (eds). Alan R. Liss: New York, (1984). , 1984, 3-18.

[22] Henderson, B. W, & Dougherty, T. J. (1992). *Photochem. Photobiol.*

[23] Figge, F. H. J. The relationship of pyrrol compounds to carcinogenesis. In AAAS Research Conf. on Cancer. F.R. Moulton. (eds). (1945). , 1945, 117-128.

[24] Figge, F. H. J. (1947). *Ann. Int. Med.*

[25] Figge, F. H. J, Weiland, G. S, & Manganiello, L. O. J. (1948). *Proc. Soc. Exp. Biol. Med.*

[26] Rasmussen-taxdal, D. S, Ward, D. E, & Figge, F. H. J. (1955). *Cancer.*

[27] Henderson, B. W, Dougherty, T. J, & Schwartz, S. et al. Historical perspective. In Photodynamic Therapy: Basic Principles and Clinical Applications. B.W. Henderson, T.J. Dougherty. (eds). Marcel Decker: New York, (1992). , 1992, 1-15.

[28] Lipson, R. L, Baldes, E. J, Olsen, A. M, & Natl, J. Cancer Inst. (1961).

[29] Arnaldo, P, Silvio, T, Von H, D, Daniel, M, & Diego, M. Paolo. Cancer Letter., (1988).

[30] Dougherty, T. J, & Clin, J. Laser Med. Surg., (1996).

[31] Dougherty, T. J, & Natl, J. Cancer Inst., (1974).

[32] De Rosa, F. S, & Vitoria, M. L.B. Bentley Pharm. Res., (2000).

[33] Nyman, E. S, Hynninen, P. H, & Photochem, J. Photobiol B: Biology, (2004).

[34] Connor, A. E. O, & Gallagher, W. M. A.T. Byrne Photochem. Photobiol., (2009).

[35] C. Abels Photochem. Photobiol. Sci., 2004, 3, 765.

[36] Favilla, I, Favilla, M. L, Gosbell, A. D, Barry, W. R, Ellims, P, & Hill, J. S. J.R. Byrne Melanoma Research, (1995).

[37] Zhou, C, & Photochem, J. Photobiol. B: Biology, (1989).

[38] Sharman, W. M, & Van Lier, J. E. C.M. Allen Adv. Drug Delivery Rev., (2004).

[39] His, R. A, Rosenthal, D. I, & Glatstein, E. Drugs, (1999).

[40] Jori, G, & Photochem, J. Photobiol. B: Biology, (1996).

[41] R. Bonnett Chem. Soc. Rev., 1995, 19.

[42] Pandey, R. K, & Porph, J. Phthal (2000).

[43] Hudson, R, Boyle, R. W, & Porph, J. Phthal. (2004).

[44] Wei, W. H, Wang, Z, Mizuno, T, Cortez, C, Fu, L, Sirisawad, M, Naumovski, L, Madga, D, & Sessler, J. L. Dalton. Trans. (2006).

[45] Chen, X, & Drain, C. M. Drug Design Rev. (2004).

[46] Allison, R, Mota, H, & Sibata, C. (2004). *Photodiangosis and Photodynamic Therapy.*

[47] Tronconi, W, Colombo, A, Decesare, M, Marchesini, R, Woodburn, K. W, Reiss, J. A, Phillips, D. R, & Zumino, F. Cancer Lett. (1995).

[48] Onuki, J, Ribas, A. V, Medeiros, M. H. G, Araki, K, Toma, H. E, & Catalini, L. H. P. Di Mascio, Photochem. Photobiol. (1996).

[49] Busetti, A, Soncin, M, Jori, G, Rodgers, M. A. J, & British, J. of Cancer (1999).

[50] Drzewiecka, A, Urbanska, K, Matuszak, Z, Pineiro, M, Arnaut, L. G, Habdas, J, & Ratuszna, A. G. Stochel Acta Bioch. Pol. (2001).

[51] Yang, S. I, Seth, J, Strachan, J. -P, Gentemann, S, Kim, D, Holten, D, Lindsey, J. S, Bocian, D. F, & Porph, J. and Phthal. (1999).

[52] Chen, X, Hui, L, Foster, D. A, & Drain, C. M. Biochem. (2004).

[53] Ko, Y. J, Yun, K. J, Kang, M. S, Park, J, Lee, K. T, Park, S. B, & Shin, J. H. (2007). *Bioorg. Med. Chem. Lett.*

[54] Zheng, X, & Pandey, R. K. Anti Cancer Agents in Med. Chem. (2008).

[55] Dabrowski, J. M, Pereira, M. M, Arnaut, L. G, Monteiro, C. J. P, Peixoto, A. F, Karocki, A, Urbanska, K, & Stochel, G. Photochem. and Photobiol. (2007).

[56] Serra, A, Pineiro, M, Santos, C. I, Rocha, A. M. d'A, Gonsalves, M, & Abrantes, M. Laranjo, M.F. Botelho, Photochem. and Photobiol. (2010).

[57] Kolarova, H, Gajgar, R, Tomankova, K, Nevrelova, P, & Mosinger, J. (2007). *Toxic. in Vitro.*

[58] Fabris, C, Vicente, M. G. H, Hao, E, Friso, E, Borsetto, L, Jori, G, Miotto, G, Colautti, P, Moro, D, Esposito, J, Ferretti, A, Rossi, C. R, Nitti, D, Sotti, G, Soncin, M, & Photochem, J. and Photobiol. B: Biology (2007).

[59] Erkkila, K. E, Odom, D. T, & Barton, J. K. Chem. Rev. (1999).

[60] (Armistead, a) P. M, & Thorp, H. H. Anal. Chem. 2001, 73, 558. (b) I.V. Yang and H.H. Thorp, Inorg. Chem. (2000). c) P.J. Carter, C.-C. Cheng, H.H. Thorp, J. Am. Chem. Soc. 1998, 120, 632. (d) C. Vialas, C. Claparols, G. Pratviel, B. Meunier, J. Am. Chem. Soc. 2000, 122, 2157.

[61] Singh, T. N, & Turro, C. Inorg. Chem. (2004).

[62] Ko, Y. J, Yun, K. J, Kang, M. S, Park, J, Lee, K. T, Park, S. B, & Shin, J. H. Bioorg. Med. Chem. Lett. (2007).

[63] Mangelli, M. T, Heinceke, J, Mayfield, S, Okyere, B, Winkel, B. S. J, Brewer, K. J, & Inorg, J. Biochem. (2006).

[64] Boerner, L. J. K, & Zaleski, J. M. Curr. Op. Chem. Bio. (2005).

[65] Gianferrara, T, Serli, B, Zangrando, E, Lengo, E, Alessio, E, & New, J. Chem. (2005).

[66] Mei, W. J, Liu, J, Chao, H, Ji, L. N, Li, A. X, & Liu, J. Z. Trans. Met. Chem. (2003).

[67] Zhao, P, Xu, L. C, Huang, J. W, Zheng, K. C, Fu, B, Yu, H. C, & Ji, L. N. Biophys. Chem. (2008).

[68] Onuki, J, Ribas, A. W, Medeiros, M. H. G, Araki, K, Toma, H. E, & Catalani, L. H. P. DiMascio, Photochem. Photobiol. (1996).

[69] Araki, K, Silva, C. A, Toma, H. E, Catalani, L. H, Medeiros, M. H. G, & Di, P. Masci, J.Inorg. Biochem. (2000).

[70] Narra, M, Elliott, P, & Swavey, S. (2006). *Inorg. Chim. Acta.*

[71] Davia, K, King, D, Hong, Y, & Swavey, S. (2008). *Inorg. Chem. Comm.*

[72] Schmitt, F, Govindaswamy, P, Suss-fink, G, Ang, W. H, Dyson, P. J, Juillerat-jeanneret, L, Therrien, B, & Med, J. Chem. (2008).

[73] Schmitt, F, Govindaswamy, P, Zava, O, Suss-fink, G, Juillerat-jeanneret, L, Therrein, B, & Biol, J. Inog. Chem. (2009).

[74] Schmitt, F, Auzias, M, Stepnicka, P, Sei, Y, Yamaguchi, K, Suss-fink, G, Therrein, B, Juillerat-jeanneret, L, & Biol, J. Inog. Chem. (2009).

[75] Schmitt, F, Barry, N. P. E, & Juillerat-jeanneret, L. B. Therrein Bioorg. and Med. Chem. Letters (2012).

[76] Rani-beeram, S, Meyer, K, Mccrate, A, Hong, Y, & Nielsen, M. S. Swavey Inorg. Chem. (2008).

[77] Sweigert, P, Xu, Z, & Hong, Y. S. Swavey Dalton Trans. (2012).

[78] Peeva, M, Shopova, M, Stoichkova, N, Michailov, N, Wohrle, D, Muller, S, & Porph, J. and Phthal. (1999).

[79] Decreau, R, Richard, M. J, Verrando, P, Chanon, M, Julliard, M, & Photochem, J. and Photobiol. B: Biology (1999).

[80] Barge, J, Decreau, R, Julliard, M, Hubaud, J. -C, Sabatier, A. -S, & Grob, J. -J. P. Verrando Exp. Dermat. (2004).

[81] Kolarova, H, Nevrelova, P, Bajgar, R, Jirova, D, & Kejlova, K. M. Strnad Toxic. in Vitro (2007).

[82] Friso, E, Roncucci, G, Dei, D, Soncin, M, Fabris, C, Chiti, G, Colautti, P, Esposito, J, De Nardo, L, Rossi, C. R, Nitti, D, Giuntini, F, & Borsetto, L. G. Jori Photochem. and Photobiol. Sciences (2006).

[83] Jiang, X. -J, Huang, J. -D, Zhu, Y. -J, Tang, F. -X, & Ng, D. K. P. J.-C. Sun Bioorg. and Med. Chem. Letters (2006).

[84] Cicillini, S. A, Prazias, A. C. L, Tedesco, A. C, & Serra, O. A. R.S. da Silva Polyhedron (2009).

[85] Camerin, M, Magaraggia, M, Soncin, M, Jori, G, Moreno, M, Chambrier, I, Cook, M. J, & Russell, D. A. (2010). *Eur. J. of Cancer*.

[86] Woodburn, K. W, Fan, Q, Kessel, D, Luo, Y, Young, S. W, & Invest, J. Dermatol. (1998).

[87] Abels, C, Fritsch, C, Bolsen, K, Szeimies, R. -M, Ruzicka, T, Goerz, G, Goetz, A. E, & Photochem, J. and Photobiol. B: Biology (1997).

[88] Zilberstein, J, Schreiber, S, Bloemers, M. C. W. M, Bendel, P, Neeman, M, Schechtman, E, Kohen, F, & Scherz, A. Y. Salomon Photochem. and Photobiol. (2001).

[89] Schreiber, S, Gross, S, Brandis, A, Harmelin, A, Rosenbach-belkin, V, Scherz, A, Salomon, Y, & Int, J. Cancer (2002).

[90] Urbanska, K, Romanowska-dixon, B, Matuszak, Z, Oszajca, J, & Nowak-sliwinska, P. G. Stochel Acta Bioch. Pol. (2002).

[91] Nagata, S, Obana, A, & Gohto, Y. S. Nakajima Lasers in Surg. and Med. (2003).

[92] Sheleg, S. V, Zhavrid, E. A, Khodina, T. V, Kochubeev, G. A, Istomin, Y. P, & Chalov, V. N. I.N. Zhuravkin Photoderm. Photoimmun. and Photomed. (2004).

[93] Schwartz, D. I, Gozlan, Y, Breenbaum, L, Babushkina, T, Katcoff, D, & Malik, Z. (2004). *British J. of Cancer*.

Chapter 12

Gene Therapy for Melanoma: Progress and Perspectives

Bryan E. Strauss and Eugenia Costanzi-Strauss

Additional information is available at the end of the chapter

http://dx.doi.org/10.5772/54936

1. Introduction

Gene therapy, the therapeutic transfer of genetic information to a target cell, continues to be a promising alternative in the fight against cancer. In the case of melanoma, the use of an experimental treatment is justified since this disease is incurable in its advanced stages. Is gene therapy a viable option for the treatment of melanoma patients? In this chapter, we will attempt to answer this question by exploring the intersection between the technology of gene therapy and the biology of melanoma, a point at which opportunities for intervention are revealed.

The technology of gene therapy depends on our ability to create a vehicle that will deliver the therapeutic payload to the target cell. Today, a variety of vectors are available that have the capacity to encode a therapeutic gene or sequences that are capable of blocking gene expression, such as RNA interference (RNAi). The technology of viral and non-viral vectors will be discussed. Viral vectors offer the benefit of using existing biological mechanisms in order to enter the target cell. However, when choosing a gene transfer vehicle, viral vectors must be carefully considered since each option will present a unique profile of advantages and disadvantages, especially as related to the efficiency of the virus in reaching the target cell and in the vector's propensity to activate an immune response. Alternatively, non-viral vectors, such as plasmids, offer the advantage of safety and ease of manipulation, but may require the use of physical or chemical agents in order to pass the through the cytoplasmic membrane and enter the cell.

With these gene transfer tools in hand, now we can turn our attention to the options for the therapeutic gene which will be inserted in the vector. Strategies for cancer gene therapy are many, but share the common goal of inhibiting or destroying the tumor cells. This may be accomplished by the use of pro-apoptic genes, tumor suppressor genes, suicide genes or immune-modulating genes (among many other options). In fact, the therapeutic sequence need not be a gene at all, but instead the RNAi system can be employed to block the expression of critical genes that contribute to tumor progression. Moreover, the gene therapy strategy need not be performed directly in the tumor cells, but may be applied to components of the immune system, such as T-cells or dendritic cells, that will then carry out the anti-tumor activity.

The biology of melanoma presents several opportunities as well as challenges for its treatment by gene therapy approaches. In particular, the high metastatic potential of late stage melanoma represents one of these challenges. Is it realistic to expect that a virus delivered to the primary treatment site will have an effect on distant or even not yet identified metastatic sites? The use of a replicating virus may overcome this barrier since these 'oncolytic' vectors, which multiply only in tumor cells, can spread from cell to cell. In addition, melanoma is considered to be an immunogenic tumor, opening the possibility of generating tumor reactive immune cells with the assistance of gene transfer technology. As an alternative to established modalities, biochemotherapy may be reincarnated in the form of gene transfer of cytokines or interferons. Some cutting edge research efforts include the development of oncolytic viruses that are armed with an immune-modulating gene, creating a double-edged anti-tumor agent.

A growing body of pre-clinical work supports the notion that gene therapy may be a valuable strategy for the treatment of melanoma. To date, quite a few clinical trials of menaloma gene therapy have been performed. With the advances in our understanding of both the technology of gene therapy and the biology of melanoma, we propose that an increasing number of these experimental approaches will reach phase III trials and be offered to a growing number of these patients who have such limited therapeutic options.

2. Gene therapy progress and pitfalls

For more than 20 years now, gene therapy has been applied in more than 1840 clinical trials for the treatment of a great variety of indications (Journal of Gene Medicine's Gene Therapy Clinical Trials Worldwide, http://www.wiley.com/legacy/wileychi/genmed/clinical). Among these trials, cancer represents the disease most commonly treated by therapies that include a gene transfer component. Currently, only a few gene therapy products have been approved for commercialization (Table 1) and the USA has yet to approve any such treatments.

The first gene therapy clinical trial was performed in the USA in 1990. This trial used an *ex vivo* approach where gammaretrovirus was employed to transfer a normal copy of the adenosine deaminase (ADA) gene to peripheral T-cells in two young patients suffering from severe combined immunodeficiency (SCID) due to the lack of ADA function (ADA-SCID) [7]. Neither of the treated patients exhibited any adverse effects and one had clinical benefit lasting well over a decade [8]. Since then, gene therapy for ADA-SCID has evolved and now uses *ex vivo* genetic modification of hematopoietic stem cells resulting in proper immune function, adenosine metabolism and no need for further treatment in 21 of 31 patients, none of whom showed adverse effects [9].

A similar approach for the treatment of SCID-X1 (SCID due to a mutated IL2RG gene, the common IL2 receptor gamma chain) and 18 of 20 patients have had their immune system restored. Unfortunately, 5 of these children developed leukemia due, in part, to the presence of the therapeutic virus in the patients' genome. Though 4 were successfully treated with chemotherapy, one patient did succumb to the leukemia [9]. Many important lessons were learned from the SCID trials, including the fact that the same vector can be innocuous in one situation (ADA-SCID), yet dangerous in another (SCID-X1). The SCID-X1 trials were more successful in achieving long term benefit (90% vs. 70%) and were less likely to provoke an adverse effect (25% vs. 50%) when comparing the traditional treatment (allogenic bone marrow transplant in particular) and gene therapy, respectively [9]. Efforts are underway to use alternative vectors, such as lentivirus, that should be safer and should not provoke the side effects seen with the gammaretroviral vectors.

Local (year/agency)	Company	Vector	Description	References
China (2003/ SFDA)	Shenzhen Gentech SiBiono	Gendicine (Ad-p53)	Non-replicating adenoviral vector expressing wild-type p53 for the treatment of head and neck cancer.	[1, 2]
China (2005/ SFDA)	Shanghai Sunway Biotech	Oncorine/H101 (Onyx-015)	Conditionally replicating adenovirus containing a mutant E1b protein which confers tumor-specific oncolysis. Approved for treatment of head and neck cancers.	[1, 2]
Phillipines (2007/ BFAD)	Epeius	Rexin-G*	Replication-incompetent retrovector targeted to the tumor matrix (collagen) and expressing a cyclin-g mutant that induces cell death. Approved for treatment of all solid tumors.	[3, 4]
European Union (2012/EMA-CHMP**)	Amsterdam Molecular Therapeutics	Glybera (alipogene tiparvovec)	Adeno-associated virus encoding the Ser(447)X variant of human lipoprotein lipase (LPL) gene for the treatment of familial LPL deficiency.	[5, 6]

*Orphan drug status approved by FDA in 2008 **Approval finalized in late 2012; orphan drug status granted in 2004.SFDA, State Food and Drug Administration of China; BFAD, Bureau of Food and Drugs; EMA-CHMP, European Medicines Agency-Committee for Medicinal Products for Human Use; FDA, Food and Drug Administration, USA

Table 1. Gene therapy products approved for commercial distribution.

Genetic modification of hematopoietic stem cells has also been explored for the treatment of β-thalessemia, Wiskott Aldrich Syndrome, adrenoleukodystrophy and chronic granulomatous disease [9, 10]. These trials were generally considered to be successful with respect to clinical benefit of the treatment, yet only the treatment of ALD was free from unwanted cellular proliferation due to the presence of the therapeutic virus. The field continues to evolve and the need for better vectors and a better understanding of their biology is warranted.

Other examples of successful gene therapy have been reported for the treatment of Leber's congenital amaurosis, a genetic alteration that leads to blindness. Several groups have transferred a normal copy of the affected gene, HPE65, to the retina using adeno-associated virus. Of the 18 patients originally treated, many have gained visual acuity and are able to identify shapes and even navigate obstacle courses that were impassable before treatment. In general, these patients first received monocular therapy, but, due to the success of the treatment, several have since been treated in the contralateral eye. The effectiveness of the second treatment was significant since clinical benefit was achieved and re-inoculation of the virus was not blocked by nor did it provoke any unwanted immune response [11].

In 1999, Jessie Gelsinger, a young patient with ornithine transcarbamylase deficiency received a massive dose of adenovirus as part of his gene therapy. Unfortunately, he suffered a strong immune reaction, entered anaphylactic shock and died [10]. Though this case did spark quite a bit of controversy and contributed to the negative public opinion of gene therapy, it does serve as a reminder of how new, experimental and unexplored aspects of gene therapy require continued re-evaluation. In this introduction, we have attempted to present a balanced description of the progress and pitfalls noted in gene therapy trials. Note that of the thousands of patients treated with gene therapy world-wide, we know of only 10 or so cases of serious adverse effects due to the gene therapy agent (the virus). When we consider the cost, time, morbidity and mortality associated with the development of many of the currently accepted ('traditional') treatments, such as bone marrow transplantation and chemotherapy, we see that gene therapy is still in its initial phases, yet many of the benefits do outweigh the risks.

3. Vectors: General concepts

The concept behind gene therapy is really quite simple: introduce genetic material into cells with the aim of inducing a clinically beneficial activity. The process of gene transfer generally requires a vector, or vehicle, to deliver the genetic payload to the target cell. In basic terms, this can be accomplished by either viral or non-viral vectors. Some 65% of clinical trials have relied on viral vectors while 35% used non-viral vectors, including plasmids and RNA (http://www.wiley.com/legacy/wileychi/genmed/clinical/). The principal advantage to using recombinant viral vectors is that their naturally occurring counterparts have already developed mechanisms for reaching and entering cells. This point is also their downfall, since our bodies have also evolved anti-viral defense mechanisms. Since plasmid vectors are essentially free of antigens and since their sequence can be carefully controlled, they are much less likely to provoke an immune response. Many cell types, but especially muscle, are quite efficiently transfected by plasmids.

Selecting a gene transfer vector depends greatly on the therapeutic approach (*ex vivo* or *in situ*), the required duration of transgene expression (for example, long term for immunodeficiencies and metabolic disorders, but short term for cancer), the disease and cell type in question (proliferating or post-mitotic, stem cell or differentiated, etc) and the characteristics of the transgene itself (the length of the cDNA, secretion of the protein product, requirement for expression in a specific tissue or under a particular physiologic condition). Some of the more popular gene transfer vectors are described in Figure 1 and Table 2.

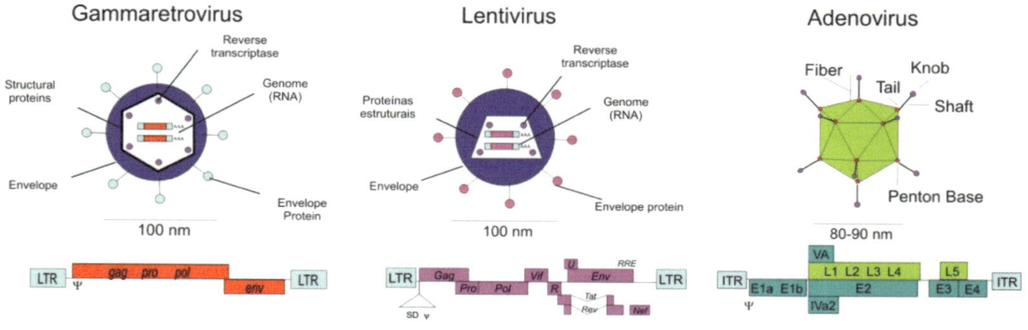

Figure 1. Schematic representation of the wild type counterpart of the typically used recombinant viral vectors. (A) Gammaretroviruses and (B) lentiviruses share similar structures, but differ greatly in their genomes and their impact on cellular function. *Gag, pro, pol* and *env* genes encode structural proteins of the capsid, protease, reverse transcriptase and envelope proteins, respectively. The additional lentiviral genes perform regulatory functions as well as alter cellular function. (C) The serotype 5 adenovirus has a protein capsid (non-enveloped) and a large, complex genome that encodes critical genes for viral replication (E1a, E1b) as well as structural and functional genes that regulate both viral and cellular activities.

In the laboratory, viral vectors are typically manipulated in the form of plasmids that encode the genome to be packaged in the viral progeny (including the gene of interest and regulatory elements that control its expression) as well as information for the generation of a functional virus particle. In general, viral vectors are engineered so that they are incapable of replicating outside of the laboratory. In other words, they can be produced in the lab, but do not form an active infection in patients, thus limiting their horizontal spread. Replication deficient viruses are capable of entering a target cell and expressing the therapeutic gene, but do not carry enough genetic information to form the next generation of virus, a process best referred to as transduction.

Plasmid vectors are much simpler from a technological point of view and come with the benefit of residing in the cell as an episome and being poorly immunogenic. Some considerations when using plasmids include vector design and delivery. Since cells do not actively take up plasmids, it would seem that their utility as a gene transfer vector would be limited. In reality, muscle cells are quite permissive to transfection even when 'naked' plasmid DNA is applied. When complexed to chemical carriers and/or in combination with physical methods of transfection, a great many tissues can be treated with plasmids (or even oligos, siRNA, RNA, etc). Non-viral vectors, therefore, offer certain advantages over recombinant viruses.

Vector targeting can be performed at either the transcriptional or transductional level. In theory, targeting would present the advantage of promoting gene transfer in the cell of interest and avoiding 'off target' effects. In this way, normal healthy cells would be spared and the treatment would be directed to the appropriate cell. Vector targeting should increase safety and efficiency of the treatment. Transductional targeting directs the virus to a specific cell type and should reduce the number of off target cells that are transduced. In other words, the virus should reach only the desired cell type. Such vectors are engineered so that that viral proteins are able to interact with specific cellular receptors present only (or principally) on the target cell. Transcriptional targeting involves the use a promoter that is active only in the desired cell type or only under specific physiologic conditions. Cancer cells offer many distinctions that benefit transcriptional targeting, such as expression of hTert or survivin, proliferation (which is typically associated with E2F1 activity) and stabilization of HIF1α under hypoxic conditions. Transcriptional targeting does not restrict which cells will be transduced, but does determine where the vector will be allowed to express the transgene. These strategies can also be combined, thus increasing the degree of specificity.

Vector	**Gammaretrovirus**	**Lentivirus**	**Adenovirus**	**Adenoassociated Virus**	**Non-viral (plasmid, naked and lipofection)**
Titer, virus particles/ml[a]	10^9	10^9	10^{12}	10^{12}	NA
Route of delivery	Ex vivo	Ex vivo	In situ	In situ	In situ
Integration in the host genome	Yes	Yes	No	Yes/No	No
Long term expression	Yes	Yes	No	Yes	No
Immune response to viral proteins	No	No	Yes	Yes, but less severe	No
Clinical trials[b]	370	55	438	92	456
Typical clinical application	Hematopoietic system	Hematopoiet ic system	Cancer, vaccines, vascular diseases	Hemophilia, cystic fibrosis	Cardiovascular, cancer, vaccines

a: titer after concentration of virus preparation

b: trials listed on http://www.wiley.com/legacy/wileychi/genmed/clinical/

NA, not applicable

Table 2. Properties of vectors commonly used in clinical gene therapy trials

http://dx.doi.org/10.5772/54936

4. Vectors: Retrovirus

Gene transfer vectors derived from retroviruses have played an important role in the development of current gene therapy approaches. As mentioned above, a retroviral vector (derived from Moloney Murine Leukemia Virus, MoMLV) was the first to be used in an FDA-sanctioned clinical trial, retroviral vectors are the second most popular viral vector and are the vector of choice for *ex vivo* gene transfer approaches (Table 2).

To be clear, we use the term 'retrovirus' to describe all viruses belonging to the retroviridae family, though we will be focusing on gammaretrovirus (the genus which includes MoMLV) and lentivirus (the genus that includes HIV). These wild-type viruses are closely related and share many features, such as a capsid that is enveloped in a lipid bilayer and which carries two copies of the viral genome in the form of single stranded RNA (Figure 1). When the virus envelope protein interacts with its cognate receptor on the cell surface, the viral and cellular membranes fuse, the capsid is internalized and the RNA strands are liberated in the cytoplasm (Figure 2). The process of reverse transcription generates a dsDNA copy of the viral genome which then must gain access to the nucleus before integrating at an essentially random position in one of the host cell's chromosomes. The DNA copy of the gammaretroviral genome gains access to the cell nucleus only upon cell division, when the nuclear envelope is dismantled. For this reason, gammaretroviruses can only infect dividing cells. In contrast, lentiviral DNA passes through the nuclear membrane by an active process that is unrelated to cell division. In other words, lentiviruses are able to infect both dividing and non-dividing cells. Once the retroviral genome has been integrated in the host DNA, it is then referred to as a provirus. Viral gene expression and viral replication result from the information encoded by the provirus. Virus progeny bud from the cell surface, a process that does not harm the host cell [12].

The recombinant versions of retroviral vectors follow the form and function of their wild-type counterparts, but modifications are engineered in the vectors to improve safety and tropism. In general terms, a plasmid (transfer vector) is used to encode the sequence (including the gene of interest) that will be encapsulated in the virus particle and separate plasmids (packaging constructs) are used to encode the proteins that make up the virus structure (Figure 3). A sequence in the viral genome, called ψ, directs encapsidation of the viral RNA. This signal is present in the transfer vector, but not in the packaging constructs, thus the information for generating a new particle is not carried by the progeny, but the gene of interest is. Since the virus progeny do not carry the genes necessary to form a new particle, viral replication does not occur in the transduced cell and serves as a safety mechanism [12].

The tropism of the retroviral vector is determined principally by its envelope protein. Through engineering of the packaging constructs, the native envelope protein can be exchanged for an alternate protein that provides adequate tropism. For gammaretroviral vectors, ample tropism is provided by the 10A1 amphotropic envelope protein, though other options do exist. For lentivirus, the native envelope proteins direct transduction of CD4 and/or CCR5 positive cells. This would be too limited for most gene transfer efforts. Instead, the lentiviral envelope is typically replaced with the envelope glycoprotein from Vesicular Stomatitis Virus (VSVg). Since VSVg interacts with heparin, a ubiquitous component of the cell membrane, such 'pseudotyped' vectors can transduce most any cell type. The VSVg envelope can also be used to pseudotype gammaretroviral vectors [12, 13].

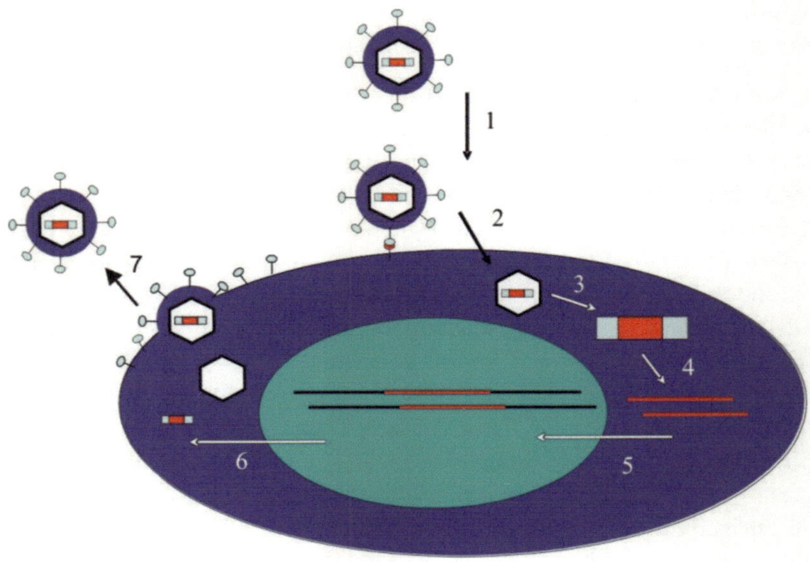

Figure 2. Schematic representation of the retroviral lifecycle. Though a gammaretrovirus is depicted, this process is quite similar for lentiviruses. (1) The retroviral envelope protein interacts with a cellular receptor and membranes are fused. (2) The capsid is internalized and (3) the viral genome, in the form of RNA, is liberated. (4) Reverse transcription results in the generation of a dsDNA copy of the viral genome which then must reach the nucleus (5), a process that for gammaretrovirus requires cell division since the viral DNA is not actively transported across the nuclear membrane, yet lentiviral DNA is and therefore does not require cell division for nuclear import. Once in the nucleus, the viral DNA is inserted in the host genome and is now referred to as a provirus. (6) Expression of the viral genes from the provirus provides all the components necessary for the assembly of progeny which then bud from the cell surface (7).

Retroviral vectors are not efficient vehicles for *in vivo* gene transfer. These vectors are quickly destroyed by complement and have a short half-life in the organism. However, the application of these vectors in cultured cells is an efficient and easy process. In addition, the integration of the provirus ensures that the viral sequence will be passed on to daughter cells after division of the host cell. These characteristics give retroviral vectors an advantage in treatments that require long term expression of the transgene and where *ex vivo* cell manipulation is anticipated, such as the case for treating SCID [13].

Retroviruses have regulatory elements, called long terminal repeats (LTRs) that act as a promoter do drive the expression of viral genes. In recombinant vectors, the LTR can be employed to drive expression of the therapeutic gene, a common practice with gammaretroviral vectors (Figure 3). For safety reasons, the LTR can be inactivated (by deletion of the enhancer sequences contained in the U3 region). Such 'self-inactivating' or 'SIN' vectors require the use of an internal heterologous promoter to drive transgene expression (Figure

3). This practice has long been employed in lentiviral vectors since it offers an additional assurance that recombination between transfer and packaging vectors will not produce a viable, replication competent progeny. An additional safety feature offered by SIN vectors is the decreased chance that the LTR will act as a promoter of host gene expression. The juxtaposition of the LTR and a host gene can result in the unwanted expression of that gene (insertional mutagenesis). In the case of a proto-oncogene, the cell would then be at risk of transformation. This is essentially the cause of the cases of leukemia seen in the SCID-X1 trials. Currently, SIN retroviral vectors are favored since they are less likely to activate the expression of cellular genes, especially if the internal promoter does not contain a strong enhancer (for example, the EF1a promoter) [13, 14].

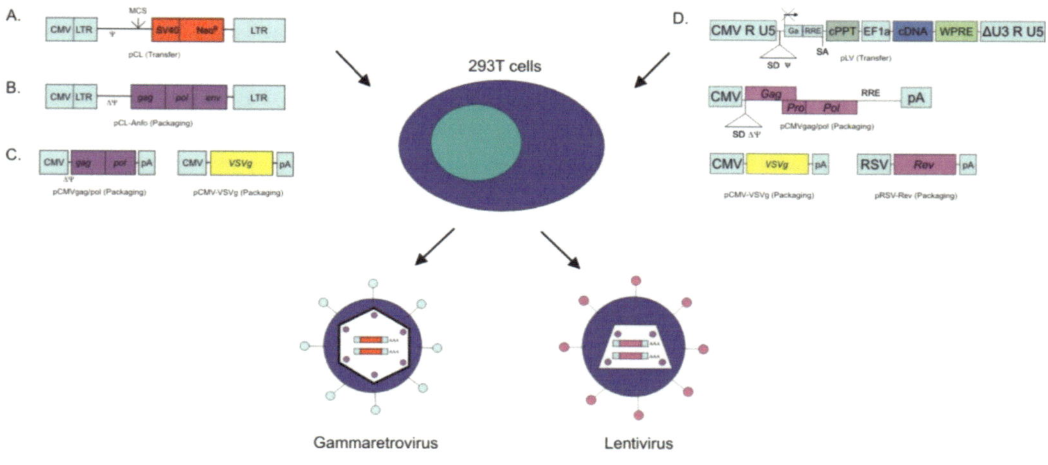

Figure 3. Schematic representation of the retroviral vectors and production. The gene of interest in cloned in a plasmid (transfer vector) that contains the retroviral regulatory elements (LTR, long terminal repeats) as well as elements to regulate the expression of the transgene. The transfer vector is co-transfected along with the necessary packaging vectors in 293T cells (an easily transfected cell line derived from HEK293) where viral progeny are formed, bud from the cell surface and accumulate in the culture medium (supernatant). For gammaretrovirus, the transfer vector (A) can be transfected along with a single packaging vector (B) or, alternatively, with two additional vectors (C) that result in a pseudotyped virus progeny. For lentivirus, third generation transfer and packaging vectors are shown (D) which are all co-transfected in 293T to form virus progeny. Note that the lentiviral vectors do not contain any viral genes associated with HIV pathogenesis. CMV, cytomegalovirus promoter; SV40, simian virus 40 promoter; Neo^R, neomycin resistance gene; *Gag*, group specific antigen (structural proteins); *Pro, pol*, viral enzymes integrase, protease and reverse transcriptase; pA, polyadenylation signal; VSVg, envelope glycoprotein of vesicular stomatitis virus; R, U5, repeat and U5 regions of the LTR; ΔU3, U3 region deleted from the LTR; SD, SA, splice donor, splice acceptor; Ψ, Psi encapsidation signal; RRE, rev-responsive element; Rev, lentiviral rev protein that regulates splicing events of the viral RNA; cPPT, central polypurine tract which facilitates nuclear importation of the lentiviral genome; WPRE, woodchuck hepatitis virus post-transcritptional regulatory element which facilitates nuclear export of the viral transcripts; EF1a, elongation factor 1-alpha promoter which is often employed in retroviral vectors.

Lentiviral vectors are thought to be safer than gammaretroviruses due mainly to their proviral integration preferences. Though neither has a specific integration site, gammaretroviruses have a greater tendency to integrate near the transcriptional start sites of cellular genes than lentivirus [15]. In other words, gammaretroviruses are thought to be more apt to promote unwanted expression of cellular genes. In the case of SCID-X1, SIN lentiviral vectors present one of the best currently available technologies for the safe transfer of the therapeutic gene [9].

Retroviral vectors play an important role in cancer gene therapy approaches. As will be described in detail, retroviral vectors are frequently used to modify components of the immune system in order to promote an anti-tumor immune response. Though the use of gammaretroviral vectors for this purpose has not met with any unwanted side effects, lentiviral vectors are gaining popularity due to their efficiency and safety.

5. Vectors: Adenovirus

Recombinant adenoviral vectors are the vehicle of choice for *in situ* gene therapy of solid tumors (Table 2). Such vectors can be produced at high concentration (10^{12} particles/mL) and are quite well equipped to mediate gene transfer *in vivo*. The genome of the adenoviral vector remains episomal, thus the issues related to provirus integration (discussed above) are rendered moot. However, adenoviral vectors are known for provoking an anti-viral immune response. In the case of cancer gene therapy, the anti-viral immune response has not been associated with serious adverse effects and may even provide a benefit of attracting the immune response to the tumor site. The episomal viral genome and anti-viral immune response limit the duration of vector function, thus making adenoviral vectors inappropriate for the long term treatment of chronic diseases, such as hemophilia or SCID. Yet, the short-lived presence of transduced cells is compatible with cancer gene therapy since the goal is to express a factor that results in the elimination of the tumor cell, a process that does not require long term expression of the transgene [16-19].

The wild-type serotype 5 adenovirus (Ad5) has a linear, dsDNA genome of approximately 36 kb surrounded by a protein capsid from which fiber proteins project (Figure 1). The fiber protein mediates interaction with the Ad5 cognate receptor, CAR (Coxsackie Adenovirus Receptor) (Figure 4). The penton base then interacts with α_v integrins and the virus particle is then internalized, travels to the nucleus via microtubules and, finally, the viral DNA is deposited in the nucleus, a process that is independent of cell division. The viral genome remains episomal while viral transcripts are expressed and progeny are formed. In this case, virus progeny accumulate within the cell eventually resulting in cell lysis and the liberation of viral progeny. Adenoviral replication requires the activity of the viral E1a and E1b proteins which inactivate Rb and p53, respectively, and are involved in transport of viral transcripts and promote the expression of other viral genes [16-19].

In the laboratory, recombinant adenoviral vectors (Ad) are manipulated in the form of plasmids (Figure 5). The transfer vector encodes the gene of interest and the viral vector encodes the remainder of the viral sequence, except that E1a and E1b are deleted. Since the viral vector is quite cumbersome (approximately 40 kb), traditional cloning methods are inefficient for inserting the gene of interest. Alternatively, recombination between the transfer vector and viral vector may be performed or the use of rare restriction sites may be employed, either method resulting in a new plasmid that contains both the gene of interest and the viral sequence.

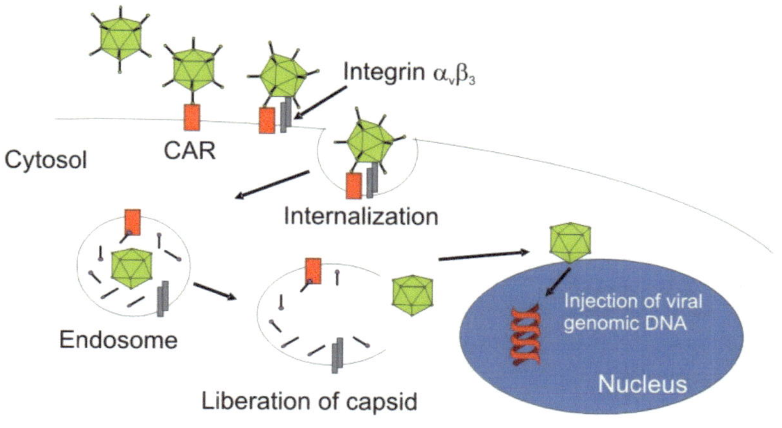

Figure 4. Schematic representation of the adenoviral life cycle. For serotype 5 adenovirus, the knob portion of the fiber protein mediates interaction with the cellular receptor, CAR (Coxsackie Adenovirus Receptor). In a second step of viral/cellular interaction, the penton base then binds with the integrin $\alpha_v\beta_3$. The virus is then internalized, partially disassembled and the capsid is carried to the nucleus my the microtubule network. The viral genome is deposited in the nucleus where expression of the viral genes results in the formation of progeny which accumulate intracellularly, eventually causing lysis and release of progeny.

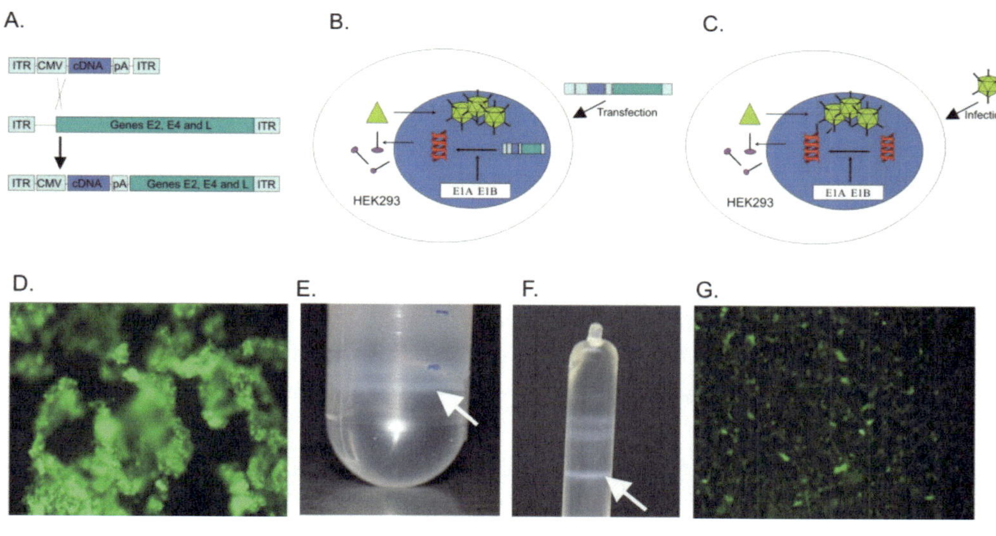

Figure 5. Schematic representation of recombinant adenoviral vectors and production. (A) The gene of interest is inserted in the small transfer vector which is then recombined with the rest of the viral genome. However, the recombinant genome is devoid of the E1a and E1b genes (thus limiting viral replication). (B) The resulting plasmid is then transfected in HEK293 cells (which harbor the E1a and E1b genes), thus initiating the production of virus. (C) The initial production is then used to infect fresh HEK293 cells, thus amplifying virus production. (D) Photomicrograph of HEK293 cells suffering from the cytopathic effect induced by the replicating adenoviral vector which, in this case, encodes eGFP (enhanced green fluorescent protein). (E) Step and (F) continuous CsCl gradient purification of the virus progeny (indicated by the arrows). (G) Cells transduced with the now purified virus progeny is evidenced by their expression of eGFP.

The new plasmid containing the gene of interest as well as the viral components is transfected into an appropriate cell line in order to initiate the production of virus particles. Since the plasmid is devoid of E1a and E1b, the vector does not provide sufficient information to promote virus production. Instead, the cell line used, HEK293, already contains the E1 genes and provides expression of E1a and E1b in *trans*. In this way, only when the plasmid is introduced in HEK293 cells is virus production initiated. The progeny viruses formed are also deficient for replication since they too lack the E1 gene. However, the progeny virus can then be used to infect fresh HEK293 cells (a process that is much more efficient than transfection) and additional virus progeny will be formed. This 'amplification' of virus is repeated until a suitable volume of viral lysate has been generated. This, in turn, must be purified (at lab scale by CsCl gradient centrifugation, at industrial scale by filtration and chromatography) to rid the virus particles of cellular debris [16-19].

Even after purification, the virus progeny will contain a mixture of viable, infectious particles and defective, incomplete virus capsids. When using the virus to transduce a target cell, only the viable particle will result in transgene expression. However, the defective particles contribute to the load of antigens that the cell/organism receives and, with increased antigen, comes an increased chance of provoking an immune response, much as was seen in the case of Jessie Gelsinger. For this reason, care should be given to distinguish between the total viral load and infectious particles used [20]. Generally, total virus load is expressed as VP/mL (virus particles per milliliter) and infectious virus as IU/mL or PFU/mL (infectious units/mL or plaque forming units/mL). Even in high quality preparations, VP/mL will be 10 to 25 times greater than IU/mL.

Adenoviral vectors have evolved since their initial use was described. First generation vectors have deletions in the E1 and E3 genes, thus limiting replication and eliminating a non-essential viral gene. In an attempt to reduce the anti-viral immune response, second generation vectors with deletion in the E4 region (gene non-critical to viral replication, but which contributes to immune activation) were developed. The third generation of adenoviral vectors is devoid of any gene encoding an adenoviral protein. Though this complicates the strategy for virus production, it does yield virus that are much less immunogenic and provide more prolonged expression of the transgene. Even with these improvements, most cancer gene therapy protocols involving adenovirus use first generation vectors [16, 17].

Expression of the transgene encoded by the adenoviral vector requires the use of an internal heterologous promoter. This provides the opportunity for transcriptional targeting or a strong, constitutively active promoter, such as CMV, may be used. In first generation adenoviral vectors, a total of 7 kb of sequence may be inserted. Especially for cancer gene therapy, this is quite adequate for a promoter, transgene (or two) and polyadenylation signal.

As mentioned above, CAR is the cellular protein that mediates the interaction with Ad5 (Figure 4). In the absence of CAR, Ad5 transduction is quite inefficient. Though many cell types express CAR, some do not, including certain types of cancer (melanoma) and some cancer stem cells. In this case, engineering of the virus may be required so that interaction with CAR is no longer necessary for successful transduction. One such approach involves the insertion of the RGD tripeptide in the H1 loop of the knob protein. In this case, the principal receptor is now α_v integrins which are widely expressed. By similar methods, the knob can also be adapted so that it interacts with specific cellular receptors of interest. That is to say, transductional targeting is achieved by altering the knob protein [17, 21].

If an adenoviral vector can be targeted at the levels of transcription and transduction, then it becomes tempting to apply the virus systemically with the expectation that it will have specificity for the target cell, such as the tumor. Unfortunately, other components of the virus, such as the fiber and the capsid, mediate interactions with heparin sulfate and factor X, both of which are highly abundant in the liver. In other words, attempts to apply the virus systemically are thwarted by viral sequestration in the liver. Even worse, the virus tends to transduce Kupfer cells (liver macrophages) that, in turn, present viral antigens to the immune system and induce an immune response. This implies that even the treatment of hepatocarcinomas by systemic administration of adenovirus will be undermined by transduction of Kupfer cells. Extensive engineering of the vector is required in order to prevent transduction of liver cells while directing transduction to the correct target [17, 22]. Though a few laboratory studies point to the viability of this approach, for now it remains quite problematic. Successful application of adenoviral vectors is typically performed by *in situ* injection of the virus into the tumor mass.

6. Vectors: Oncolytic adenovirus

Up to this point we have described vectors that are deficient for replication. However, viral replication can also be used to benefit the treatment of cancer. Such oncolytic or virotherapies rely on the viral replication to cause lysis of the tumor cell. The resulting progeny can then infect additional tumor cells and repeat the process, in theory, until all tumor cells have been eliminated. Clearly, such an approach requires extensive engineering of the vector such that replication is permitted only in the tumor cell, thus sparing normal cells [23].

An additional benefit to the oncolytic approach is that cell death does not depend on apoptosis. A fundamental feature of tumor cells is their resistance to cell death even in response to signals that would, in a normal cell, be fatal. Since oncolytic activity is not dependent on cellular genes, there is a greatly reduced chance that the cell would develop resistance to the viral activity. The same cannot be said for many pharmacologic approaches [23].

Several viruses, such as Herpes Simplex, Vaccinia and even retroviral vectors have been developed into oncolytics. However, for simplicity, we will focus on conditionally replicating adenoviruses (CRAds). The key to controlling CRAds lies in the E1 genes. As mentioned above, adenoviral replication requires the function of the E1a and E1b proteins (encoded by the E1 genes). If E1a and/or E1b function is permitted only in tumor cells, then the virus will replicate only in tumor cells. One approach uses a tumor-specific promoter to drive expression of the E1 gene. Promoters such as hTert, E2F1 and survivin are much more active in tumor cells than in differentiated adult tissues. The use of one of these promoters to drive E1 gene expression creates a degree of tumor specificity [23].

Another approach involves the use of a mutant version of the E1a gene. Adenoviral replication is not supported in the presence of wild type Rb and, for this reason, E1a has evolved to interrupt Rb activity. Since Rb is typically inactivated in tumor cells, E1a is no longer required to provide this function. Deletion of the 24 amino acids from E1a which mediate its interaction with Rb results in an altered E1a protein that no longer blocks Rb function. In a normal cell, the persistence of Rb function blocks viral replication. In a tumor cell, the typical loss of Rb activity creates a condition where viral replication is supported. CRAds that combine transductionoal and transcriptional targeting as well as the E1a deletion mutant have been created and tested with promising results [23-25].

A classic example of an oncolytic adenovirus was originally known as Onyx-015. In this vector, the E1b gene was mutated with the intention of permitting viral replication in p53-deficient cells, but normal cells, with wild-type p53, should not allow viral replication. This vector has been widely studied and even approved for commercialization in China (Table 1). However, it was later noted that the underlying mechanism that controls Onyx-015 replication is not related to the p53 status, but instead to the RNA export functions of the E1b protein [26, 27].

In addition to the sophisticated engineering of the CRAds, some these vector also carry a therapeutic gene. Such vectors are referred to as armed CRAds. For example, the expression of GM-CSF or interferon-β together with the activity of the CRAd should promote an anti-tumor immune response. Alternatively, the vector may be armed with additional death-inducing factors, such as the thymidine kinase gene (TK) derived from herpes simplex virus. In this case, the application of the prodrug ganciclovir induces cell killing and augments the effect of the CRAd. Another approach involves the use of the TNF-related apoptosis-inducing ligand (TRAIL) which, when cleaved into a soluble form, induces apoptosis in tumor, but not normal, cells [24, 25, 28].

In all, oncolytic viruses can combine tumor specific activities in order to bring about cell death independent of apoptosis, but can also be armed to induce apoptosis, immune activation and interrupt cellular DNA replication.

7. Vectors: Non-viral

The typical non-viral vector is a recombinant plasmid, though oligos, siRNA and RNA fall into this category. Recombinant plasmids are derived from their wild-type counterpart, a small circle of episomal dsDNA found in a variety of bacteria. In the lab, we need only maintain regulatory sequences that control the replication of the plasmid in their bacterial host as well as an antibiotic resistance gene that facilitates the manipulation and maintenance of the plasmid in the lab. The therapeutic gene of interest is then inserted along with appropriate regulatory sequences (such as a promoter and polyadenylation site). Once constructed, the production of the vector is performed using well established techniques involving large volumes of bacterial cultures and purification of the plasmid by filtration and chromatography [29-31].

Though the use of plasmid vectors is quite routine and performed in a great many research labs on a daily basis, some considerations of vector design and delivery should be taken into account. The vector itself should not contain extraneous sequences that are not part of the treatment. That is to say, the vector delivered to the patient should not contain antibiotic resistance genes or regulatory sequences of bacterial origin. Such sequences could provide expression of unwanted peptides or even contain GC rich sequences, both known to provoke immune responses. However, production of plasmids requires the presence of just such regulatory sequences. To overcome this, the plasmids are often engineered such that once the bacteria and the plasmids they contain have been expanded to the necessary volume, recombination can be induced such that the unwanted sequences are eliminated and only the small circular DNA containing the gene of interest remains. It is this small circular DNA that is then purified and delivered to the patient, free of non-essential sequences [31].

Plasmid delivery can be performed by direct injection of 'naked' DNA with or without physical methods to promote transfection, such as the gene gun, electroporation or microbubbles. Alternatively, the plasmid may be complexed with chemical compounds that facilitate its passage across the cell membrane. Such complexes may include lipids, polyethylene glycol, polyethyleneimine or other compounds can both secure the DNA molecules as well as mediate cellular uptake. Such approaches are often referred to as 'nanotechnology' since these virus-sized particles can be engineered to achieve high levels of transfection and can even include targeting strategies (such as described for transductional targeting) [30, 32-35].

While non-viral gene transfer may be relatively efficient, simple and safe, the episomal nature of the plasmid and limited half-lives of oligos and mRNA often result in short lived expression of the therapeutic gene. As the cell divides or as the transfected material degrades, the therapeutic gene is lost. Such an approach may be inappropriate for the treatment of chronic illnesses, such as immune deficiencies or metabolic disorders. However, non-viral gene transfer is an interesting option when limited transgene expression is sufficient or desirable, such as for the induction of angiogenesis in ischemic tissues or, in the case of cancer, induction of cell death and/or a tumor-specific immune response.

Recently, a new approach was described for non-viral gene transfer to the skin. This new technology involves the use of an array of very small needles that breakdown over time and has been termed dissolvable protrusion array device (PAD) [36, 37]. For this, an array of pins is dipped in a polyvinyl alcohol polymer solution and slowly raised while drying; essentially creating hollow core stalagmites that can be filled with a solution of nucleic acid, such as siRNA. The array of microneedles can then be applied to the skin, penetrating the stratum corneum barrier and depositing the material where it dissolves and locally releases the therapeutic payload. As a demonstration of this technology, human skin xenografts were treated with PAD loaded with an siRNA againt CD44 and significant reduction in target gene expression was observed [36, 37]. In theory, the PAD can be loaded with more than one therapeutic sequence or even with chemotherapeutic drugs, so it is easy to imagine the administration of genetic and pharmacologic therapies directly to the cutaneous tumor mass.

8. Strategies of melanoma gene therapy

Melanoma has played an important part in the history and development of gene therapy. The first clinical trial to use gene therapy to treat cancer was performed at the US National Institute of Health (NIH) Clinical Center in February of 1991, lead by Steven Rosenberg of the National Cancer Institute (NCI). When the results were published, they affirmed that " attempts at gene therapy for cancer are underway ...." [38].

In fact, the milestone study was based on work initiated several years before. Since 1986, Rosenberg had increasing success in treating intractable melanomas with TIL cells (tumor infiltrating lymphocytes) that are surgically removed from a patient's cancer and cultured for 4 to 6 weeks in the laboratory along with interlekin-2 (IL-2), a growth factor that stimulates the immune system, and then the cells are re-infused into the patient. The TILs have a selective affinity for the tumors from which they came, so the TIL-IL2 cells can infiltrate the primary tumors and their metastases [39]. However, as with many new therapies, TIL-IL2 only works a fraction of the time. The question was why? Are the cells reaching their target? A gene transfer experiment was proposed in an attempt to answer that.

The experimental strategy was relatively simple. The first step was to genetically modify human TILs through the introduction of a foreign marker gene in the laboratory (*ex vivo*). The gene for a bacterial enzyme encoding neomycin phosphotransferase (neo^R), which transmits resistance to the antibiotic G418, was chosen. Using a gammaretrovirus to deliver the neo gene, a population of TILs were marked *ex vivo*. Rosenberg, Blaese and Anderson succeeded in getting more than 5% of TILs to take up the neo gene. After administration, these modified TILs can be easy identified in patients' pheripheral blood and tumor biopsies. In 1989, the first of ten patients with end-stage melanoma was treated with infusion of TILs transduced with gammretrovirus and, by following the neo-marker, the research team could follow the TILs. This initial study was designed to determine the long-term traffic patterns and distribution of TILs in the body. It was not expected to offer any medical benefit, yet this clinical experiment demonstrated that gammaretrovirus-mediated transduction could be used to safely modify human lymphocytes which were subsequently administered to the patient. This trial led to additional gene transfer protocols utilizing therapeutic genes with potential for clinical benefit [40].

This and other early gene marking studies suggested that recombinant gene transfer could be achieved in a selected subpopulation of cells. These pioneering trials also helped address important regulatory concerns and stimulated research into delivery vehicles with applications for inherited and acquired diseases. Interestingly, in parallel, M. Blaese and F. Anderson used a similar approach where the gene for adenosine deaminase was transferred by gammaretrovirus into lymphocytes of children with severe combined immunodeficiency disease and is regarded as the first therapeutic gene therapy trial, as mentioned above [7].

Since Rosenberg knew that TILs localize at tumor sites and that TILs can be safely modified with gammaretrovirus, he then attemped to introduce TNF (tumor necrosis factor-alpha) into TILs and use these genetically modified cells as vehicles to deliver TNF, a potent antitumor protein, directly into the tumor. This trial represents the first time a candidate therapeutic gene was introduced into human cells with the goal of treating cancer [41]. Three late-stage melanoma patients were treated with unselected TILs that had been transduced with the TNF gammaretrovirus, but the subsequent seven patients received modified TILs that were selected for G418 resistance in order to increase the fraction of tranduced cells present in the TIL cultures. The modified TILs were expected to accumulate at the tumor sites and produce local concentrations of TNF high enough to mediate tumor death, yet without exposing the patient to high systemic doses of TNF. The treatment was well tolerated and, as often seen in phase I safety trials, clinical benefit was not profound [38]. However, this trial paved the way for future cancer gene therapy efforts.

To date, some 1186 cancer gene therapy trials have been cited, representing approximately 65% of all gene therapy clinical protocols (http://www.wiley.com/legacy/wileychi/genmed/clinical/). A great many approaches have been attempted with the fundamental goal of eliminating the tumor cells by direct induction of cell death or by induction of an anti-tumor immune response. Specifically in the case of melanoma, some 161 trials have been cited (Figure 6). In fact, melanoma is the most frequent indication seen in cancer gene therapy trials, even more than prostate, lung or breast. Among these melanoma gene therapy trials, 7 phase III protocols have been cited. These include transfer of the B7.1 gene (5 trials) and GM-CSF (2 trial).

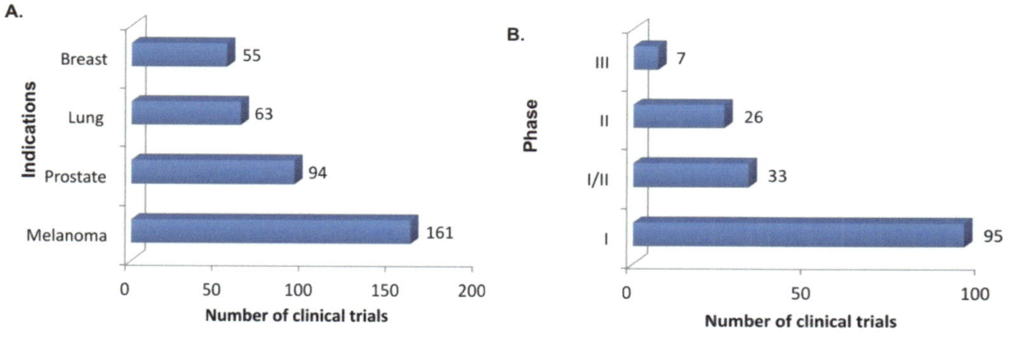

Figure 6. Progress in clinical trials of melanoma gene therapy. (A) Distribution of more frequent indications for cancer gene therapy. (B) Distribution of clinical trials of melanoma gene therapy by phase. Data extracted from Journal of Gene Medicine Clinical Trial Database (current as of June 2012).

These clinical trials highlight the variety of approaches that have been attempted (Figure 7). These include strategies of viral gene transfer (62% of trials), where adenovirus and gammaretrovirus are the most used. Non-viral vectors (38% of trials) have been used as naked DNA or in conjunction with physical and chemical means of improving their efficiency. Strategies have included the transfer of seven principal gene families, including interleukins, tumor associated antigens, suicide genes and genes for the modulation of the immune response (GM-CSF, B7.1 and type I interferon). In the following discussion we present some illustrative examples from pre-clinical to phase III trials.

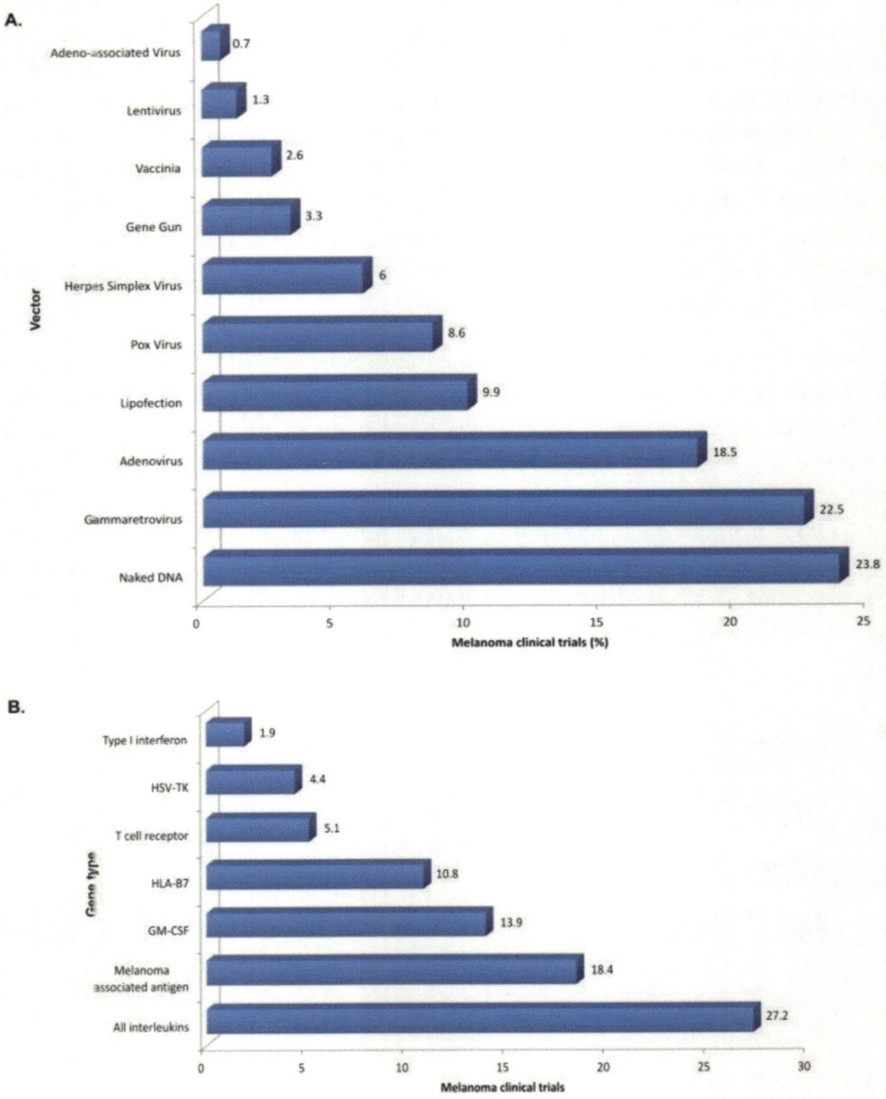

Figure 7. Strategies of melanoma gene therapy tested in the clinic. (A) Frequency of vector usage. (B) Therapeutic gene type used. Data extracted from Journal of Gene Medicine Clinical Trial Database (current as of June 2012).

9. Suicide genes

A classic cancer gene therapy approach involves the transfer of a 'suicide gene' or 'gene directed enzyme prodrug therapy'. In this scenario, an enzyme is introduced in the target cell by gene transfer. This enzyme alone does not have an effect on the cell, but when an appropriate prodrug is administered, the enzyme converts the innocuous prodrug into an active, death inducing compound. Two of the better known examples are the thymidine kinase gene derived from herpes simplex virus (HSV-TK) which promotes phosphorylation of the prodrug ganciclovir and the bacterial cytosine deaminase (CD) gene which converts the prodrug 5-fluorocytidine (5FC) into the chemotherapeutic agent 5-fluorouracil (5FU). In both cases, the compound produced by the enzyme/prodrug interaction blocks DNA replication and, as a result, induces cell death. The advantages of suicide gene therapy include very limited reaction to the enzyme or prodrug in isolation, yet their combination results in a localized concentration of an anti-neoplastic agent. Since DNA replication is a prerequisite for the action of the modified prodrug, this approach has specificity for dividing cells and spares post-mitotic cells even in the case that they should be transduced. Suicide gene therapy is aided by the 'by-stander' effect where the modified prodrug may be passed from a transduced cell to a non-transduced neighbor, killing it only if it is actively dividing. In addition, at least in the case of HSV-TK/ganciclovir, a significant tumor-specific immune response may be elicited, thus amplifying the effects of the gene therapy even further [42].

Specifically in the case of melanoma, a few examples of clinical application of suicide genes have been reported. For example, a phase I/II study utilized a gammaretroviral vector for the transfer of the HSV-tk gene to melanoma patients. However, these authors actually implanted cells that were actively producing the vector in the patients. In this way, the tumor cells would receive a constant supply of virus until administration of the prodrug which would then bring about the death of both the tumor cells and the virus producing cells. These treatments were associated with well tolerated inflammatory skin reactions and moderate fever. During ganciclovir treatment, the tumors did show signs of shrinkage, but increased in size upon drug withdrawal. These results are quite encouraging given that the treatment was well tolerated and showed signs of clinical benefit, at least during the prodrug treatment [43].

In a separate trial, 13 melanoma patients were treated with gammaretrovirus by direct injection of the virus particles into the tumor mass followed by ganciclovir administration. The gene transfer protocol was well tolerated with only one patient showing grade III pain at the injection site. The treatment with the prodrug was associated with some side effects, including dyspnea, pain and poor appetite. However, no response was detected when comparing injected and non-injected tumors. Though the desired result was no observed, the gene therapy procedure was well tolerated [44].

Laboratory assays using CD have yielded some promising results and also exemplify interesting technologies. For example, Kucerova et al [45] have used mesenchymal stem cells to infiltrate melanoma tumors in a mouse model. In this case, the mesenchymal stem cells offer the advantage of migration to and within the tumor mass, an inherent property of these cells. The human fat-derived mesenchymal cells were transduced with a gammaretrovirus encoding the CD gene and delivered i.v. or i.p. in nude mice bearing a tumor derived from a human melanoma cell line (A375). Significant inhibition of tumor progression was seen with the i.v. injection of the CD-expressing mesenchymal cells plus 5FC treatment [45].

In another example involving CD/5FC, an adenoviral vector was targeted to tumor vascular endothelial cells at both the transductional and transcriptional levels. For this, the adenoviral vector displayed the RGD tripeptide in the H1 loop of a mutated fiber knob protein (so that transduction depends on $\alpha_v\beta_3$ integrins instead of CAR) and also used the endothelial cell-specific Tie2 receptor promoter to drive expression of the CD gene. B16 tumors were established in nude mice and the modified adenovirus was administered i.v., but only after pre-treatment with hetastarch, a reagent that effectively blocks hepatic uptake of adenovirus. The authors report that only endothelials, pericytes and tumor monocytes were transduced, but not the tumor cells themselves. Administration of 5FC resulted in significant inhibition of tumor progression [46].

10. Adoptive cell transfer

One of the most promising frontiers of cancer therapy is the use of adoptive cell transfer (ACT). Especially in the case of metastatic melanoma, where few options exist, ACT may overcome some of the limitations seen with even the most promising treatments (including high-dose IL-2 and anti-CTLA-4). In addition, a naturally occurring, tumor specific T cell response is seen in a large percentage of melanoma patients, suggesting that these tumors are immunogenic and that T cells can be made to recognize them. ACT utilizes the patients' own T cells where they are activated *ex vivo*, expanded, and returned to the patient to carry out tumor-specific cytolysis. Since gene transfer is the theme of this chapter, we will focus on approaches that involve genetic modification of either the T cells themselves or of the dendritic cells (DC) used to activate them. At its core, ACT is used to generate T cells that are tumor reactive, though several approaches have been described [47, 48].

Tumor infiltrating lymphocytes (TILs) can be isolated from melanoma biopsies and the T cells expanded *ex vivo*. This approach, which does not involve genetic modification, relies on two critical factors, the ability to isolate T cells and expanding them to clinically significant numbers. Over time, alternatives to this approach have been explored, such as preconditioning by lymphodepletion, the use of young TILs (cells that have not undergone extensive expansion *ex vivo*) or enrichment for CD8+ TILs. Isolation of T cell clones from TILs that are specific for melanoma associated antigens (such as MART1/MelanA, NY-ESO-1 or gp100) can also be performed, but this process requires 3 to 5 months and the clinical outcome (50% objective response) does not surpass that seen with polyclonal TILs [47, 48].

The above argument points to considerable success with ACT, however there is room for improvement, especially with respect to tumor regression. Genetic modification of T cells as a form of ACT has been developed and tested clinically. For example, the T cells may be transduced with a retrovirus that provides expression of a cytokine, such as IL-2, IL-12 or IL-15 or may be modified to resist the effects of immunoregulatory factors. The aim here is to preserve the function of the ACT, but does not necessarily assist in tumor reactivity of the T cells. Thus far, IL-12 and IL-15 expressing cells are still being tested, while IL-2 expressing cells did not show any advantage over non-modified ACT [47-50].

Since the role of the T cell receptor (TCR) is to mediate, in part, the recognition of and response to specific antigens, the patients' T cells may be modified by the introduction of a recombinant

TCR with specificity for a tumor associated antigen. This is a time consuming process and the clinical response rate is less than ideal, though this approach is often seen as an alternative for those patients that failed to provide TILs from biopsies. In the ground-breaking work of Morgan et al, peripheral blood lymphocytes from melanoma patients were transduced with a gammaretrovirus encoding the alpha and beta chains of the MART-1-specific TCR. The lymphodelpeted patients received an infusion of the genetically modified, autologous cells. The persistence of these cells was variable and related to experimental conditions of each cohort, but modified cells found even after 90 days. Two (out of 15) patients with progressive metastatic melanoma showed full clinical regression with this treatment [51]. In a later trial conducted by this group, they used improved versions of the TCR and observed a response rate of 30% [52]. Though the response rate was low, these studies show the feasibility of this approach and the importance of fine tuning the TCR.

In a related approach, T cells are modified to express a chimeric antigen receptor (CAR). CARs are engineered molecules that consist of an antigen-recognizing domain derived from an antibody (single-chain variable fragment) fused to a component of the TCR complex (CD3 zeta chain) and, sometimes, also fused to a costimulatory molecule (such as CD28) [47, 48]. This arrangement assures that antigen recognition is sufficient to activate T cell cytolytic function, an interaction that is not HLA restricted and requires only low levels of antigen, thus streamlining and amplifying the T cell response. The lack of HLA restriction implies that the CAR modified T cells need not be autologous and a supply of cells may be generated and maintained at the ready.

Treatment of melanoma with CAR-modified T cells has been performed only in preclinical models, but these show promising results. For example, a CAR specific for ganglioside GD2 was developed in the Brenner laboratory, inserted in a gammaretroviral vector and used to modify T cells. When these cells were exposed to melanoma cells expressing GD2, cytokines were released and melanoma cells were eliminated both *in vitro* and *in vivo* [53]. In a similar fashion, the Rosenberg and Morgan group has developed a high molecular weight melanoma associated antigen (HMW-MAA or CSPG4)-specific CAR. Both CD4 and CD8 T cells expressing this recombinant receptor were reactive and induced target cell cytolysis in an HLA-independent manner [54].

Clinical trials with CAR-modified T cells have been performed for other tumor types, including ovarian cancer, neuroblastoma, leukemia and lymphoma and some clinical benefit has been reported [47, 48]. Unfortunately, a patient being treated with ERBB2-targeted, CAR-modified T cells suffered an adverse reaction and died when these cells lodged in the lung due to low level expression of ERBB2 and initiated a cytokine storm [55]. In a separate trial, a patient treated with CD19-targeted cells also succumbed due, it is believed, to a T cell response [56]. These unanticipated events should not detract from the potential of CAR-modified T cells. Clearly, continued study of the CAR design and T cell response is required and, no doubt, is forthcoming. Nor should this event reflect on the field of gene therapy since safety issues related to the vector itself were not involved in the function of the CAR and subsequent cellular responses.

11. Vaccines

Since melanoma is well known to be an immunogenic tumor, there have been a great many efforts to develop vaccines that induce an anti-melanoma response. Many approaches using peptides, whole proteins, whole cell lysates delivered directly to the patient have been attempted. Also, the introduction of GM-CSF in melanoma cells provides a vaccine that promotes the immune response. Alternatively, dendritic cells themselves may be introduced in the patient, a process that relies on the availability of such cells as well as their ability to recruit and activate T cells in the cancer patient. Currently, much emphasis has been given to the target specific approach of blocking CTLA-4 or PD1 with monoclonal antibodies, thus promoting T cell function, for the treatment of melanoma [57]. Future hopes involve the combination of these vaccine and targeted modalities.

GM-CSF acts by recruiting and promoting the maturation of DCs, a process that is crucial to mounting an effective immune response. Many studies have explored the genetic modification of tumor cells with gammaretroviral vectors expressing GM-CSF, irradiation of these cells and subsequent use of these cells as a tumor vaccine. Soiffer et al [58, 59] observed that metastatic lesions in 11 of 16 treated patients had a dense infiltrate of T cells and extensive tumor destruction, a phenomenon not seen in the absence of this treatment. Vaccination sites showed adverse effects, such as erythema and induration and occasional hemorrhaging, otherwise the treatment was well tolerated [58]. In a later trial, this group used adenovirus instead of the gammaretroviral vector for GM-CSF gene transfer to patient-derived metastatic melanoma cells, followed by irradiation and vaccination. The vaccine was successfully produced for 34 of 35 patients and toxicities included only grade 1 to 2 local skin reactions. Again, infiltration and necrosis of metastatic sites was observed (10 of 16 patients). After 36 months of follow-up, 29% of patients were still alive, four of whom showed no evidence of disease [59].

Though the GM-CSF secreting cells provided some measure of improvement, the successful vaccine requires an abundance of functional T cells to carry out cytolysis. One factor that blocks T cell function in many cancer patients is the CTLA-4 gene. By blocking CTLA-4 function, T cell activity is liberated. Ipilumimab, a monoclonal antibody that binds to and blocks CTLA-4 function was recently approved by the FDA for the treatment of late stage melanoma [57]. Studies by the Dranoff group applied ipilumimab in melanoma patients that had previously been treated with the GM-CSF secreting cellular vaccine [60, 61]. The observations included only low grade inflammatory toxicities, though high level ipilumimab treatment is known to cause high grade toxicity in 15 to 25% of melanoma patients. Though not designed to reveal clinical benefit, evidence of tumor shrinkage was observed in some patients. Since ipilumimab also increases the number of Tregs, proper T cell function may require a specific balance between effector and regulatory cells. A future direction may be to combine the vaccine, ipilumimab and an inhibitor of Tregs [60].

As an alternative, DCs can be modified *ex vivo* with antigens or a vector or mRNA encoding tumor associated antigens. These professional antigen presenting cells can then be introduced in the patient as an immunotherapy. For example, the work of Steele et al

[62] describes the transfection of a plasmid encoding both melan-A and gp100 into DC derived from the patients' own PBMCs followed by delivery of these gene-modified cells in the stage IV melanoma patients (n=27). The number of rounds of vaccination was variable, between 1 and 14, though 15 patients received 4 rounds of treatment. In all, partial response or stable disease was seen in seven patients and treatment-related adverse events were quite mild (flu-like symptoms or mild erythema at the injection site). As with many early phase trials, these results show that the treatment was well tolerated and that a positive response was seen in a few patients [62].

12. Oncolytic viruses (virotherapy)

As described above, oncolytic vectors use the lytic virus life cycle in order to destroy cancer cells. These vectors are engineered so that replication can occur only in tumor cells and, in some cases, are armed with a gene to aide in tumor cell killing. The engineering may include transductional and transcriptional targeting, alteration of viral replication genes and the insertion of a functional transgene.

Some interesting examples of conditionally replicating adenoviruses for virotherapy of mouse models of melanoma have been reported. For example, the group of Albert Deisseroth has developed an oncolytic vector where expression of E1a is controlled by the tyrosinase promoter. Tyrosinase, a melanoma associated antigen, is an important factor in melanogenesis and may even have additional regulatory functions [63]. In this way, E1a expression from the vector should be melanoma-specific. In addition, the vector was modified with the insertion of the RGD tripeptide in the H1 loop of the fiber knob protein, much as was discussed above. This vector showed increased infectivity in melanoma cells and suppressed growth of xenograft tumor models [64].

In an alternative approach, an oncolytic adenovirus was developed where the SPARC (secreted protein acidic and rich in cysteines) promoter was used to drive expression of E1a. In this case, the SPARC promoter should support viral replication not only in the tumor cells, but also in tumor associated stromal cells. Though this approach was beneficial for a model of pancreatic carcinoma, the authors observed that the stromal cells in the melanoma model actually hampered virus performance [65]. This study is interesting since it points out the importance and complexity of the tumor microenvironment on the gene therapy approach.

In a final pre-clinical example, an oncolytic adenovirus was developed which was armed with IL-24 (MDA-7, melanoma differentiation-associated gene-7) as well as arrestin. IL-24, a secreted protein, inhibits melanoma by autocrine and paracrine effects, including inhibition of angiogenesis, immune stimulation and radiosensitization. Arrestin also inhibits angiogenesis and tumor growth. With this doubly-armed oncolytic vector, it was shown that melanoma cells were significantly inhibited both *in vitro* and *in vivo*, the latter being associated with reduced angiogenesis and increased apoptosis [66].

Oncolytic vectors have also been tested clinically. We start by describing a second generation HSV (herpes simplex virus) oncolytic that was developed by deleting not only the ICP34.5

gene (typical of first generation vectors), but also the ICP47 gene which impedes antigen expression. In addition, early expression of another viral factor, US11, promotes tumor-specific virus replication. Finally, this vector was armed with GM-CSF (which promotes dendritic cell maturation and, thus, anti-tumor immune response) and termed OncoVEX^{GM-CSF}. In a phase I dose escalation trial, viral treatments were generally well tolerated, but side effects were more pronounced in patients who were HSV-seronegative before receiving treatment. Of the 26 evaluable patients, 3 showed stable diseaes (including 2 melanoma cases) and 6 showed flattening of the treated tumors. Some notable aspects of this study were the relatively low frequency of viral treatments, low viral dose and lack of chemotherapy required to induce a response [67]. In phase II trials treating stage IIIc and IV melanoma, treatment with OncoVex^{GM-CSF} induced tumor specific (MART-1) CD8-positive T cells and reduced Tregs [68] and, in a separate trial, resulted in a 26% response rate [69]. Currently, a phase III trial, 'OPTIM: Oncovex^{GM-CSF} pivotal trial in melanoma' is underway [70].

The vaccinia virus, best known for its role in eradicating smallpox, has also been developed into an oncolytic vector [71]. These vectors have a rapid lytic cycle, enter cells by membrane fusion (and not a specific receptor) and the enveloped progeny are protected from immune destruction, all factors that enable poxviruses to spread within the organism. Tumor specific poxviruses rely on reduced type I intereferon response, increased rate of cell division, decreased rate of apoptosis and immune evasion seen in tumor cells. In addition, the epidermal growth factor receptor (EGFR)-Ras signaling pathway, which is typically active in tumor cells, promotes poxvirus replication. Since tumor cells are naturally permissive for poxvirus replication, viral transformation genes can be eliminated from the vector. In this way, the vector will replicate only in tumor cells and leave normal cells unharmed. The oncolytic poxvirus can also be armed, such as with the GM-CSF gene and with the bacterial β-galactosidase (LacZ) gene, serving as a marker for transduction as well as an antigen against which antibodies can be generated and measured [71]. The JX-594 poxvirus possesses these features and has been tested clinically.

In a proof of principle trial, 10 melanoma patients were enrolled and treated with no significant side effects, mainly grade 1-2 flu-like symptoms. Post-treatment biopsies showed necrosis and/or intense perivascular lymphocytic infiltration and radiographic tumor assessment, possible in only 5 of the patients, all of which showed stable disease in the treated tumor and 3 patients also showed stable disease at distant, non-treated sites [72].

The oncolytic vectors discussed above were delivered intratumorally. Intravenous delivery, on the other hand, is quite challenging due to the multiple impediments that prevent the virus from successfully reaching its target. However, JX-594 has been delivered i.v. and showed clinical benefit. In this dose escalation study, 23 patients with solid tumors, including melanoma, were treated and adverse effects were limited to grade 1-2 flu-like symptoms. Staining for the β-galactosidase protein revealed the presence of the virus in tumor tissues. In addition, anti-β-galactosidase antibodies were measured and revealed a dose-dependent relationship with the viral load used to treat the patients. GM-CSF was detected in patient blood samples only after treatment. Evidence of anti-tumor activity was noted, including >25% descrease in

http://dx.doi.org/10.5772/54936

FDG-PET. This is study was the first to show dose-related delivery, replication and transgene expression upon i.v. delivery [73].

13. B7.1

Tumor cells often escape detection by the immune system even when anti-tumor immune cells are generated [74]. Among the many possible mechanisms for this phenomenon, metastatic melanoma cells are quite often deficient for B7-1 and B7-2, factors that are essential for full T cell activation. The lack of even one of these factors leads to T cell anergy, inactivation of the T cell after encountering an antigen, essentially generating self-tolerance. In other words, the lack of these factors actually teaches the T cells to ignore the melanoma. This implies that using gene therapy to replace at least one of these missing factors should initiate tumor specific T cell mediated cytolysis.

In 1993, Gary Nabel showed that a plasmid vector encoding HLA-B7 could be safely introduced into patients' melanoma tumors by means of a liposome. One of the five patients showed reduced tumor mass [75]. A subsequent trial by this group revealed T cell infiltration and TIL reactivity was enhanced in treated patients. In addition, two patients showed local inhibition of tumor growth [76]. The concept was then expanded upon by transfer of the β2-microglobulin gene along with HLA-B7 in a single plasmid vector/liposome complex, a treatment now known as Allovectin-7. In this way, Allovectin-7 provides an allogeneic MHC class I protein, essential for antigen presentation and T cell activation [77].

Several phase II studies of Allovectin-7 have been completed. For example, Stopeck et al [78] reported a regimen where 6 intratumoral injections of 10 μg of Allovectin-7 were performed over a 9 week period. The treatment was well tolerated and regression of the injected lesion was seen in 18% of patients, including a complete response and three partial responses [78]. A few years later, a phase II trial was described where 77 patients were treated with the same Allovectin-7 regimen; 9.1% had complete or partial responses with 4.8 months median duration of the response. Interestingly, this trial showed that the treatment was beneficial even in lesions distant to the treatment site [79].

More recently, a phase II dose escalation study was reported [80]. In this study, 127 patients received a total of 2 mg of plasmid DNA, some 10-times more than was used in the previous trials. Complete response was seen in four patients, 11 achieved partial response and the overall response rate was 11.8%. Stable disease was seen in 32 patients. Interestingly, the duration of response was quite extensive, 13.8 months, and evidence of a systemic effect, such as vitiligo and shrinkage of lesions distant to the treatment site, was seen in some patients. No toxicities above grade 2 were noted, but adverse effects were consistent with the expected pro-inflammatory response triggered by Allovectin-7 [80].

Variations of the HLA-B7 gene transfer strategy have also been explored. For example, the B7.1 cDNA has been inserted in a vaccinia virus. In this way, the virus introduces the HLA-B7 gene to a large number of tumor cells and the vector itself may participate in the anti-tumor immune response. In a phase I trial involving 12 patients, intratumoral injection of the B7.1-armed vaccinia virus, termed rV-B7.1, yielded no serious adverse effects, 2 patients with vitiligo, partial objective response was seen in 1 patient and disease stabilization in 2. Patients developed an anti-vaccinia antibody response and 5 of 6 patients showed increase in gp100-specific T cells and 4 of 6 showed increase in MART-1-specific T cells. A patient with >59-month survival post-treatment showed an increase in both of the T cell subsets [81].

The Kaufman group also established a vaccinia vector encoding not only B7.1, but also the costimulatory molecules ICAM-1 and LFA-3 (intracellular adhesion molecule-1 and leukocyte function-associated antigen-1, respectively). This new vector was termed rV-TRICOM. In a phase I trial, side effects were limited to low grade reactions at the site of injection, yet there was a 20.7% objective clinical response. One patient showed a complete response over a 22 month period. Due to the lack of HLA-A*0201 patients, anti-tumor immune responses were not measured, yet anti-vaccinia responses were seen [82].

14. Interferon and interleukin gene transfer

Biochemotherapy, such as treatment with recombinant IL-2 or type I interferon, has shown some degree of success. However, these approaches are hampered by the high doses needed to overcome the short half-life of these proteins. Often, these high doses are come with unwanted systemic toxicities [83, 84]. As an alternative approach, gene therapy may offer the advantage of high concentrations of the therapeutic agent, but only localized to the tumor, thus avoiding systemic toxicity.

Clinical trials with adenoviral vectors expressing IL-2 have been performed. For example, Stewart et al [85] reported a lack of conventional clinical response, yet 24% of patients did show incomplete local tumor regression. They also noted increased CD3 and CD8-positive TILs [85]. In another example, a phase I/II trial included 25 metastatic melanoma patients and 10 patients with other solid tumors. Objective clinical responses, including 2 complete responses, were seen in 5 of the melanoma patients who received the higher dosage of vector. Serum levels of IL-2 were increased after treatment and were proportional to the vector dose used. Side effects were limited to flu like symptoms [86].

IL-24 (or MDA-7, melanoma differentiation associated gene-7) has been extensively reviewed and tested in a variety of pre-clinical models. IL-24 was isolated from human metastatic melanoma cells previously treated by the combination of interferon-beta and mezerein, a protein kinase C activator. This treatment induces a differentiated state that is associated with the differential expression of a number of interesting genes, IL-24 among them. IL-24 is a novel member of the IL-10 gene family and has been shown to depress growth and induce apoptosis specifically in transformed, but not normal or immortalized, cells. In addition, IL-24 has been associated with a potent bystander effect, implying that, in a gene therapy scenario, even non-transduced tumor cells may be killed [87, 88].

To the best of our knowledge, two phase I clinical trial has been reported involving IL-24 gene transfer to melanoma patients. In these studies, a non-replicating adenoviral vector encoding IL-24, termed INGN 241, induced a systemic TH1 cytokine response. Objective responses, including complete response, was seen at higher vector dosages [89, 90]. Despite the melanoma origin of the IL-24 gene, it has been more extensively studied for other tumor types [87].

Gene therapy of melanoma with interferons has not been extensively explored, even though biochemotherapy with type I interferon is well known. One of the few examples includes adenovirus mediated transfer of the interferon-gamma gene. In this trial, 11 patients were treated with increasing vector doses. One grade 3 toxicity was observed and one patient showed stable disease [91]. Matsumoto et al [92] report the use of cationic liposomes complexed with a plasmid encoding the human interferon-beta gene in patients with metastatic melanoma. There were no recognized adverse events and 1 (of 5) patients showed mixed response [92].

Our own laboratories are actively developing novel tools for gene therapy of cancer, including melanoma. Since some 90% of melanoma cases retain wild type p53 [93], we reason that the endogenous p53 protein may be re-activated and induced to participate in the treatment scheme. To this end, we have developed viral vectors where the expression of the transgene is regulated by the transactivation function of p53. We have shown that these vectors offer superior levels of transgene expression [94-96] and the use of p53 or its functional partner, Arf (p14Arf in humans, p19Arf in mice) creates a positive feedback loop [95, 97]. That is to say, transgene function elevates p53 activity which, in turn, promotes expression from the vector and so on. Our published data show that p19Arf, when delivered by our p53-responsive vector, resulted in the sensitization of B16 mouse melanoma cells to pharmacologic agents both *in vitro* and *in vivo* [97]. In our unpublished data, we have combined the activities of the p53/Arf axis with intereferon-β. Though studies are ongoing, we have seen that the combined, but not individual, gene therapies induce massive cell death both *in vitro* and *in vivo*. In addition, immune protection is induced by either *in situ* tumor treatment or by a whole cell vaccine transduced by the gene combination.

15. Conclusion

We have cited several, but certainly not all, examples of how gene therapy is advancing for the treatment of melanoma. Though much has been learned, a long road remains before major successes can be had. As with any experimental approach, progress is incremental and may rely on joining distinct technologies. For example, the history of melanoma gene therapy actually coincides with therapies for immune disorders. But, by daring to test new therapeutic strategies, gene therapy of melanoma has paved the way for cancer gene therapy in general.

The future advances in melanoma gene therapy may come from combining pharmacologic and genetic approaches. For example, the vectors mentioned above may be used in combination with monoclonal antibodies (such as ipilumimab), small molecule inhibitors (such as vermuafenib, PLK4032, the inhibitor of BRAF) and chemotherapies (such as dacarbazine). Though much work remains to be done, it stands to reason that maximizing cell death and the anti-tumor immune response should offer hope for future treatments of melanoma.

Acknowledgements

We are grateful for the efforts of Juliana G. Xande (ICB-USP) for mining the gene therapy clinical trial database. Our work is supported by grants from FAPESP (Fundação de Amparo À Pesquisa do Estado de São Paulo) and fellowships from CNPq (Conselho Nacional de Desenvolvimento Científico e Tecnológico).

Author details

Bryan E. Strauss[1] and Eugenia Costanzi-Strauss[2]

*Address all correspondence to: bryan.strauss@icesp.org.br

1 Cancer Institute of Sao Paulo, University of Sao Paulo School of Medicine, Brazil

2 University of Sao Paulo, Biomedical Sciences Institute, Brazil

References

[1] Jia, H. and J. Kling, *China offers alternative gateway for experimental drugs.* Nat Biotechnol, 2006. 24(2): p. 117-8.

[2] Peng, Z., Q. Yu, and L. Bao, *The application of gene therapy in China.* IDrugs, 2008. 11(5): p. 346-50.

[3] Gordon, E.M. and F.L. Hall, *Noteworthy clinical case studies in cancer gene therapy: tumor-targeted Rexin-G advances as an efficacious anti-cancer agent.* Int J Oncol, 2010. 36(6): p. 1341-53.

[4] Gordon, E.M. and F.L. Hall, *Rexin-G, a targeted genetic medicine for cancer.* Expert Opin Biol Ther, 2010. 10(5): p. 819-32.

[5] Miller, N., *Glybera and the future of gene therapy in the European Union.* Nat Rev Drug Discov, 2012. 11(5): p. 419.

[6] Burnett, J.R. and A.J. Hooper, *Alipogene tiparvovec, an adeno-associated virus encoding the Ser(447)X variant of the human lipoprotein lipase gene for the treatment of patients with lipoprotein lipase deficiency.* Curr Opin Mol Ther, 2009. 11(6): p. 681-91.

[7] Blaese, R.M., et al., *T lymphocyte-directed gene therapy for ADA- SCID: initial trial results after 4 years.* Science, 1995. 270(5235): p. 475-80.

[8] Muul, L.M., et al., *Persistence and expression of the adenosine deaminase gene for 12 years and immune reaction to gene transfer components: long-term results of the first clinical gene therapy trial.* Blood, 2003. 101(7): p. 2563-9.

[9] Fischer, A., S. Hacein-Bey-Abina, and M. Cavazzana-Calvo, *Gene therapy for primary adaptive immune deficiencies.* J Allergy Clin Immunol, 2011. 127(6): p. 1356-9.

[10] Sheridan, C., *Gene therapy finds its niche.* Nat Biotechnol, 2011. 29(2): p. 121-8.

[11] Cideciyan, A.V., *Leber congenital amaurosis due to RPE65 mutations and its treatment with gene therapy.* Prog Retin Eye Res, 2010. 29(5): p. 398-427.

[12] Coffin, J.M., S.H. Hughes, and H.E. Varmus, *Retroviruses.* 1997, Plainsview, New York: Cold Spring Harbor Laboratory Press.

[13] Dropulic, B., *Lentiviral vectors: their molecular design, safety, and use in laboratory and preclinical research.* Hum Gene Ther, 2011. 22(6): p. 649-57.

[14] Baum, C., et al., *Retrovirus Vectors: Toward the Plentivirus?* Mol Ther, 2006. 13(6): p. 1050-1063.

[15] Wu, X., et al., *Transcription start regions in the human genome are favored targets for MLV integration.* Science, 2003. 300(5626): p. 1749-51.

[16] Ahi, Y.S., D.S. Bangari, and S.K. Mittal, *Adenoviral vector immunity: its implications and circumvention strategies.* Curr Gene Ther, 2011. 11(4): p. 307-20.

[17] Khare, R., et al., *Advances and future challenges in adenoviral vector pharmacology and targeting.* Curr Gene Ther, 2011. 11(4): p. 241-58.

[18] Russell, W.C., *Update on adenovirus and its vectors.* J Gen Virol, 2000. 81(Pt 11): p. 2573-604.

[19] Russell, W.C., *Adenoviruses: update on structure and function.* J Gen Virol, 2009. 90(Pt 1): p. 1-20.

[20] Nyberg-Hoffman, C., et al., *Sensitivity and reproducibility in adenoviral infectious titer determination.* Nat Med, 1997. 3(7): p. 808-11.

[21] Everts, M. and D.T. Curiel, *Transductional targeting of adenoviral cancer gene therapy.* Curr Gene Ther, 2004. 4(3): p. 337-46.

[22] Khare, R., et al., *Generation of a Kupffer cell-evading adenovirus for systemic and liver-directed gene transfer.* Mol Ther, 2011. 19(7): p. 1254-62.

[23] Yamamoto, M. and D.T. Curiel, *Current issues and future directions of oncolytic adenoviruses.* Mol Ther, 2010. 18(2): p. 243-50.

[24] Hernandez-Alcoceba, R., *Recent advances in oncolytic virus design.* Clin Transl Oncol, 2011. 13(4): p. 229-39.

[25] Eager, R.M. and J. Nemunaitis, *Clinical development directions in oncolytic viral therapy.* Cancer Gene Ther, 2011. 18(5): p. 305-17.

[26] O'Shea, C.C., et al., *Late viral RNA export, rather than p53 inactivation, determines ONYX-015 tumor selectivity.* Cancer Cell, 2004. 6(6): p. 611-23.

[27] Crompton, A.M. and D.H. Kirn, *From ONYX-015 to armed vaccinia viruses: the education and evolution of oncolytic virus development.* Curr Cancer Drug Targets, 2007. 7(2): p. 133-9.

[28] Kaur, B., T.P. Cripe, and E.A. Chiocca, *"Buy one get one free": armed viruses for the treatment of cancer cells and their microenvironment.* Curr Gene Ther, 2009. 9(5): p. 341-55.

[29] Wang, T., J.R. Upponi, and V.P. Torchilin, *Design of multifunctional non-viral gene vectors to overcome physiological barriers: dilemmas and strategies.* Int J Pharm, 2012. 427(1): p. 3-20.

[30] Tiera, M.J., et al., *Polycation-based gene therapy: current knowledge and new perspectives.* Curr Gene Ther, 2011. 11(4): p. 288-306.

[31] Schleef, M., et al., *Production of non viral DNA vectors.* Curr Gene Ther, 2010. 10(6): p. 487-507.

[32] Vinogradov, S. and X. Wei, *Cancer stem cells and drug resistance: the potential of nanomedicine.* Nanomedicine (Lond), 2012. 7(4): p. 597-615.

[33] Elsabahy, M., A. Nazarali, and M. Foldvari, *Non-viral nucleic acid delivery: key challenges and future directions.* Curr Drug Deliv, 2011. 8(3): p. 235-44.

[34] Geusens, B., et al., *Lipid-mediated gene delivery to the skin.* Eur J Pharm Sci, 2011. 43(4): p. 199-211.

[35] Geis, N.A., H.A. Katus, and R. Bekeredjian, *Microbubbles as a vehicle for gene and drug delivery: current clinical implications and future perspectives.* Curr Pharm Des, 2012. 18(15): p. 2166-83.

[36] Lara, M.F., et al., *Inhibition of CD44 Gene Expression in Human Skin Models, Using Self-Delivery Short Interfering RNA Administered by Dissolvable Microneedle Arrays.* Hum Gene Ther, 2012. 23(8): p. 816-23.

[37] Gonzalez-Gonzalez, E., et al., *Silencing of reporter gene expression in skin using siRNAs and expression of plasmid DNA delivered by a soluble protrusion array device (PAD).* Mol Ther, 2010. 18(9): p. 1667-74.

[38] Rosenberg, S.A., et al., *The development of gene therapy for the treatment of cancer.* Ann Surg, 1993. 218(4): p. 455-63; discussion 463-4.

[39] Rosenberg, S.A., P. Spiess, and R. Lafreniere, *A new approach to the adoptive immunotherapy of cancer with tumor-infiltrating lymphocytes.* Science, 1986. 233(4770): p. 1318-21.

[40] Rosenberg, S.A., et al., *Gene transfer into humans--immunotherapy of patients with advanced melanoma, using tumor-infiltrating lymphocytes modified by retroviral gene transduction.* N Engl J Med, 1990. 323(9): p. 570-8.

[41] Gershon, D., *Gene therapy. Cancer trial starts.* Nature, 1991. 349(6309): p. 445.

[42] Ardiani, A., et al., *Enzymes to die for: exploiting nucleotide metabolizing enzymes for cancer gene therapy.* Curr Gene Ther, 2012. 12(2): p. 77-91.

[43] Klatzmann, D., et al., *A phase I/II dose-escalation study of herpes simplex virus type 1 thymidine kinase "suicide" gene therapy for metastatic melanoma. Study Group on Gene Therapy of Metastatic Melanoma.* Hum Gene Ther, 1998. 9(17): p. 2585-94.

[44] Singh, S., et al., *Toxicity assessment of intratumoral injection of the herpes simplex type I thymidine kinase gene delivered by retrovirus in patients with refractory cancer.* Mol Ther, 2001. 4(2): p. 157-60.

[45] Kucerova, L., et al., *Cytosine deaminase expressing human mesenchymal stem cells mediated tumour regression in melanoma bearing mice.* J Gene Med, 2008. 10(10): p. 1071-82.

[46] Li, P., et al., *Use of adenoviral vectors to target chemotherapy to tumor vascular endothelial cells suppresses growth of breast cancer and melanoma.* Mol Ther, 2010. 18(5): p. 921-8.

[47] Rosenberg, S.A. and M.E. Dudley, *Adoptive cell therapy for the treatment of patients with metastatic melanoma.* Curr Opin Immunol, 2009. 21(2): p. 233-40.

[48] Bernatchez, C., L.G. Radvanyi, and P. Hwu, *Advances in the treatment of metastatic melanoma: adoptive T-cell therapy.* Semin Oncol, 2012. 39(2): p. 215-26.

[49] Kerkar, S.P., et al., *Tumor-specific CD8+ T cells expressing interleukin-12 eradicate established cancers in lymphodepleted hosts.* Cancer Research, 2010. 70(17): p. 6725-34.

[50] Kalbasi, A., et al., *Prevention of interleukin-2 withdrawal-induced apoptosis in lymphocytes retrovirally cotransduced with genes encoding an antitumor T-cell receptor and an antiapoptotic protein.* J Immunother, 2010. 33(7): p. 672-83.

[51] Morgan, R.A., et al., *Cancer regression in patients after transfer of genetically engineered lymphocytes.* Science, 2006. 314(5796): p. 126-9.

[52] Johnson, L.A., et al., *Gene therapy with human and mouse T-cell receptors mediates cancer regression and targets normal tissues expressing cognate antigen.* Blood, 2009. 114(3): p. 535-46.

[53] Yvon, E., et al., *Immunotherapy of metastatic melanoma using genetically engineered GD2-specific T cells.* Clinical Cancer Research, 2009. 15(18): p. 5852-60.

[54] Burns, W.R., et al., *A high molecular weight melanoma-associated antigen-specific chimeric antigen receptor redirects lymphocytes to target human melanomas.* Cancer Research, 2010. 70(8): p. 3027-33.

[55] Morgan, R.A., et al., *Case report of a serious adverse event following the administration of T cells transduced with a chimeric antigen receptor recognizing ERBB2.* Mol Ther, 2010. 18(4): p. 843-51.

[56] Brentjens, R., et al., *Treatment of chronic lymphocytic leukemia with genetically targeted autologous T cells: case report of an unforeseen adverse event in a phase I clinical trial.* Mol Ther, 2010. 18(4): p. 666-8.

[57] Weber, J., *Immune checkpoint proteins: a new therapeutic paradigm for cancer--preclinical background: CTLA-4 and PD-1 blockade.* Semin Oncol, 2010. 37(5): p. 430-9.

[58] Soiffer, R., et al., *Vaccination with irradiated autologous melanoma cells engineered to secrete human granulocyte-macrophage colony-stimulating factor generates potent antitumor immunity in patients with metastatic melanoma.* Proc Natl Acad Sci U S A, 1998. 95(22): p. 13141-6.

[59] Soiffer, R., et al., *Vaccination with irradiated, autologous melanoma cells engineered to secrete granulocyte-macrophage colony-stimulating factor by adenoviral-mediated gene transfer augments antitumor immunity in patients with metastatic melanoma.* J Clin Oncol, 2003. 21(17): p. 3343-50.

[60] Hodi, F.S., et al., *Immunologic and clinical effects of antibody blockade of cytotoxic T lymphocyte-associated antigen 4 in previously vaccinated cancer patients.* Proc Natl Acad Sci U S A, 2008. 105(8): p. 3005-10.

[61] Hodi, F.S., et al., *Biologic activity of cytotoxic T lymphocyte-associated antigen 4 antibody blockade in previously vaccinated metastatic melanoma and ovarian carcinoma patients.* Proc Natl Acad Sci U S A, 2003. 100(8): p. 4712-7.

[62] Steele, J.C., et al., *Phase I/II trial of a dendritic cell vaccine transfected with DNA encoding melan A and gp100 for patients with metastatic melanoma.* Gene Ther, 2011. 18(6): p. 584-93.

[63] Slominski, A., M.A. Zmijewski, and J. Pawelek, *L-tyrosine and L-dihydroxyphenylalanine as hormone-like regulators of melanocyte functions.* Pigment Cell Melanoma Res, 2012. 25(1): p. 14-27.

[64] Liu, Y., et al., *Conditionally replication-competent adenoviral vectors with enhanced infectivity for use in gene therapy of melanoma.* Hum Gene Ther, 2004. 15(7): p. 637-47.

[65] Lopez, M.V., et al., *Tumor associated stromal cells play a critical role on the outcome of the oncolytic efficacy of conditionally replicative adenoviruses.* PLoS One, 2009. 4(4): p. e5119.

[66] Chai, L., et al., *A novel conditionally replicating adenoviral vector with dual expression of IL-24 and arresten inserted in E1 and the region between E4 and fiber for improved melanoma therapy.* Cancer Gene Ther, 2012. 19(4): p. 247-54.

[67] Hu, J.C., et al., *A phase I study of OncoVEXGM-CSF, a second-generation oncolytic herpes simplex virus expressing granulocyte macrophage colony-stimulating factor.* Clinical Cancer Research, 2006. 12(22): p. 6737-47.

[68] Kaufman, H.L., et al., *Local and distant immunity induced by intralesional vaccination with an oncolytic herpes virus encoding GM-CSF in patients with stage IIIc and IV melanoma.* Ann Surg Oncol, 2010. 17(3): p. 718-30.

[69] Senzer, N.N., et al., *Phase II clinical trial of a granulocyte-macrophage colony-stimulating factor-encoding, second-generation oncolytic herpesvirus in patients with unresectable metastatic melanoma.* J Clin Oncol, 2009. 27(34): p. 5763-71.

[70] Kaufman, H.L. and S.D. Bines, *OPTIM trial: a Phase III trial of an oncolytic herpes virus encoding GM-CSF for unresectable stage III or IV melanoma.* Future Oncol, 2010. 6(6): p. 941-9.

[71] Kirn, D.H. and S.H. Thorne, *Targeted and armed oncolytic poxviruses: a novel multi-mechanistic therapeutic class for cancer.* Nat Rev Cancer, 2009. 9(1): p. 64-71.

[72] Hwang, T.H., et al., *A mechanistic proof-of-concept clinical trial with JX-594, a targeted multi-mechanistic oncolytic poxvirus, in patients with metastatic melanoma.* Mol Ther, 2011. 19(10): p. 1913-22.

[73] Breitbach, C.J., et al., *Intravenous delivery of a multi-mechanistic cancer-targeted oncolytic poxvirus in humans.* Nature, 2011. 477(7362): p. 99-102.

[74] Gajewski, T.F., *Failure at the effector phase: immune barriers at the level of the melanoma tumor microenvironment.* Clinical Cancer Research, 2007. 13(18 Pt 1): p. 5256-61.

[75] Nabel, G.J., et al., *Direct gene transfer with DNA-liposome complexes in melanoma: expression, biologic activity, and lack of toxicity in humans.* Proc Natl Acad Sci U S A, 1993. 90(23): p. 11307-11.

[76] Nabel, G.J., et al., *Immune response in human melanoma after transfer of an allogeneic class I major histocompatibility complex gene with DNA-liposome complexes.* Proc Natl Acad Sci U S A, 1996. 93(26): p. 15388-93.

[77] Bedikian, A.Y. and M. Del Vecchio, *Allovectin-7 therapy in metastatic melanoma.* Expert Opin Biol Ther, 2008. 8(6): p. 839-44.

[78] Stopeck, A.T., et al., *Phase II study of direct intralesional gene transfer of allovectin-7, an HLA-B7/beta2-microglobulin DNA-liposome complex, in patients with metastatic melanoma.* Clinical Cancer Research, 2001. 7(8): p. 2285-91.

[79] Gonzalez, R., et al., *Phase 2 trial of Allovectin-7 in advanced metastatic melanoma.* Melanoma Res, 2006. 16(6): p. 521-6.

[80] Bedikian, A.Y., et al., *A phase 2 study of high-dose Allovectin-7 in patients with advanced metastatic melanoma.* Melanoma Res, 2010. 20(3): p. 218-26.

[81] Kaufman, H.L., et al., *Targeting the local tumor microenvironment with vaccinia virus expressing B7.1 for the treatment of melanoma.* Journal of Clinical Investigation, 2005. 115(7): p. 1903-12.

[82] Kaufman, H.L., et al., *Local delivery of vaccinia virus expressing multiple costimulatory molecules for the treatment of established tumors.* Hum Gene Ther, 2006. 17(2): p. 239-44.

[83] Atkins, M.B., *Cytokine-based therapy and biochemotherapy for advanced melanoma.* Clinical Cancer Research, 2006. 12(7 Pt 2): p. 2353s-2358s.

[84] Hamm, C., et al., *Biochemotherapy for the treatment of metastatic malignant melanoma: a systematic review.* Cancer Treat Rev, 2008. 34(2): p. 145-56.

[85] Stewart, A.K., et al., *Adenovector-mediated gene delivery of interleukin-2 in metastatic breast cancer and melanoma: results of a phase 1 clinical trial.* Gene Ther, 1999. 6(3): p. 350-63.

[86] Dummer, R., et al., *Intralesional adenovirus-mediated interleukin-2 gene transfer for advanced solid cancers and melanoma.* Mol Ther, 2008. 16(5): p. 985-94.

[87] Dent, P., et al., *MDA-7/IL-24 as a cancer therapeutic: from bench to bedside.* Anticancer Drugs, 2010. 21(8): p. 725-31.

[88] Fisher, P.B., et al., *Melanoma differentiation associated gene-7/interleukin-24 (mda-7/IL-24): novel gene therapeutic for metastatic melanoma.* Toxicol Appl Pharmacol, 2007. 224(3): p. 300-7.

[89] Tong, A.W., et al., *Intratumoral injection of INGN 241, a nonreplicating adenovector expressing the melanoma-differentiation associated gene-7 (mda-7/IL24): biologic outcome in advanced cancer patients.* Mol Ther, 2005. 11(1): p. 160-72.

[90] Cunningham, C.C., et al., *Clinical and local biological effects of an intratumoral injection of mda-7 (IL24; INGN 241) in patients with advanced carcinoma: a phase I study.* Mol Ther, 2005. 11(1): p. 149-59.

[91] Khorana, A.A., et al., *A phase I trial of immunotherapy with intratumoral adenovirus-interferon-gamma (TG1041) in patients with malignant melanoma.* Cancer Gene Ther, 2003. 10(4): p. 251-9.

[92] Matsumoto, K., et al., *A pilot study of human interferon beta gene therapy for patients with advanced melanoma by in vivo transduction using cationic liposomes.* Jpn J Clin Oncol, 2008. 38(12): p. 849-56.

[93] Giglia-Mari, G. and A. Sarasin, *TP53 mutations in human skin cancers.* Hum Mutat, 2003. 21(3): p. 217-28.

[94] Bajgelman, M.C. and B.E. Strauss, *Development of an adenoviral vector with robust expression driven by p53.* Virology, 2008. 371(1): p. 8-13.

[95] Strauss, B.E., M.C. Bajgelman, and E. Costanzi-Strauss, *A novel gene transfer strategy that combines promoter and transgene activities for improved tumor cell inhibition.* Cancer Gene Ther, 2005. 12(12): p. 935-46.

[96] Strauss, B.E. and E. Costanzi-Strauss, *pCLPG: a p53-driven retroviral system.* Virology, 2004. 321(2): p. 165-72.

[97] Merkel, C.A., et al., *Activation of endogenous p53 by combined p19Arf gene transfer and nutlin-3 drug treatment modalities in the murine cell lines B16 and C6.* BMC Cancer, 2010. 10: p. 316

Chapter 13

The Potential Importance of K Type Human Endogenous Retroviral Elements in Melanoma Biology

Jianli Dong, Gengming Huang,
Rasheen Imtiaz and Fangling Xu

Additional information is available at the end of the chapter

http://dx.doi.org/10.5772/55264

1. Introduction

Human endogenous retroviruses (HERVs) are thought to be germline-integrated genetic remnants of exogenous retroviral infections and comprise approximately 8% of the human genome [1, 2]. Similar to exogenous retroviruses such as human immunodeficiency virus (HIV) and human T cell leukemia virus (HTLV), a complete HERV sequence is composed of GAG, POL, and ENV genes flanked by two long terminal repeats (LTRs). Although most HERVs are degenerated with disruptive open reading frames, a few proviruses have retained intact genes, and the corresponding proteins can thus be expressed [1, 3]. HERVs have been implicated in the etiology of cancer, chronic inflammation, and other diseases [2], and emerging data support a role of HERV-K in melanomagenesis. For example, HERV-K is activated in melanomas but not in melanocytes [4, 5], and inhibition of HERV-K by RNA interference (RNAi) suppresses the *in vivo* growth of melanoma cells [6-9]. We have demonstrated recently that expression of K-type human endogenous retrovirus (HERV-K) correlates with ERK activation and p16 loss in human melanoma specimens, and that inhibition of MEK and CDK4 in combination, suppresses HERV-K expression [10, 11]. Importantly, if HERV-K drives melanomagenesis downstream of the BRAF-MEK-ERK and p16/CDK4 pathways, when HERV-K is already turned on, cells may be resistant to therapies targeting BRAF-MEK-ERK and p16-CDK4. Triple therapies, such as simultaneous targeting of HERV-K, BRAF/MEK and CDK4, may be necessary to produce more effective and long-lasting therapeutic effects. This strategy is analogous to HIV "cocktail" therapy that disrupts human immunodeficiency virus (HIV) at different stages of viral replication and has brought many acquired immune deficiency syndrome (AIDS) patients from near death to fairly normal and productive lives.

2. The K type Human Endogenous Retroviral Element (HERV-K)

HERVs are thought to be germline-integrated genetic remnants of exogenous retroviral infections and comprise approximately 8% of the human genome [1,2]. They are transmitted vertically by Mendelian inheritance [12]. HERVs can be classified into over 20 families based on transfer RNA (tRNA) specificity of the primer binding site used to initiate reverse transcription; thus, HERV-K would use lysine and HERV-W tryptophan if they were replicating viruses [13]. Through millions of years of evolution, HERVs have become indispensible parts of the human genome. For example, syncytin-1, encoded by the envelope (ENV) gene of HERV-W, mediates intercellular fusion of trophoblast cells to form syncytiotrophoblast as well as preventing maternal immune attack against the developing embryo, thereby facilitating implantation of the embryo [1,2]. Similar to exogenous retroviruses such as human immunodeficiency virus (HIV) and human T cell leukemia virus (HTLV), a complete HERV sequence is composed of group-specific antigen (GAG), polymerase (POL), and ENV genes flanked by two long terminal repeats (LTRs) (Fig. 1). Although most HERVs are degenerated with disruptive open reading frames, a few proviruses have retained intact genes, and the corresponding proteins can thus be expressed [1, 3]. Increased HERV expression has been found under pathological conditions, particularly in cancer and inflammatory disease [12, 14]. Unlike most HERVs that harbor defective mutations, the HML-2 group of HERV-Ks has open reading frames that code for functional viral proteins, which may form noninfectious particles [15, 16]. HERV-K proteins and virus-like particles have been demonstrated in human cell lines of teratocarcinoma [17], breast cancer [18], placenta [19], and melanoma [5].

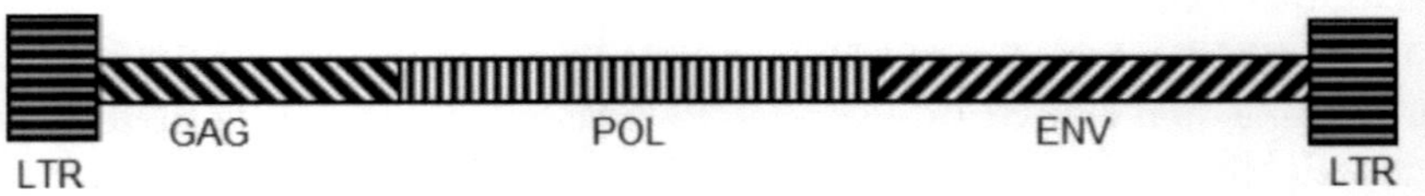

Figure 1. HERV-K genome organization. An intact HERV-K genome is approximately 9700 nucleotides long, like other retrovirus. HERV-K has several genes, mutated so unable to encode functional viral proteins to produce infectious virus. However, pieces of protein domains can be produced by HERV-K sequences. In wild-type retroviral sequences, the group-specific antigen (GAG) codes for the Gag polyprotein. Gag protein provides the basic physical infrastructure of retrovirus; Polymerase (POL) codes for viral enzyme reverse transcriptase, integrase, and protease; envelope (ENV) codes for proteins embedded in the viral envelope which enable the virus to attach to and fuse with target cells. Flanking functional genes are long terminal repeat (LTR) regions that play important roles in initiating viral DNA synthesis and its integration as well as regulating transcription of the viral genes.

HERVs have been implicated in the etiology of cancer, chronic inflammation, and other diseases [2], and emerging data support a role of HERV-K in melanomagenesis. For example, HERV-K is activated in melanomas but not in melanocytes [4, 5], and inhibition of HERV-K by RNAi suppresses the *in vivo* growth of melanoma cells [6-9]. Putative pathogenic mechanisms for HERV-K include mutagenesis by retro-transposition [8, 20], regulation of gene transcription downstream of the insertion sites [21], HERV-K mediated intercellular fusion [Huang et al., in preparation], subversion of immune surveillance by viral proteins [6], as well as direct influences on cell proliferation, differentiation, and anchorage-dependent growth [7, 9].

http://dx.doi.org/10.5772/55264

Like functional retrovirus, HERV-K transcripts can retro-transpose and insert back to the host genome, depending on the insertion sites, may lead to mutagenesis. The enzymes encoded by HERV-K may also induce retro-transposition of Long-interspersed nuclear element-1 (LINE-1) elements, as in the case of HIV-1 [22]. We designed experiment to determine HERV-K genomic integration sequences by HERV-K anchored polymerase chain reaction (PCR). The PCR amplicons can be sequenced after subcloning of individual sequences or next generation sequencing (NGS).

We designed and performed preliminary experiments as shown in Fig. 2. DNA was extracted from human cells using QIAamp® DNA Mini kit (Qiagen, Valencia, CA) following manufacturer's procedures. The optical density (OD) values of DNA were measured before samples were stored at -80°C for further use. Primers used (based on HERV-K108, accession # AF164614) were: 5'3': GCG GTC CCA AAA GGG TCA GTN NNN NNN NNN; 5'ERV (nucleotide 2156-): TTT GCC AGA ATC TCC CAA TC; 3'ERV (nucleotide 4063-): TTG AGC CTT CGT TCT CAC CT; 5'Tag: GCG GTC CCA AAA GGG TCA GT. To perform PCR, about 75ng DNA from human cells was amplified with 0.3 μM 5'3' and 5'ERV or 3'ERV primers, 0.4 mM dNTPs, 1X Pfx Buffer, 1mM MgSO4, and 1.25 unit Platinum® Pfx DNA Polymerase (Invitrogen, Carlsbad, CA). The PCR reaction was carried out in a 9700 thermocycler (Applied Biosystem, Carlsbad, CA). Initial denaturing was at 94°C for 5 minutes, then 94°C for 15 seconds, 36°C for 30 seconds, and 68°C for 4 minutes, for 35 cycles, with an extension at 68°C for 10 minutes after the last cycle. Then 10 μl of the PCR products were used for the 2nd PCR using 5'Tag and 5'ERV or 3'ERV primers with the same amplification conditions except 55°C for annealing. The 2nd PCR products were purified using the QIAquick PCR Purification Kit (Qiagen Inc., Valencia, CA). The resulting templates can be sequenced after subcloning or directly by next generation sequencing.

In a recent study, Macfarian etc shown that during embryogenesis, transcripts of embryonic and extraembryonic tissues are initiated from long terminal repeats derived from endogenous retroviruses [21]. It is conceivable that HERV-K LTR may also regulate gene transcription during melanomagenesis, a hypothesis that can be tested in future studies. The experimental strategy used in Fig. 2 may also apply to determine transcripts downstream of HERV-K sequences.

As with some other viruses, syncytium formation is a characteristic of retroviral infection. As shown in Fig. 3B, pleomorphic cells with features of nuclear atypia, multinuclear/nuclear syncytia are characteristic of malignant cells. We hypothesize that HERV-K mediated intercellular fusion contributes to the formation of pleomorphic cells in tumor specimens.

We performed experiments to identify fusogenic domains and epitopes in HERV-K ENV protein, and to generate HERV-K ENV monoclonal antibodies and evaluate for ability to block ENV mediated intercellular fusion. The fusogenic activity of syncytin has been located to its N-terminus [23]. To map fusogenic domains of HERV-K ENV protein, we will generate a series of C-terminal truncations of HERV-K ENV by PCR using HERV-K108 sequence as template. PCR amplicons will be cloned into pcDNA 3.3-TOPO TA Mammalian Expression Vector using TA Cloning Kit (Invitrogen, Grand Island, NY). The ENV expression constructs will be transfected into melanoma cells and examined for activities to rescue fusogencity inhibited by HERV-K inhibition.

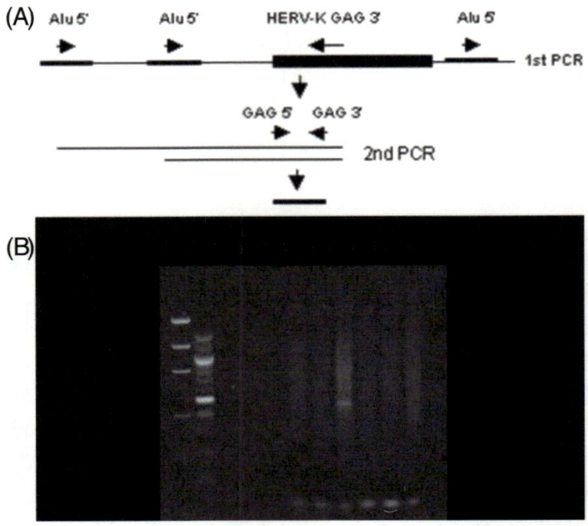

Figure 2. Experimental design to detect HERV-K genome insertion sites. A. HERV-K and Alu elements are bolded. Alu is a short stretch of approximately 300 bp originally characterized by the action of the Alu (*Arthrobacter luteus*) restriction endonuclease. There are over one million Alu elements interspersed throughout the human genome, and it is estimated that about 10.7% of the human genome consists of Alu sequences. PCR is designed to amplify HERV-K and flanking Alu sequneces. Amplicon sequences flanking HERV-K can be determined by subcloning or NGS. B. Gel electrophoresis of 1st PCR products. 1 and 2, molecular weight markers; 3-11 1st round PCR amplicons of genomic DNA extracted from different clones of cultured A375 melanoma cells. Sample 8 may have a unique insertion site captured by the PCR assay (arrow).

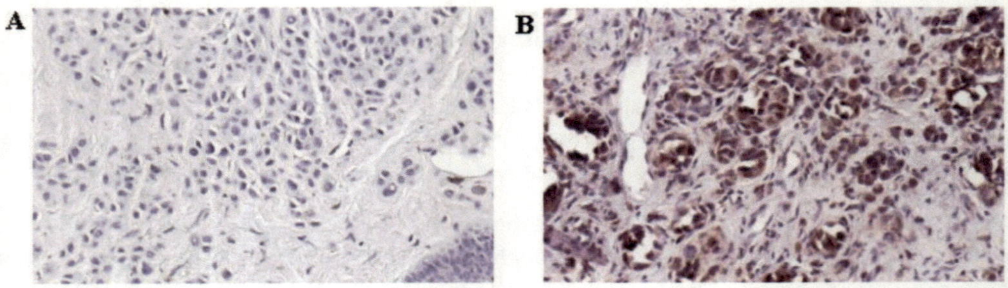

Figure 3. HERV-K may contribute to the generation of pleomorphic tumor cells. Formalin-fixed, paraffin embedded microscopic sections of nevus (A) and melanoma (B) were analyzed to examine cell morphology. Pleomorphic cells with features of nuclear atypia, multinuclear/nuclear syncytia were easily detected in melanoma (B) but not in nevus (A) cells. In an unpublished study, we have shown that such pleomorphic cells in melanomas express HERV-K (Huang et al., submitted). Magnification: x 200.

3. Possible regulation of HERV-K by BRAF-MEK and p16-CDK4

We noticed that the growth characteristics of melanoma cells that can be modified by HERV-K activation (e.g., changes in cell shape, loss of melanin, anchorage-independent growth) [9] overlap with those that can be blocked by suppression of BRAF-MEK-ERK signaling pathway, especially with simultaneous restoration of p16 or inhibition of CDK4 [23-26]. This observation, together with the knowledge that aberrations in BRAF-MEK-ERK and p16-CDK4 pathways are early events and often co-exist during melanomagenesis, and the evidence that RAF-MEK-ERK signaling pathway is required for the completion of HIV-1 reverse transcription [27], prompted us to hypothesize that HERV-K is regulated by BRAF-MEK-ERK and p16-CDK4 pathways. We have reported that expression of HERV-K GAG and ENV proteins correlates with ERK activation and p16 loss in a panel of melanocytic specimens, and that inhibition of MEK and CDK4, especially in combination, suppresses HERV-K protein expression in cultured melanoma cells [11].

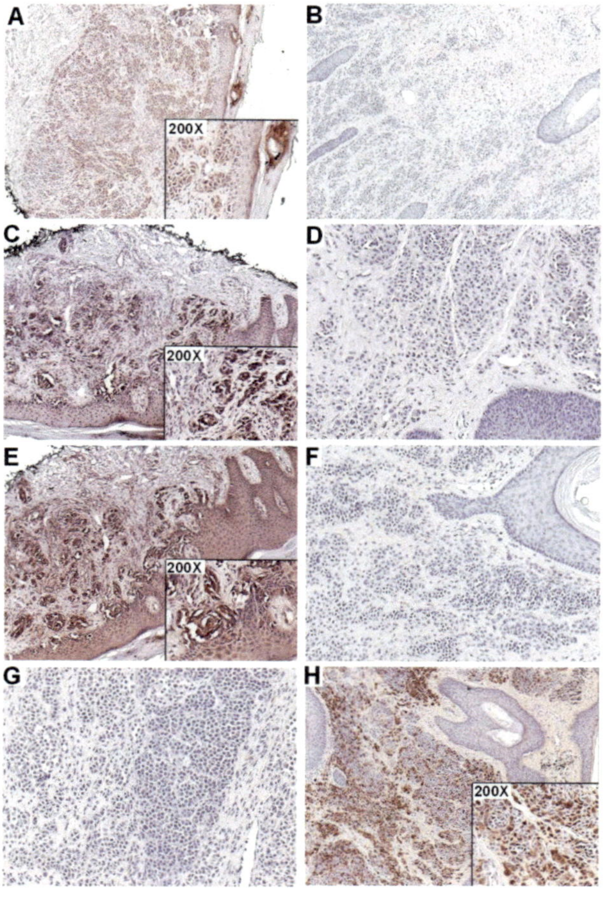

Figure 4. Expression of HERV-K GAG and ENV, p-ERK and p16 in neval and melanoma specimens [8]. Formalin-fixed and paraffin-embedded routine pathology specimens of melanoma (A, C, E, G) and nevus (B, D, F, H) were analyzed by immunohistochemical staining using HERV-K GAG (A, B), ENV (C, D), p-ERK (E, F), and p16 (G, H) specific antibodies. Shown is a representative staining pattern. HERV-K GAG and ENV were mainly detected in melanoma cells (A and C), but rarely expressed in neval cells (B and D). p-ERK was mainly detected in melanoma cells (E) but rarely found in neval cells (F). p16 was rarely expressed in melanoma (G) but prominently expressed in neval cells (H). Magnification: ×100 and ×200 (insets).

Seventy two formalin-fixed, paraffin-embedded pathological specimens were available from the archives at the University of Texas Medical Branch (UTMB). The samples included 38 nevi (11 junctional, 3 compound, and 24 dermal) and 34 melanomas (10 Lentigo maligna, 10 superficial spreading, 7 nodular, and 7 metastatic). The study was approved by the UTMB institutional review board (IRB) for the protection of human subjects. Immunohistochemical staining was modified from the protocol of All-in-One Kit for Immunohistochemical Staining for Tissues with Antibodies (Invitrogen, Carlsbad, CA). Four-micron-thick sections of paraffin blocks were dewaxed in three changes of xylene and rehydrated through a graded series of alcohol concentrations into water. Sections were washed with PBS Tween (PBST) (Sigma, St Louis) three times, each for 5 minutes, then blocked with horse serum for 30 minutes at room temperature. For antigen retrieval, sections were heat-treated in a microwave oven for 20 minutes in 0.01 M citrate buffer (pH 6.0, 100 mM stock), and cooled for 20 minutes in a beaker. For immunostaining the slides were incubated at 4 ℃ overnight with primary antibodies including phospho-p44/42 ERK (Thr202/Tyr204,Cat. #9101, Cell Signaling Technology, Danvers, MA), p16 (Cat. #MS-887 NeoMarkers, Fremont, CA), HERV-K GAG and ENV (Cat. #s 1841-5 and 1811-5, respectively, Austral Biologicals, San Ramon, CA) following the manufacturer's instructions. The slides were incubated with horseradish peroxidase (HRP)-conjugated secondary antibodies, followed by signal development, counterstaining and mounting using All-in-One Kit for Immunohistochemical Staining for Tissues with Antibodies (Invitrogen, Carlsbad, CA). As described previously [28], blood vessel were stained distinctly for p-ERK and used as an internal control for p-ERK antibody. Epidermal keratinocytes and adnexal glands were internal controls for p16 [28]. Melanoma cell line A375 was reported positive for HERV-K using the same HERV-K antibodies [9], and was used as positive control for HERV-K GAG and ENV antibodies, as described [11].

As shown in Fig. 3 [11], we examined the expression of HERV-K GAG and ENV proteins, the active form of ERK (phospho-ERK, p-ERK), and p16 in a panel human melanocytic specimens including 38 benign nevi and 34 melanomas. Both HERV-K GAG and ENV proteins were largely cytoplasmic, but occasional nuclear staining was observed, whereas p-ERK was typically co-expressed in cytoplasm and nucleus. It has been reported that wild-type *INK4A* is expressed in both nucleus and cytoplasm, whereas mutant p16, if expressed, is either nuclear or cytoplasmic [29]. HERV-K GAG cytoplasmic staining was over 10-fold more frequent in melanoma than in nevus (38% of melanomas vs. 3% of nevi, $p < 0.001$) (Table 1). Similarly, HERV-K ENV immunoreactivity was detected in the cytoplasm in 44% of melanomas and 11% of neval specimens (a 4-fold difference, $p = 0.003$). The nuclear staining of GAG and ENV were infrequently detected in both nevi and melanomas, and the differences did not reach statistical significance (Table 1). p-ERK staining was 5-fold more often positive in melanomas than in nevi (68% and 13%, respectively, $p < 0.001$). p16 staining, both in the cytoplasm and nucleus, was more frequently observed in nevi than in melanomas (cytoplasmic, 79% vs. 50%, $p = 0.014$; nuclear, 79% vs. 15%, $p < 0.001$) (Table 1). Figure 3 demonstrates representative staining pattern of HERV-K GAG, HERV-K ENV, p-ERK and p16 in melanoma and neval specimens.

Antigen	Positivity (%)		p value
	Nevi [n=38]	Melanoma [n=34]	
HERV-K GAG, cytoplasmic	3	38	$p < 0.001$**
HERV-K GAG, nuclear	0	6	$p = 0.493$
HERV-K ENV, cytoplasmic	11	44	$p = 0.003$**
HERV-K ENV, nuclear	8	12	$p = 0.7$
p-ERK, cytoplasmic and nuclear	13	68	$p < 0.001$**
p16, cytoplasmic	79	50	$p = 0.014$*
p16, nuclear	79	15	$p < 0.001$**

Protein immunoreactivity, cytoplasmic or nuclear, was dichotomized as negative/decreased (<30% of cells staining positively) and positive (>30% of cells staining positively).

** Difference is significant at the ≤0.01 level (2-tailed)

* Difference is significant at the ≤.05 level (2-tailed).

Table 1. Expression of HERV-K GAG and ENV, p-ERK and p16 in neval and melanoma specimens [8]

Further analysis showed that the expression of HERV-K GAG in the cytoplasm of melanoma was positively correlated with p-ERK ($p = 0.005$), and negatively correlated with p16 cytoplasmic expression ($p = 0.012$) (Table 2). The expression of HERV-K ENV in the cytoplasm of melanomas was positively correlated with p-ERK ($p < 0.001$), and negatively correlated with p16 nuclear expression ($p = 0.046$) (Table 2).

	HERV-K GAG cytoplasmic	HERV-K GAG nuclear	HERV-K ENV cytoplasmic	HERV-K ENV nuclear
p-ERK, cytoplasmic and nuclear	$p = 0.005$**	$p = 0.093$	$p < 0.001$**	$p = 0.2$
p16, cytoplasmic	$p = 0.012$*	$p = 0.058$	$p = 0.114$	$p = 0.608$
p16, nuclear	$p = 0.123$	$p = 0.378$	$p = 0.046$*	$p = 0.251$

Note: ** Correlation is significant at the 0.01 level (2-tailed).

* Correlation is significant at the 0.05 level (2-tailed).

Table 2. Associations of the expression of p-ERK, p16, and HERV-K GAG and HERV-K ENV[8]

As described [11], human melanoma cell lines 624Mel, A101D, A375, and OM431 were kindly provided by Dr. Stuart Aaronson (Mount Sinai School of Medicine, New York, NY). Cells were maintained in Dulbecco's modified Eagle medium (DMEM, Mediatech, Herndon, VA) supplemented with 10% heat-inactivated fetal bovine serum (FBS; Sigma, St. Louis, MO) and 50 units/mL penicillin-streptomycin (Invitrogen, Carlsbad, CA) in a humidified incubator at 37 °C with 5% CO_2. Total RNA was extracted from cultured melanoma cells using an RNA extraction kit ToTALLY RNA (Ambion, Austin, TX) according to the manufacturer's instructions, and purified with RNase free DNase Set (Qiagen, Valencia, CA). RNA concentration was assessed spectrophotometrically at 260/280 nm. Two μg of total RNA was reverse transcribed and amplified by One-Step RT-PCR (Qiagen, Valencia, CA) using 50 pmol of primer pairs specific for HERV-K POL, ENV genes and GAPDH for control as described [9]. Briefly, samples were reverse transcribed at 50 C for 30 min, then heat-activated by incubation at 95 C for 15 min. Samples were subjected to 30 cycles of PCR amplification as described [9] in MasterCycler® Personal (Eppendorf, Hamburg, Germany). Each cycle consisted of 1 min at 95 C, 1 min at 56 C and 1 min at 72 C. After the final cycle, samples were incubated at 72 °C for 10 min. PCR products were inspected by separation through 1% agarose gels. PCR products were purified using QIAquick PCR Purification Kit (Qiagen, Valencia, CA). The purified PCR products were directly sequenced on both strands using a 3100 Capillary Array Sequencer and Big Dye Terminator Chemistry (Applied Biosystems, Foster City, CA). NCBI BLAST search of the human genome was performed to identify the amplified sequences [11].

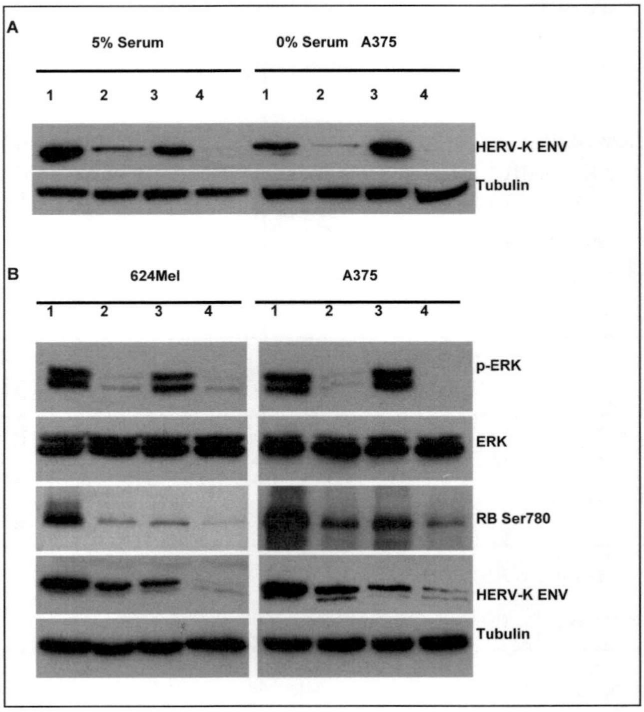

Figure 5. MEK and CDK4 inhibitors suppress HERV-K ENV protein expression [8]. A. 624Mel (1), A101D (2), A375 (3), and OM431 (4) melanoma cells were cultured in DMEM with 5% serum or serum starved overnight, and cell lysates collected for Western blotting. B. 624Mel and A375 melanoma cells were treated with solvent vehicle control (1), 25 μg MEK inhibitor PD98059 (2), 1 μg CDK4 inhibitor 219476 (3), and 25 μg PD98059 plus 1 μg 219476 (4) for 48 h under serum starvation, and cell lysates collected for Western blotting. Western blotting was performed using 50 μg total cell extracts and commercially available HERV-K ENV antibody that recognized a 37 Kd spliced transmembrane domain of ENV protein. Tubulin was used as loading control.

http://dx.doi.org/10.5772/55264

Western blots were performed as described [24, 11]. Briefly, harvested cells were lysed in Lysis Solution (Cell Signaling, Danvers, MA) supplemented with Complete Mini Protease Inhibitor Cocktail Tablets (Roche Diagnostics Corporation, Indianapolis, IN). Protein concentration of lysates was determined using the Quick Start Bradford 1 x Dye Reagent (Bio-Rad, Hercules, CA). Lysates were separated in 10% SDS-polyacrylamide gel, electrophoretically transferred to Immobilon-P membrane (Millipore Corp, Billerica, MA), and probed with primary antibodies followed by incubation with horseradish peroxidase-conjugated secondary antibodies. The following antibodies were used: phospho-p44/42 ERK (Thr202/Tyr204) and p44/42 ERK (Cell Signaling, Danvers, MA), PhosphoPlus(R) RB (Ser780, Ser795, Ser807/811) Antibody Kit (Cell Signaling, Boston, MA), HERV-K GAG and ENV (Cat. #s1841-5 and 1811-5, respectively, Austral Biologicals, San Ramon, CA), and HRP-conjugated secondary antibodies (Jackson Immunoresearch, West Grove, PA). Immunoreactive bands were visualized with SuperSignal chemiluminescence substrate (Pierce, Rockford, IL). The blots were exposed to blue sensitive blue x-ray film (Phenix Research, Candler, NC).

MEK inhibitor PD98059 (Calbiochem, San Diego, CA) was dissolved in DMSO as a 50 mM stock solution, aliquoted and stored in –20 °C. CDK4 inhibitor 219476 (Cat. #219476, Calbiochem, San Diego, CA) was dissolved in DMSO as a 2 mM stock solution and stored at 4 °C. 1×10^6 melanoma cells were seeded in a cell culture dish in DMEM containing 10% FBS and antibiotics. On the second day, cells were treated with PD98059 and 219476 in DMEM without serum for 48 h and then harvested. Statistical analyses were performed by using SPSS 13.0 software (SPSS Inc., Chicago, IL). Fisher exact test was used to detect the differences in immunostaining between melanomas and nevi. Pearson Correlation was used to test the correlations of immunostaining (HERV-K GAG, HERV-K ENV, p-ERK, and p16).

The expression of HERV-K has been reported in several melanoma cell lines [4, 5, 9, 30]. We examined HERV-K in four melanoma cell lines, 624Mel, A375, A101D, and OM431 that have constitutive activation of p-ERK, and loss of wild-type p16 with corresponding hyperphosphorylation of RB protein [24, 25, 26]. As previously reported [11], HERV-K expression was detected using a specific HERV-K ENV antibody as described [5, 9], that recognizes a 37 Kd spliced transmembrane domain of ENV protein [4, 5, 30]. HERV-K ENV protein was prominently expressed in 624Mel and A375 cells, weakly positive in A101D cells, but barely detectable in OM431 cells (Fig. 4A). We extracted total cellular RNA from all the four cell lines and performed conventional RT-PCR using specific HERV-K POL and ENV primers as described [9]. Direct sequencing of RT-PCR amplicons and NCBI BLAST analysis showed that the expressed sequences share 96%-98% overall homology with Group N HERV-K [31] (data not shown), as reported in other melanoma cells [32].

We have established experimental conditions (including time course and dose-response curve) of treating several melanoma cells with PD98059 and 219476, to respectively inhibit MEK and CDK4, alone and in combination [26]. 624Mel and A375 lines were used to test whether HERV-K EVE expression was suppressed by the MEK and CDK4 inhibitors. As expected, treatment with PD98059 inhibited ERK phosphorylation in both 624Mel and A375 cells (Fig. 4B, lane 2). It is worth noting that we consistently observed somewhat further reduced levels of p-ERK by PD98059 when combined with CDK4 inhibition (Fig. 4B, p-ERK, lane 4 vs. lane 2; also in Li et al., 2009, Fig. 1a, lane 4 vs. lane 2); which may contribute to the observed functional interaction between BRAF-MEK-ERK and p16-CDK4-RB pathways [25, 26]. Phosphorylation of serine 780, a CDK4 target in the RB protein, was reduced by PD98059 and 219476, especially in combination in both cell lines (Fig. 4B). Similarly, HERV-K ENV expression was inhibited by either PD98059 or 219476, especially when used in combination (Fig. 4B). The results were consistent with findings of the association between HERV-K expression and p-ERK and p16 in melanocytic specimens (Table 2).

Multiple endogenous and exogenous factors have been linked to the activation of HERVs including hormones, cytokines, and cytotoxic chemicals [33]. To our knowledge, a direct association between ERK and p16-CDK4 pathways and HERV expression has only been reported by our group [11]. It has been shown that HERV-K sequences, as other host genes, are regulated by DNA methylation in the promoter/enhancer sequences located in the 5′-LTR regions [34]. Since RB protein, a downstream mediator of BRAF-MEK-ERK and p16-CDK4 signaling pathways, is a key regulator of DNA methylation [35], it is conceivable that the observed association between HERV-K, p-ERK and p16-CDK4 may act through RB, a notion that will surely prompt further investigation. It is worth noting that the four melanoma cell lines examined, 624Mel, A375, A101D and OM431, all have *BRAF* T1799A mutation, constitutive activation of ERK, loss of wild-type p16, and over-expression of phospho-RB protein [24]. However, only 624Mel and A375 cells express high levels of HERV-K ENV protein (Fig. 4A), suggesting that HERV-K ENV protein is regulated by mechanisms in addition to ERK and p16-CDK4 pathways.

HERV-K may prove to be a key mediator of BRAF-MEK-ERK and p16-CDK4-RB pathways during melanoma pathogenesis. Activation of BRAF/ERK was recently shown to drive chromosome abnormality and aneuploidy in melanocytes [36]. It is conceivable that the effect may be mediated, at least partly, through HERV-K sequences that are capable of jumping around by retro-transposition leading to mutagenesis and chromosomal abnormalities [8, 20]; HERV-K proteins have been shown to suppress the host immune system [6]. Activation of HERV-K by BRAF-MEK-ERK and CDK4 signaling may facilitate tumor progression especially in the blood/lymph stream when circulating tumor cells are under attack by the immune system, thus providing a critical survival/escape mechanism for invasion and metastasis [12, 37]. Alternatively, it is possible that the observed growth promotion and anti-apoptotic effects of activated ERK and CDK4 [25, 26] can be mediated, at least in part, by HERV-K since HERV-K has been shown to directly affect melanoma cell proliferation, differentiation, and anchorage related survival [7, 9].

4. Combined inhibition of CDK4 potentiate the effect of MEKi

Constitutive dysregulation of MEK-ERK and p16-CDK4-RB pathways both occur at high frequencies in melanoma. We found that simultaneous inhibition of both MEK and CDK4 generated more potent and dramatic lethal effects than individual inhibition in melanoma cells [10, 25, 38]. We also found that the expression of K- type human endogenous retrovirus (HERV-

K) correlates with ERK activation and p16 loss in melanoma cells and that inhibition of MEK and CDK4 can block HERV-K expression [11]. As shown in Fig. 5, if HERV-K drives tumor progression downstream of RAF-MEK-ERK and p16/CDK4, when HERV-K is already turned on, cells may escape the inhibitory effects of therapies targeting RAF-MEK-ERK and p16/CDK4. Given that HERV may drive malignant growth downstream of MEK and CDK-4, we hypothesized that cells with activated HERV may not respond to the therapeutic effects of MEK and CDK4 blockers and that triple therapy, such as targeting HERV-K, MEK and CDK4, may be necessary to produce more effective and long-lasting therapeutic effects than single or, as we have proposed previously, double inhibition of MEK-ERK and CDK4 [25, 26]. This strategy is analogous to HIV "cocktail" therapy that disrupts HIV at different steps of replication and brought many AIDS patients from death to fairly normal and productive lives [39].

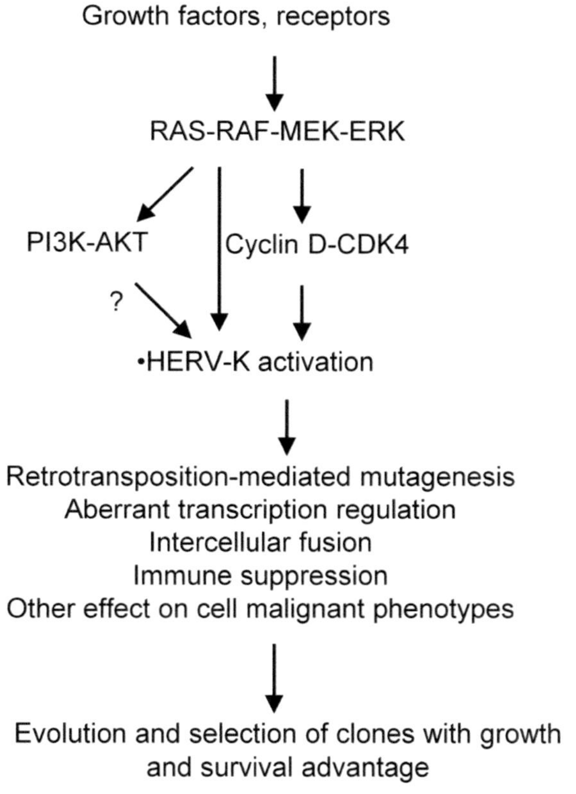

Figure 6. Potential regulation and activity of BRAF-MEK-ERK, CDK4, and HERV-K in carcinogenesis and tumor progression. Constitutive activation of RAS-RAF-MEK-ERK and cyclin D-CDK4 are common paradigm of cancer biology. We have reported that that simultaneous inhibition of both BRAF-MEK and CDK4 generated more potent and dramatic lethal effects than individual inhibition in melanoma cells [10, 25, 38]. We have also shown that the expression of HERV-K correlates with ERK activation and p16 loss in melanoma cells and that inhibition of MEK and CDK4 can block HERV-K expression [11]. When HERV-K is already turned on by MEK, CDK4 or alternative pathways, cells may escape the inhibitory effects of therapies targeting RAF-MEK-ERK and p16/CDK4. Triple inhibition of BRAF-MEK, CDK4, and HERV-K may stop the evolution and selection of cell clones with growth and survival advantage.

Group	Treatment
1	solvent control
2	solvent control + BRAFi/MEKi
3	solvent control + CDK4i
4	solvent control + BRAFi/MEKi + CDK4i
5	HERV-Ki + solvent control
6	HERV-Ki + BRAFi/MEKi
7	HERV-Ki + CDK4i
8	HERV-Ki + BRAFi/MEKi + CDK4i

The triple inhibition experiment (Table 3) can be performed using cultured melanoma cells or in mouse melanoma xenograft, as described [10, 24, 25, 38]. Inhibition of BRAF (BRAFi), MEK (MEKi), CDK4 (CDK4i), and HERV-K (HERV-Ki) can be achieved using either RNA interference (RNAi) or small molecular inhibitors that are in active clinical development (http://clinicaltrials gov/).

Table 3. Triple Therapy Treatment Groups

We designed experiments to examine the effects of combined inhibition of HERV-K, BRAF/MEK, and CDK4 in melanoma cells (Table 3). Human melanoma cell lines MeWo, A101D and A375 that harbor wild-type, heterozygote, and loff of heterozygosity (LOH) *BRAF* T1799A alleles, respectively [24, 40] can be used. These cell lines express HERV-K transcripts and/or proteins, have constitutive activation of MEK-ERK signaling pathway, and high levels of phospho-RB (p-RB) [24, 25, 3840, 41] (and data not shown). Stable suppression of HERV-K, BRAF, or CDK4 can be achieved by stable expression of HERV-K short hairpin RNA (shRNA) [7, 9], *BRAF* shRNA, or *INK4A* cDNA [24], or using small molecular inhibitors of BRAF inhibitor (BRAFi), including Vemurafenib (PLX4032, RO5185426, Hoffmann-La Roche) that has been U.S. Food and Drug Administration (FDA) approved for treatment of melanoma, Dabrafenib (GSK2118436, GlaxoSmithKline), PLX3603 (RO5212054) (Hoffmann-La Roche); MEK inhibitor (MEKi), including PD-325901 (Pfizer), GSK1120212 (GlaxoSmithKline), MSC1936369B (EMD Serono), ARRY-438162 (MEK162) (Array BioPharma), AZD6244 (AstraZeneca), and BAY86-9766 (Bayer); CDK4 inhibitor (CDK4i), including PD-0332991 (Pfizer), LY2835219 (Eli Lilly and Company), LEE011 (Novartis Pharmaceuticals). All are in active clinical development (http://clinicaltrials.gov/).

We performed experiments to simultaneously inhibit MEK and CDK4 using known pharmacological inhibitors PD98059 and 219476, respectively, along with using azidothymidine (AZT) to target HERV-K reverse transcription activity as described [42]. AZT (also called ZDV) is a nucleoside analog reverse-transcriptase inhibitor (NRTI), a type of antiretroviral drug used for the successful treatment of HIV infection. It is a therapeutic analog of thymidine. Optimal results were obtained when cultured A101D and 624Mel cells were treated for a period of 48 hours (Fig. 6). A decrease in the number of viable cells was observed for both A101D and 624Mel cells. The data from this study provided preliminary data of the effect AZT has on melanoma cells in combination with inhibitors of MEK and CDK4, in support of our hypothesis

http://dx.doi.org/10.5772/55264

and our rationale for using AZT as a complementary treatment. Several follow-up studies will be performed. The effects of the chemical treatment on melanoma cells, e.g., cell proliferation, apoptosis, and cell cycle progression will be measured using established methods [10, 38]. Molecular mediators of the effects (phospho-ERK, phospho-RB, HERV proteins) will be measured using commercial available antibodies by Western blotting. Future studies are also necessary to further investigate the regulation and activities of HERV-K in melanoma pathogenesis.

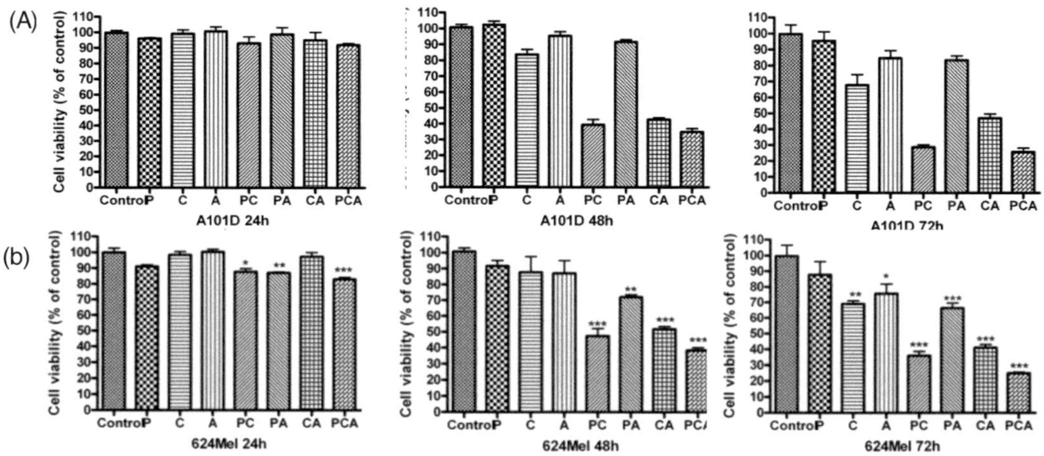

Figure 7. Combined use ofMEK, CDK4, and HERV-K inhibitors enhances the therapeutic effect in cultured melanoma cells. A101D (A) and 624Mel (B) human melanoma cell lines were grown in culture as described [10, 38]. CellTiter 96 Aqueous One Solution Cell Proliferation Assay (MTS, Promega, Madison, WI) was used to measure total viable cells following manufacture's instructions. 5,000 melanoma cells were seeded in each well of 96-well plates, and were grown for 24 hrs in media with 10% Fetal Bovine Serum (FBS). Afterward, media were aspirated and various combinations (Table 3) of treatment chemicals were added to each well in media without serum. Based on dose-response analyses, the final concentrations used were: PD90895 (P) at 25 μM; 219476 (C) at 1 μM; AZT (A) at 1000 μM. The plates were incubated for a period of 24 hrs, 48hrs, and 72 hrs, respectively. Subsequently, MTS solution was added to each well according to the manufacturers protocol. The plates were then incubated for 2-4 hrs, afterward absorbance was measured at 490nm. Data were analyzed and compared for treatment efficiency. Triple inhibition (PCA) generated more inhibitory effects in control solvent, single, or double combination.

We have learnt the significance of "contaminating DNA" in the measurement of HERV-K expression from our recent investigation of the correlation between HERV-K expression and HIV-1 viral load in plasma specimens [Esqueda et al., in press]. We performed RNA extraction using HIV-1 ViroSeq RNA preparation method (Abbott Molecular, Des Plaines, IL). According to the manufacturer this RNA preparation kit extracts total nucleic acid including RNA plus DNA (Dr. Gavin Cloherty, personal communication). According to Qiagen, "The QIAamp Viral RNA Mini Kit is not designed to separate viral RNA from cellular DNA, and both will be purified in parallel if present in the sample" (page 9, QIAamp Viral RNA Mini Handbook, 04/2010). We used DNase I digestion to effectively remove contaminating cellular DNA in the RNA samples. As demonstrated in Fig. 7, without DNase I digestion, HERV-K RT-PCR was uniformly positive in all five HIV-1 positive plasma specimens, whereas only samples #3 and #5 were positive after DNase I digestion. The results emphasize that optimized methodology in the laboratory is essential to the accurate assessment of HERV-K activation.

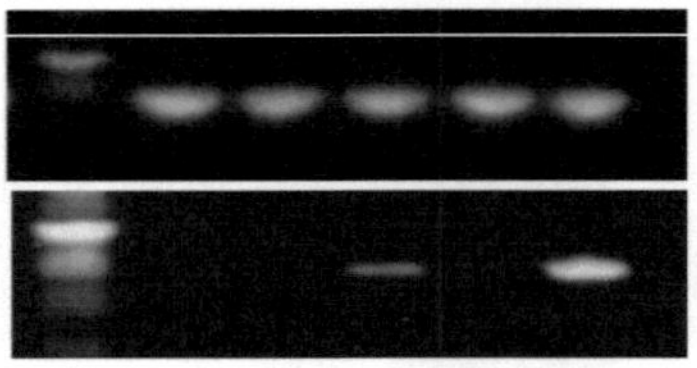

Figure 8. DNase I digestion affects HERV-K RT-PCR results. Viral RNA was extracted from five HIV-1 positive specimens using HIV-1 ViroSeq kit. Without DNase I digestion, HERV-K RT-PCR was uniformly positive in all the 5 cases, whereas only samples #3 and #5 remained positive after DNase I digestion. MW, molecular weight marker.

5. Conclusion

Constitutive dysregulation of MEK-ERK and p16-CDK4-RB pathways both occur at high frequencies in melanoma. We found that simultaneous inhibition of both MEK and CDK4 generated more potent and dramatic lethal effects than individual inhibition did, in melanoma cells. It has been shown recently that the K-type human endogenous retroviral sequence (HERV-K) is expressed in melanoma cells but not in melanocytes. HERVs are germline-integrated genetic remnants of retroviral infections that are transmitted vertically by Mendelian inheritance. It is estimated that 8% of the human genome consists of retroviral elements including HERVs (4). HERVs can be classified to over 20 families based on tRNA specificity of the primer binding site used to initiate reverse transcription. HERV sequences are similar to the HIV sequence. HERV-K activation was observed to be correlated with changes in growth characteristics of melanoma cells (e.g., changes in cell shape, loss of melanin, anchorage-independent growth. We have shown that the expression of HERV-K correlates with ERK activation and p16 loss in melanoma cells and that inhibition of MEK and CDK4 can block HERV-K expression. Given that HERV may drive malignant growth downstream of MEK and CDK-4, we hypothesized that cells with activated HERV may not respond to the therapeutic effects of MEK and CDK4 blockers and that triple inhibition of MEK, CDK4, and HERV should be more effective than double treatment, a hypothesis supported by our preliminary data. Additional studies are necessary to further examine the regulatory relationship between aberrant MEK-ERK and p16-CDK4-RB pathways and HERV-K activation, the roles and mechanisms of HERV-K in carcinogenesis and clonal evolution of malignant cells. The potential therapeutic efficacy of triple inhibition of BRAF-MEK, CDK4, and HERV-K need to be further explored in our fight against melanoma and other malignancies.

http://dx.doi.org/10.5772/55264

Nomenclature

AIDS: acquired immune deficiency syndrome

Alu: *Arthrobacter luteus*

BRAF: v-raf murine sarcoma viral oncogene homolog B1

BRAFi: BRAF inhibitor

CDK4: cyclin-dependent kinase 4

CDK4i: CDK4 inhibitor

DMEM: Dulbecco's modified Eagle medium

DNA: deoxyribonucleic acid

ENV: envelop

ERK: extracellular-signal-regulated kinase

FBS: fetal bovine serum

FDA: Food and Drug Administration

FGF: fibroblast growth factor

FISH: fluorescent *in situ* hybridization

GAG: group-specific antigen

HERV: human endogenous retroviruse

HERV-K: K-type human endogenous retrovirus

HIV: human immunodeficiency virus

HTLV: human T cell leukemia virus

IHC: immunohistochemical staining

INK4A: inhibitor of cyclin-dependent kinase 4A; part of cyclin-dependent kinase inhibitor 2A gene (*CDKN2A*), also known as multiple tumor suppressor 1 (*MTS1*)

LINE-1: long-interspersed nuclear element-1

LOH: loss of heterozygosity

LTR: long terminal repeatRs

MEK: mitogen-activated protein kinase/ERK kinase

MEKi: MEK inhibitor

NGS: next generation sequencing

OD: optical density

PAGE: polyacrylamide gel electrophoresis

PARP: poly (ADP-ribose) polymerase

PBS: phosphate buffered saline

PCR: polymerase chain reaction

p-ERK: phopho-ERK

PI3K: phosphatidylinositol 3-kinase

POL: polymerase

RAF: v-raf murine sarcoma viral oncogene homolog. Human has three RAF: CRAF, BRAF, and ARAF

RAS: rat sarcoma viral oncogene homolog. Human has three RAS: HRAS, NRAS, and KRAS (KRAS4A and KRAS4B proteins arise from alternative splicing)

RB: retinoblastoma proteins including pRB, p107, and p103

RNA: ribonucleic acid

RNAi: RNA interference

RT-PCR: reverse transcription polymerase chain reaction

SDS: sodium dodecyl sulfate

shRNA: short hairpin RNA

tRNA: transfer RNA

Acknowledgements

We thank Dr. Stuart Aaronson for human melanoma cell lines. This work was supported by Bill Walter III Melanoma Research Fund, Harry J. Lloyd Charitable Trust, and Cancer and Leukemia Group B Foundation (to J.D.).

Author details

Jianli Dong*, Gengming Huang, Rasheen Imtiaz and Fangling Xu

*Address all correspondence to: jidong@utmb.edu

Department of Pathology, Sealy Center for Cancer Biology, University of Texas Medical Branch at Galveston, Galveston, TX, USA

http://dx.doi.org/10.5772/55264

References

[1] De Parseval, N, & Heidmann, T. *Human endogenous retroviruses: from infectious elements to human genes.* Cytogenet Genome Res, (2005). , 318-332.

[2] Kurth, R, & Bannert, N. *Beneficial and detrimental effects of human endogenous retroviruses.* Int J Cancer, (2009).

[3] Ahn, K, & Kim, H. S. *Structural and quantitative expression analyses of HERV gene family in human tissues.* Mol Cells, (2009). , 99-103.

[4] Buscher, K, et al. *Expression of human endogenous retrovirus K in melanomas and melanoma cell lines.* Cancer Res, (2005). , 4172-4180.

[5] Muster, T, et al. *An endogenous retrovirus derived from human melanoma cells.* Cancer Res, (2003). , 8735-8741.

[6] Mangeney, M, et al. *Endogenous retrovirus expression is required for murine melanoma tumor growth in vivo.* Cancer Res, (2005). , 2588-2591.

[7] Oricchio, E, et al. *Distinct roles for LINE-1 and HERV-K retroelements in cell proliferation, differentiation and tumor progression.* Oncogene, (2007). , 4226-4233.

[8] Pothlichet, J, Mangeney, M, & Heidmann, T. *Mobility and integration sites of a murine C57BL/6 melanoma endogenous retrovirus involved in tumor progression in vivo.* Int J Cancer, (2006). , 1869-1877.

[9] Serafino, A, et al. *The activation of human endogenous retrovirus K (HERV-K) is implicated in melanoma cell malignant transformation.* Exp Cell Res, (2009). , 849-862.

[10] Dong, J, & Schwab, C. L. *Simultaneous knockdown of mutant BRAF and expression of INK4A in melanoma cells leads to potent growth inhibition and apoptosis.* Treatment of Metastatic Melanoma, ed. R.M. R. (2011). InTech. , 149-182.

[11] Li, Z, et al. *Expression of HERV-K correlates with status of MEK-ERK and 16INK4A16ICDK4pathways in melanoma cells.* Cancer Invest, (2010). p. 1031-7.

[12] Voisset, C, Weiss, R. A, & Griffiths, D. J. *Human RNA "rumor" viruses: the search for novel human retroviruses in chronic disease.* Microbiol Mol Biol Rev, (2008). table of contents., 157-196.

[13] Blomberg, J, et al. *Classification and nomenclature of endogenous retroviral sequences (ERVs): problems and recommendations.* Gene, (2009). , 115-123.

[14] Lee, E, et al. *Landscape of somatic retrotransposition in human cancers.* Science, (2012). , 967-971.

[15] Beimforde, N, et al. *Molecular cloning and functional characterization of the human endogenous retrovirus K113.* Virology, (2008). , 216-225.

[16] Turner, G, et al. *Insertional polymorphisms of full-length endogenous retroviruses in humans.* Curr Biol, (2001). , 1531-1535.

[17] Lower, R, et al. *Identification of human endogenous retroviruses with complex mRNA expression and particle formation.* Proc Natl Acad Sci U S A, (1993). , 4480-4484.

[18] Seifarth, W, et al. *Comprehensive analysis of human endogenous retrovirus transcriptional activity in human tissues with a retrovirus-specific microarray.* J Virol, (2005). , 341-352.

[19] Kalter, S. S, et al. *Brief communication: C-type particles in normal human placentas.* J Natl Cancer Inst, (1973). , 1081-1084.

[20] Tchenio, T, & Heidmann, T. *Defective retroviruses can disperse in the human genome by intracellular transposition.* J Virol, (1991). , 2113-2118.

[21] Macfarlan, T. S, et al. *Embryonic stem cell potency fluctuates with endogenous retrovirus activity.* Nature, (2012). , 57-63.

[22] Jones, R. B, et al. *HIV-1 infection induces retrotransposition of LINE-1 elements.* Retrovirology, (2009). suppl 2: , 43.

[23] Drewlo, S, et al. *C-Terminal truncations of syncytin-1 (ERVWE1 envelope) that increase its fusogenicity.* Biol Chem, (2006). , 1113-1120.

[24] Rotolo, S, et al. *Effects on proliferation and melanogenesis by inhibition of mutant BRAF and expression of wild-type INK4A in melanoma cells.* Int J Cancer, (2005). , 164-169.

[25] Zhao, Y, et al. *Simultaneous knockdown of BRAF and expression of INK4A in melanoma cells leads to potent growth inhibition and apoptosis.* Biochem Biophys Res Commun, (2008). , 509-513.

[26] Li, J, et al. *Simultaneous Inhibition of MEK and CDK4 Leads to Potent Apoptosis in Human Melanoma Cells.* Cancer Invest, (2009).

[27] Mettling, C, et al. *Galphai protein-dependant extracellular signal-regulated kinase-1/2 activation is required for HIV-1 reverse transcription.* Aids, (2008). , 1569-1576.

[28] Richmond-sinclair, N. M, et al. *Histologic and epidemiologic correlates of P-MAPK, Brn-2, pRb, 53and p16 immunostaining in cutaneous melanomas.* Melanoma Res, (2008). p. 336-45.

[29] Ghiorzo, P, et al. *Expression and localization of mutant 16proteins in melanocytic lesions from familial melanoma patients.* Hum Pathol, (2004). p. 25-33.

[30] Buscher, K, et al. *Expression of the human endogenous retrovirus-K transmembrane envelope, Rec and Np9 proteins in melanomas and melanoma cell lines.* Melanoma Res, (2006). , 223-234.

[31] Romano, C. M, Ramalho, R. F, & Zanotto, P. M. *Tempo and mode of ERV-K evolution in human and chimpanzee genomes.* Arch Virol, (2006). , 2215-2228.

[32] Hirschl, S, et al. *Sequence variability of retroviral particles derived from human melanoma cells melanoma-associated retrovirus.* Virus Res, (2007). , 211-215.

[33] Taruscio, D, & Mantovani, A. *Factors regulating endogenous retroviral sequences in human and mouse.* Cytogenet Genome Res, (2004). , 351-362.

[34] Lavie, L, et al. *CpG methylation directly regulates transcriptional activity of the human endogenous retrovirus family HERV-K(HML-2).* J Virol, (2005). , 876-883.

[35] Montoya-durango, D. E, et al. *Epigenetic control of mammalian LINE-1 retrotransposon by retinoblastoma proteins.* Mutat Res, (2009). , 20-28.

[36] Cui, Y, et al. *Oncogenic B-Raf(600Einduces spindle abnormalities, supernumerary centrosomes, and aneuploidy in human melanocytic cells.* Cancer Res, (2010). , 675-684.

[37] Singh, S, et al. *The role of human endogenous retroviruses in melanoma.* Br J Dermatol, (2009).

[38] Li, J, et al. *Simultaneous inhibition of MEK and CDK4 leads to potent apoptosis in human melanoma cells.* Cancer Invest, (2010). , 350-356.

[39] Henkel, J. *Attacking AIDS with a'cocktail' therapy?* FDA Consum, (1999). , 12-17.

[40] Estrada, Y, Dong, J, & Ossowski, L. *Positive crosstalk between ERK and 38in melanoma stimulates migration and in vivo proliferation.* Pigment Cell Melanoma Res, (2009). p. 66-76.

[41] Li, Z, et al. *Expression of HERV-K Correlates With Status of MEK-ERK and 16INK4A16ICDK4Pathways in Melanoma Cells.* Cancer Invest, (2010).

[42] Lee, Y. N, & Bieniasz, P. D. *Reconstitution of an infectious human endogenous retrovirus.* PLoS Pathog, (2007). , e10.

Chapter 14

Emerging GM3 Regulated Biomarkers in Malignant Melanoma

Pu Wang*, Peipei Guan*, Su Xu, Zhanyou Wang,
Sadako Yamagata and Tatsuya Yamagata

Additional information is available at the end of the chapter

http://dx.doi.org/10.5772/54941

1. Introduction

Gangliosides, GSLs, are expressed in the outer leaflet of the plasma membrane of animal cells and involved in a variety of functions, including serving as antigens, receptors for bacterial toxins, mediators of cell adhesion, and mediators and modulators of signal transduction. Moreover, the accumulated lines of evidence have shown that gangliosides play pivotal roles in cancer metastasis. As the first and simplest member in the metabolic series of the ganglioside family, GM3 is a metabolic precursor of more complex natural gangliosides, which in turn determines their contents and biological functions in cells and tissues. GM3 has been demonstrated to be involved in regulation of various processes including cell proliferation, differentiation, apoptosis, embryogenesis and oncogenesis, etc. However, it is difficult to understand the defined functional concepts of GM3 in cancer metastasis because GM3 indirectly exert their effects via regulating target genes.

Target genes indicated in cellular transformation and tumor progression have been divided into two categories: proto-oncogenes and tumor suppressor genes. In cancer, it can thus be speculated that an altered balance of tumor suppressor genes towards proto-oncogenes may contribute to tumor transformation. Alterations in proto-oncogenes and tumor suppressor genes are largely dependent on point mutation, amplification or translocation. Consequently, the normal control mechanisms that constrain the expression of genes are undermined, and thus the oncogene is continually expressed, resulting in tumor transformation [1]. Similarly, genetic transformation has been linked to melanoma genesis and progression. These genes encompass many signaling pathways, including the RTK, PI3-K, Rb, p53, Wnt, and NF-κB pathways [2]. Further evidence implicated the downstream oncogenes of these pathways in melanoma ranges from Ras, B-Raf, Kit,

Mitf, Cyclin D1, CDK4 to HDM2 [1], [3]. Although genetic discoveries related to melanoma transformation have been accelerated greatly in recent years, the involvement of GM3 in melanoma metastasis via these proto-oncogenes or tumor suppressor genes has not yet been clearly established.

The present chapter was aimed to give insights into the mechanisms that GM3 regulates melanoma metastasis via its target genes. To keep the discussion focused, we will discuss the relationship between GM3 contents and their abilities to regulate proto-oncogenes or tumor suppressor genes, which in turn mediate melanoma metastasis. To screen GM3 target genes, we obtained cells (CSSH-1) that overexpressed B4galt6 cDNA and cells (CAH-3) that suppressed its expression, which in turn result in GM3 modulation [4], [5]. In the CSSH-1 cells, GM3 contents were doubled, but in the CAH-3 cells, GM3 expression was halved compared with vector transfectant control, SM-1 and CM-1, respectively [4], [5]. To further confirm the roles of GM3 in melanoma cells, St3gal5 silenced cells were established by transfecting B16 cells with St3gal5 siRNA and it was found that the introduction of St3gal5 siRNA to B16 cells resulted in GM3 depletion as compared with the scrambled siRNA transfectant control [4], [5]. Moreover, we would elucidate the mechanism that GM3 regulate melanoma metastasis via the genes, such as Ly-GDI, TNF-α, MMP-9, MMP-2, Caveolin-1 and Plaur, etc. and the functions of these genes on the phenotypes of melanoma cells, such as invasive proliferation, adhesion, migration and invasion would be finally addressed based on our and others' publications (Table 1) [6].

2. Materials and methods

2.1. Cell lines and culture

Murine melanoma B16 cells were kindly provided by Dr. Kiyoshi Furukawa of Nagaoka University of Technology, Japan. The cells were maintained in medium containing Dulbecco's modified Eagle's medium (DMEM; Gibco, Invitrogen Corporation, NY, USA) supplemented with 10% fetal bovine serum (TBD; Tianjin Hao Yang Biological Company, Tianjin, China), 100 U/ml penicillin, and 100 μg/ml streptomycin and incubated in a humidified (37°C, 5% CO2 and 95% air) incubator (Sanyo, Toyota, Japan). The cells were usually grown in a 60-mm culture dish (BD Falcon, CA, USA) and passaged once they reached 75% confluence. To observe the effects of pharmacological inhibitors on genes expression, cells were treated with pharmacological inhibitors for 24 h before analyzing genes expression by RT-PCR.

2.2. Chemicals and antibodies

LY294002 and LY303511 were purchased from Sigma-Aldrich (St. Louis, MD, USA). The Rneasy mini kit to extract total RNA was obtained from Qiagen (Hilden, Germany). The RT-PCR kit was from Takara Biotechnology Corporation (Dalian, China). All other reagents were from Invitrogen (Carlsbad, CA, USA), unless otherwise specified.

Regulation Manner	Gene Name	CSSH-1/SM-1	CAH-3/CM-1	B11/B16	Biological Functions
Positive	Caveolin-1	1.378	0.321	0.146	(1)[7], (4)[7], (5)[7]
	Ly-GDI	2.156	0.423	0.387	(5)[8]
	PKN-1	1.658	0.626	0.495	(4)[9]
	E-cadherein	1.875	0.695	0.721	(1)[10], (3)[11], (5)[12], (6)[13]
	Gelsolin	1.841	0.543	0.502	(4)[14]
	MMP-9	1.915	0.174	0.282	(4)[15], (5)[16]
	MMP-2	1.532	0.534	0.472	(4)[17], (5)[18]
	Apaf1	1.350	0.608	0.509	(2)[19]
	Rho B	2.247	0.427	0.318	(5)[20], (6)[20], (8)[20]
	Midkine	1.403	0.518	0.417	(1)[21]
	Lymphotoxin α	2.245	0.475	0.497	(6)[22]
	Tnf α	2.188	0.349	0.292	(4)[23], (5)[23]
	Plau	1.453	0.397	0.750	(5)[24], (6)[24]
	Plaur	2.209	0.543	0.720	(2)[25]
Negative	Integrin β5	0.783	1.465	1.754	(1)[26, 27], (2)[28], (3)[29], (4)[30]
	Vimentin	0.111	1.984	2.089	(7)[31]
	TGF-β1	0.571	2.124	3.309	(1)[32], (4)[33], (5)[33]
	TGFBR 2	0.716	1.453	1.903	(1)[34]
	N-Cam	0.282	2.901	2.223	(3)[35]
	Src	0.639	1.347	1.925	(1)[36], (3)[36], (4)[37], (5)[36]

(1) Invasive Proliferation; (2) Apoptosis; (3) Adhesion; (4) Motility; (5) Invasion; (6) Metastasis; (7) Tumor marker; (8) Transformation

Table 1. GM3 involved in regulating cancer related genes in melanoma.

2.3. RNA extraction and RT-PCR

RNA extraction and analysis of amplified DNA were described in our previous work [4], [5], [9], [38-40]. The primers used in this study were designed with primer 3 software and syntehsized by Shanghai Genebase Biotechnology Corporation (Shanghai, China). Primer sequences used for the PCR in this study were as follows: Plau, Sense 5′-GCCCACAGA CCTGATGCTAT and Antisense 5′-TAGAGCCTTCTGGCCACACT; Plaur, Sense 5′-AGGTGGTGACAAGAGGCTGT and Antisense 5′-AGCTCTGGTCCAAAGAGGTG; gelsolin, Sense 5′-TCCAACAAGGTGCCAGTGGA and Antisense 5′- CAGCACAAAGGCATCGTTGG; Caveolin-1, Sense 5′-CTACAAGCCCAACAACAAGGC and Antisense 5′- AGGAAGCTCTTGATGCACGGT; Ly-GDI and Eef sequences are provided in our previous publications [5], [40]. The mRNA levels of the genes under consideration, using Eef mRNA as an internal control, were determined by RT-PCR semiquantitatively, as described previously [4, 5, 9, 38-40]. Candidate mRNA values are expressed as a ratio of candicate mRNA to Eef mRNA and are usually expressed as unity for control experiments.

2.4. siRNA and cDNA constructs

Target sequences were designed and synthesized as previously described [4, 5, 9, 38-40]. Effective siRNA sequence targeting Ly-GDI can be found in our previous publications [5, 40]. For ectopic expression of Caveolin-1 or Ly-GDI, total RNA was isolated from mouse FBJ-S1 cells. After the first-strand cDNA was synthesized, a Caveolin-1 or Ly-GDI transcript was amplified using the following sense and antisense primers: Caveolin-1, Sense 5'-GCTAG-CATGTCTGGGGGCAAATACGT and Antisense 5'-GGATCCTCA-TATCTCTTTCTGCGTGC; Ly-GDI, 5'- GCTAGCATGACGGAGAAGGATGCACAGCCA and Antisense 5'- GGATCCTCATTCTGTCCAATCCTTCT. The coding sequence of Caveolin-1 or Ly-GDI was inserted between NheI and BamHI digestion sites for sense expression in a pITES-puro3 expression vector with puromycin resistance (Clonetech, USA). The plasmids were prepared and confirmed by sequencing analysis.

2.5. Transfection

In RNA interference experiments, B16 cells were transfected as previously described [4, 5, 9, 38-40]. In brief, B16 cells were transfected with Ly-GDI siRNA for 3 days and the stably transfected cells were further selected by G418 treatment. In control experiments, cells were transfected with scramble siRNA and also selected with G418. For ectopic expression experiments, B16 cells were transfected with Caveolin-1 or Ly-GDI cDNA contructs before analysing the mRNA expression of corresponding genes after 3 days. Control cells were transfected with empty vector.

3. Involvement of GM3 targeted genes in mediating melanoma metastasis

Accumulating evidence using thin-layer chromatography techniques has shown that the gangliosides GM3 and GD3 are predominantly expressed in melanoma cells and are present in relatively higher concentrations than the more complicated gangliosides GT1, GD1 and GM1 in adult brain tissue [41]. In line with this report, GM3 has been detected in both human and murine melanoma cells by MAb M2590 [42], [43]. Although GM3 has been identified several decades ago, the progress on the mechanism of GM3 in mediating melanoma metastasis is slow. Prior works have shown that GM3 facilitates melanoma B16 cells to metastasize in C57BL/6 mice [44], [45], but the mechanism remains unknown. In view of the complicated steps of melanoma metastasis and multiple biological functions of GM3, it is necessary to address the targets molecules through which GM3 exerts its functions on melanoma metastasis.

3.1. Ly-GDI

Ly-GDI, a Rho GTPase dissociation inhibitor beta, is also known as RhoGDI2, Arhgdib or D4-GDI. It belongs to a family of RhoGDIs including RhoGDI1 and RhoGDI3. The family is named for its ability to inhibit the dissociation of bound GDP from its partner Rho GTPase, which regulates interactions with regulatory guanine nucleotide exchange factors, GAP, and the effector targets [46]. Among GDIs, Ly-GDI differs substantially at the structural level from the other two GDIs and is regarded as an invasive and metastatic suppressor gene in human bladder cancer cells [47], [48]. In line with these findings, Ota *et al.* [49] also reported that truncated Ly-GDI promotes metastasis of mouse colon cancer. Along with these prior works, our recent data demonstrate that Ly-GDI expression was positively regulated by GM3, which in turn suppresses anchorage-independent growth in mouse melanoma B16 cells [5]. As anchorage-independent growth has been previously regarded as one of the most important oncogenic properties of tumor cells, it is important to describe the signal transduction pathway between GM3 and Ly-GDI, leading to suppress melanoma invasive proliferation in soft agar medium.

As a first step, we evaluated the effect of endogenous GM3 on Ly-GDI mRNA expression. Our data reveal that Ly-GDI mRNA expression is always proportional to endogenous GM3 contents (Table. 1), which suggests possible roles of GM3 in Ly-GDI regulation. To further confirm the notion that GM3 is responsible for Ly-GDI regulation, GM3 was exogenously added in the culture medium of GM3-depleted cells, such as B11 clone and CAH-3 cells, as well as B16 parental cells. Our data reveal that exogenous GM3 significantly bound to biological membranes, which resulted in upregulation of Ly-GDI expression in three cell lines [5]. Reciprocally, GM3 depletion was carried out by incubating cells with D-PDMP, which in turn suppresses Ly-GDI expression. Collectively, our data demonstrated that GM3 contents play pivotal role in regulating Ly-GDI expression [5].

To keep the discussion focused, we next aimed to characterize the signaling pathway of GM3 in regulating Ly-GDI expression. In light of the possible role of PI3-K pathway in GM3 signaling cascade [4], [40], we examined the effects of PI3-K inhibitor, LY294002, on Ly-GDI mRNA expression in the absence or presence of GM3. Treatment of B16 and CSSH-1 cells with LY294002 not only suppressed Ly-GDI mRNA expression, but also reversed the effects of GM3 on increasing Ly-GDI mRNA expression. Similarly, this pharmacological intervention was also effective in suppressing Akt phosphorylation at Ser 473 and Thr 308 without altering total Akt levels. To further exclude the possible non-specific effects of PI3-K inhibitors, we transfected B16 cells with Akt1 or Akt2 siRNA. Our results revealed that Akt1 or Akt2 knock down decreases Ly-GDI expression at mRNA level and the effects of suppression are more profound in Akt1/2 doubly silenced cells. It is noteworthy that GM3 are not able to upregulate Ly-GDI expression in Akt1/2 double knock down cells. Collectively, our results demonstrate that GM3 regulate Ly-GDI expression via PI3-K/Akt pathway [5].

Although we had found that PI3-K/Akt pathway plays pivotal role in regulating Ly-GDI expression, the question is easily raised whether GM3 directly activates PI3-K pathway or not. In view of the important role of Pdpk1 and mTOR complexes in PI3-K signaling cascade [50], we determined their expression in B11 cells. Our data revealed that GM3 knock down concurrently reduces Pdpk1 and Raptor expression, whereas induces Rictor expression. Taking the advantage of siRNA technique, we further found that Pdpk1 and Raptor, but not Rictor knock down abolished GM3 effects on Ly-GDI induction via blocking Akt phosphorylation at Thr 308 [5]. From these observations, we demonstrate that GM3 induces Ly-GDI expression via PI3-K, Pdpk1, Akt^{Thr308} and mTOR/Raptor pathway in melanoma B16 cells (Fig.

1). More importantly, the experiments were also carried out to determine if Ly-GDI is the key molecule in mediating melanoma B16 cells anchorage-independent growth. Our data demonstrate that Ly-GDI knock down significantly increased the proliferating ability of B16 cells in soft agar or serum free medium [5]. It is noteworthy that expression of GM3 is gradually increased during the progression of melanoma malignancy. For instance, GM3 was not detected in normal or naevi skin, but 60% of primary and 75% of metastatic melanoma expressed GM3 [51]. Our data along with previously published results [51] suggest that relatively lower levels of GM3 and Ly-GDI at the early stage of melanoma facilitate melanoma cells to undergo invasive proliferation in vigorous environment. These observations also provide insights into the molecular basis of GM3 on augmenting melanoma invasive proliferation at the early stage of pathology.

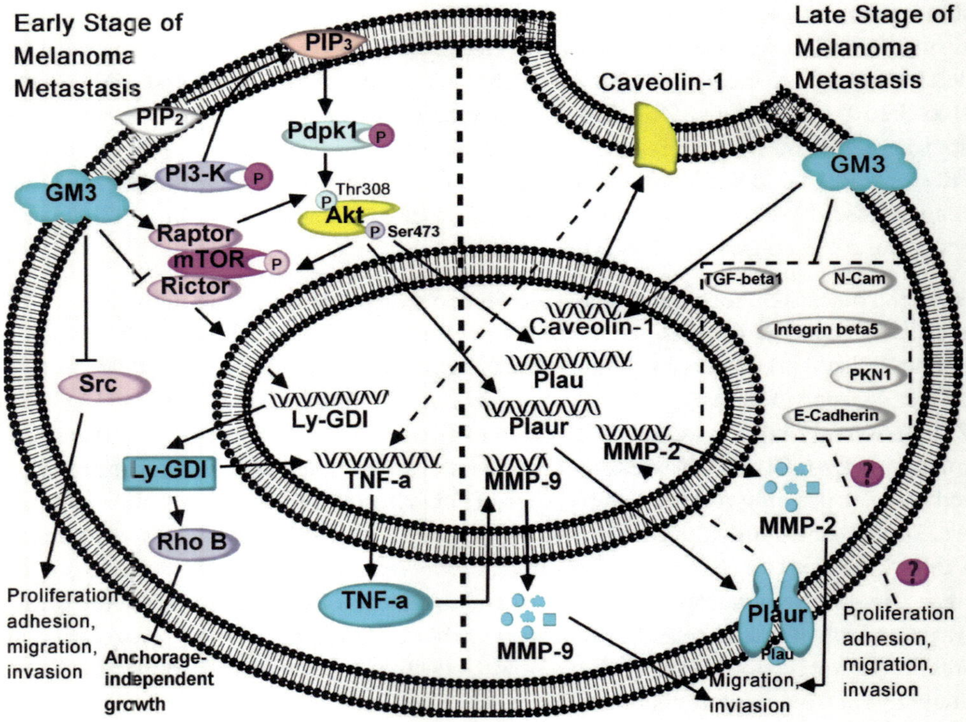

Figure 1. Proposed cascade of GM3 signaling events in murine melanoma B16 cells metastasis. In melanoma B16 cells, GM3 is gradually increased during the progression of melanoma malignancy and facilitates melanoma cells to metastasize. We here found that GM3 signals are transduced via PI3-K, Pdpk1, Akt and the mTOR/Raptor pathway, leading to the expression of Ly-GDI and RhoB, which in turn suppresses mouse melanoma cell proliferation in soft agar or serum deprived medium. In addition, GM3 is able to suppress melanoma cell proliferation, adhesion, migration and invasion by inhibiting Src mRNA expression. It is noted that the above mechanisms will result in cell invasive proliferation, migration and invasion because of relatively lower level of GM3 at early stage of melanoma progression. In contrast, higher level of GM3 at late stage of melanoma metastasis will trigger cell migration and invasion via MMP-2, MMP-9 and Caveolin-1 etc, although the signaling transduction pathway is the same as the above discussion. These *in vitro* observations not only decipher the codes of GM3 in regulating melanoma metastasis *in vivo*, but also help find new therapeutic strategies to treat melanoma disorders.

3.2. TNF-α

TNF-α is a multifunctional cytokine, which is synthesized as a 26kDa (233 amino acids) membrane-bound propeptide (pro-TNF-α) and is secreted upon cleavage by TNF-α converting enzyme [52]. Studies on the effects of TNF-α using experimental models of invasion and metastasis have shown that it can often act as a tumor promoting factor [53]. More specifically for melanoma, TNF-α has been reported to upregulate the expression of integrin subunits, which in turn enhance the interaction of human melanoma cells with ECM substrates [54], [55]. The more recent study from this laboratory showed that TNF-α induces integrin expression, cell attachment and invasion via fibronectin in human melanoma cells [55]. In light of these prior works, our recent data demonstrate that TNF-α located downstream of Ly-GDI to mediate melanoma metastasis (Fig. 4) [4], [39], [40]. To verify that TNF-α follows the same GM3 signaling cascade as Ly-GDI, we carried out the same experiments as above Ly-GDI. In line with GM3 regulating Ly-GDI signaling pathway [5], our results revealed that GM3 regulates TNF-α mRNA and protein expression via PI3-K, Akt and mTOR pathway [4], [40], suggesting that TNF-α is indeed the downstream target of Ly-GDI through which mediate biological functions of GM3 and Ly-GDI in melanoma metastasis. Once TNF-α was found to be a link in the chain of GM3 signaling, we focused on its biological effects on melanoma metastasis. The results demonstrate that TNF-α is able to enhance melanoma migration via inducing MMP-9 expression and activity [39], which will be further discussed in "MMP-9 and MMP-2" part (Fig. 1). On the other hand, Venessa *et al.* [56] proposed that TNF-α protect melanoma cells from apoptosis by BRAF inhibition. In contrast, Andrea *et al.* [57] reported that TNF-α exhibited antiproliferative effects on four melanoma cell lines. In line with this report [57], accumulating evidence demonstrates that TNF-α suppresses melanoma metastasis in patients or murine models [58]. Although TNF-α shows its effects on suppressing melanoma metastasis, we still could not negate its ability to induce melanoma migration and invasion. Since the debating is still going on and the multiple biological functions of TNF-α, we are not able to arbitrarily judge that TNF-α induces or reduces melanoma metastasis until now. It would be finally decided by the mechanism that TNF-α predominantly exerts.

3.3. MMP-9 and MMP-2

As above discussion, TNF-α is able to enhance melanoma migration via inducing MMP-9 expression and activity [39], we next aimed to elucidate its mechanism. In order to determine the role of MMP-9 in cell migration, we examined the effects of an MMP-9 agonist and antagonist on cell migration, as stimulation of MMP-9 expression by TNF-α has been reported in several studies [59], [60]. We therefore used TNF-α as a positive control against the MMP-9 inhibitor GM6001. RT-PCR results demonstrate that TNF-α markedly induces MMP-9 expression and activity, which is reversed by GM6001 treatment [39]. Furthermore, cell migration tested by transwell experiments showed that the numbers of cells migrating were consistent with MMP-9 expression [39]. This finding is in accordance with previously published data showing that TNF-α increases human melanoma cell invasion and migration *in vitro*, whereas they could not further extend their investigation to MMP-9 [23]. Bianchini *et al.* [59] proceed to find that invasive phenotype of murine melanoma cells stimulated with

TNF-α was characterized by an enhanced MMP-9 expression. More importantly, we extended their investigations to GM3 and further reveal that GM3 also regulate MMP-9 expression and activity via PI3-K, Akt, Ly-GDI and TNF-α pathway [39]. Therefore, our findings [39] along with the prior works [23], [59] demonstrate that TNF-α induces melanoma migration and invasion via augmenting MMP-9 expression.

In addition to MMP-9, it is noteworthy that MMP-2 is also induced by endogenous GM3 (Table. 1). Although we are still not figure out the mechanism that GM3 positively regulates MMP-2 expression in melanoma B16 cells, MMP-2 has been implicated to be associated with progression of the melanoma [61]. In more detail, although all skin and nodal metastasis were negative for MMP-2, higher MMP-2 concentrations were observed in patients with metastatic disease (stage IV) than in those with primary melanoma (stage I) or in controls [61]. In addition, Liu *et al.* [62] recently published research showing that d-GM3, a derivative of ganglioside GM3, stimulates melanoma cell migration and invasion by increasing the expression and activation of MMP-2. To keep the discussion focused, it should be also noted that expression of GM3 is gradually increased during the progression of melanoma malignancy [51]. Once GM3 was markedly induced at the late stage of melanoma, MMP-9 and MMP-2 would be activated by GM3, which in turn mediating migration and invasion in melanoma progression. Therefore, multiple biological functions and stage dependent expression manner of GM3 make it possible to induce invasive proliferation of melanoma at early stage and stimulate melanoma cell migration and invasion at late stage of melanoma progression (Fig.1).

3.4. Plau and Plaur

During the course of MMP-9 and MMP-2 investigations, experimental evidence had led to the recognition of Plau and Plaur [59], [62]. Indeed, Plau and Plaur are highly expressed in advanced stages of primary and metastatic melanoma progression [63]. In addition, Bianchini *et al.* [59] proposed that costimulation with TNF-α and IFNγ enhancing murine melanoma B16 cells metastasis via inducing Plaur mRNA and protein expression. Moreover, Liu *et al.* [62] extended the above findings to exogenous d-GM3 treatment, the results suggested that d-GM3 promotes melanoma cell migration and invasion through Plaur signaling dependent pathway, which in turn mediating melanoma cell migration and invasion via MMP-2. Along with these prior works [59], [62], our data revealed that endogenous GM3 is able to positively regulate Plau and Plaur mRNA expression in mouse melanoma B16 cells (Table. 1). Although the mechanism that GM3 regulates Plau and Plaur mRNA expression is still going on in our lab, we already found that PI3-K/Akt pathway plays key roles in regulating Plau and Plaur mRNA expression in B16 cells (Fig. 2). To elucidate the biological functions of Plau and Plaur, Bianchini *et al.* [59] already found that Plaur monoclonal antibody treatment caused a significant reduction of invasiveness in TNF-α/IFNγ stimulated melanoma cells. In addition, targeting Plaur has practical implications in treating cancer. For example, 1) downregulating Plaur expression leads to dormancy of cancer cells [64]; 2) administrating Plaur antagonists markedly inhibits metastatic ability, including that of melanomas [65]; 3)deficiency of plasminogen/Plau in mice slows tumor growth and progression [65]; and 4) inhibiting Plau and/or its binding with Plaur prevents metastasis in animal models [66]. Collectively, the additional role of Plau/

Plaur signaling in mediating GM3 function [67] makes Plau/Plaur system as an attractive target for cancer therapy.

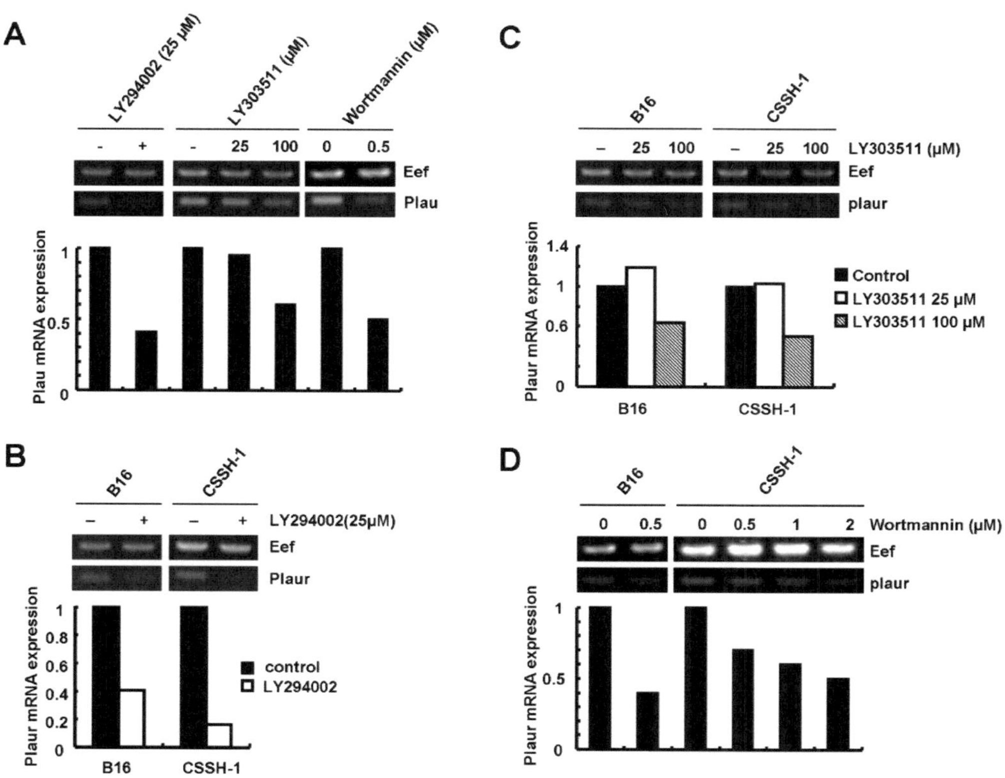

Figure 2. Involvement of PI3-K signaling pathway in Plau and Plaur synthesis in mouse melanoma B16 cells. B16 (A-D) or CSSH-1 (B-D) cells were incubated with either LY294002, LY303511 or Wortmannin for the indicated concentrations. Plau (A) and Plaur (B-D) mRNA expressions were determined by RT-PCR after 24h incubation. Eef served as internal control. The intensity of bands was analyzed relative to Eef for each treatment using the Bio-Profile Bio ID gel image system at 312nm.

3.5. Gelsolin

Gelsolin is a representative actin-regulatory protein with an 82kDa mass and is present in most vertebrate tissues. Gelsolin controls the length of actin polymers *in vitro* by a variety of mechanisms [68], [69]. Since actin filament reorganization is important for cell shape and motility, gelsolin has crucial roles in the control of these cellular functions [70], [71]. Accumulating evidence has shown that gelsolin expression is frequently downregulated in several types of human cancers, such as gastric, bladder, colon and lung [72]- [75]. In addition, ectopic expression of wild-type gelsolin resulted in suppression of tumorigenicity of both bladder and colon carcinoma cell lines [73], [76]. However, a new 85kDa truncated gelsolin (GSNp85), co-expressed with wild-type gelsolin, was frequently expressed in vertical growth phase melanomas (Clark level II-IV) and metastatic growth phase melanomas [77]. Moreover, Litwin *et al.* [78] recently found that downregulation of gelsolin expression in melanoma A375 cells significantly reduce their migratory potential. These disparate observations might be attributed to different species of cancer cells. Consistent with the prior works [77], [78], we newly found that endogenous GM3 has ability to regulate gelsolin mRNA expression (Table. 1). In addition, PI3-K/Akt signaling pathway was found to exert critical role in mediating gelsolin mRNA induction (Fig. 3A). Moreover, gelsolin is found to be downstream targets of Ly-GDI in melanoma B16 cells by the experiments of Ly-GDI knock down (Fig. 3B). This observation not only demonstrates the critical role of Ly-GDI, but also provides new insights in melanoma metastasis (Fig. 1). More importantly, it is also indicating that alterations in the expression level of gelsolin and its subcellular distribution may be directly responsible for determining migration capacity of melanoma.

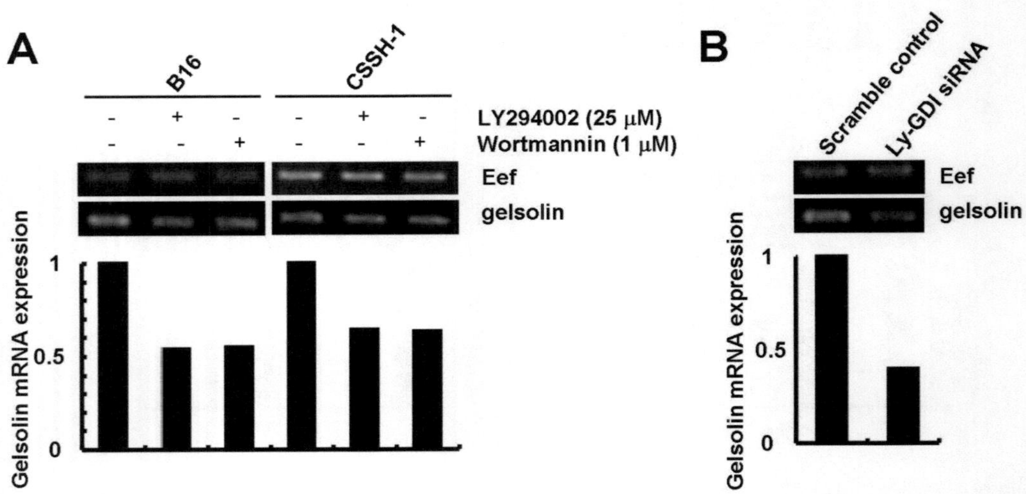

Figure 3. Involvement of PI3-K signaling pathway in gelsolin synthesis in mouse melanoma B16 cells. B16 (A, left panel) or CSSH-1 (A, right panel) cells were incubated with either LY294002 (25 μM) or Wortmannin (1 μM) for 24 h. In selected experiments, B16 cells were transfected with Ly-GDI siRNA and further established Ly-GDI knocking down cell lines by G418 selection (B). Gelsolin mRNA expression was determined by RT-PCR after 24h incubation. Eef served as internal control. The intensity of bands was analyzed relative to Eef for each treatment using the Bio-Profile Bio ID gel image system at 312nm.

3.6. Caveolin-1

Caveolin-1 is a 22-24 KDa protein originally identified as a structural component of caveolae, specialized invagination of the plasma membrane. These caveolae represent compartments in which key signaling transduction molecules are concentrated to provide an efficient system for cellular cross talk. However, relatively little information is available concerning the role of Caveolin-1 in melanomas. Early studies demonstrate that increased Caveolin-1 expression was associated with enhanced malignancy in a non-cutaneous, retinal melanoma [79]. An even more recent study identified exosomes in the plasma of melanoma patients with high levels of Caveolin-1.In this particular case, exosomes are associated with malignant tumor progression as a small vesicle secreted by both normal and tumoral cells [80]. These prior works demonstrate that Caveolin-1 are relevant to function in melanoma metastasis.

Additional studies support the notion that presence of Caveolin-1 helps melanoma metastasis. Felicetti et al. proposed that Caveolin-1 expression is associated with increased metastatic potential in different human melanoma cell lines. Specifically, Caveolin-1 expression increased cell proliferation, anchorage-independent growth, migration and invasion in WM983A melanoma cell line. Alternatively, Caveolin-1 down-regulation in metastatic Caveolin-1 overexpressing melanomas reduces their proliferation, as well as their tumorigenicity [7]. Consistent with prior works [7], we further found that Caveolin-1 was regulated by endogenous GM3 (Table. 1). More importantly, our recent data revealed that Caveolin-1 is able to regulate TNF-α (Fig. 4), which in turn mediates melanoma migration or invasion through MMP-9 as discussed above [39]. Our data along with previous reports [7] further implicated the important role of GM3-enriched membrane subdomain, especially Caveolae, in melanoma metastasis.

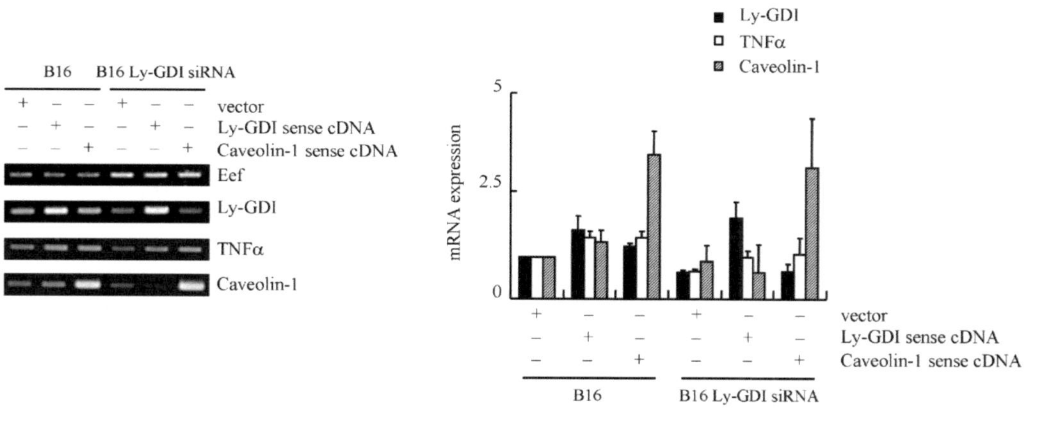

Figure 4. Ly-GDI overexpression induces TNF-α mRNA expression in mouse melanoma B16 cells. B16 or Ly-GDI knocking down cells were transfected with Ly-GDI or Caveolin-1 cDNA construct. Ly-GDI, TNF-α and Caveolin-1 mRNA expressions were determined by RT-PCR after 3 days transfection. Eef served as internal control. The intensity of bands was analyzed relative to Eef for each treatment using the Bio-Profile Bio ID gel image system at 312nm.

3.7. Src

Over the past few decades, studies of Src and the SFKs have given new insights into the role of these proteins in regulating cell adhesion, invasiveness and motility in cancer cells and in tumor vasculature, rather than directly influencing cell proliferation [81]. Src expression and activity are increased in melanoma cell lines and in melanoma tumors *in vivo* [82]. Src activity was detected in the following cell lines: LOX, IMVI, MALME-3M, SK-MEL-2, SK-MEL-5, SK-MEL-28, M19-MEL, UACC-62 and UACC-257. The highest activity was that in the M14 melanoma cell lines.

Src can activate STAT3, STAT5 and other downstream targets in melanoma [83]. The expression of STAT3 is highly expressed in both primary and metastatic melanoma in humans, although the expression level is variable [81]. In addition, STAT3 is activated in human melanoma, but not in melanocytic or in benign melanocytic neoplasms [84]. Moreover, blocking STAT3 signaling in mouse B16 melanoma cells resulted in the release of soluble factors capable of inducing apoptosis and cell-cycle arrest [85]. *In vivo*, inerfering with STAT3 signaling suppressed growth of syngeneic murine melanoma B16 tumor [86]. In addition to STAT3, it was recently found that STAT5 signaling in melanoma cell lines is mediated by the EGFR tyrosine kinase and by intracellular non-receptor tyrosine kinase, such as Src and JAK1. The expression of STAT5 is increased in melanoma metastasis compared with normal human melanocytes and STAT5 is activated in 62% of human melanoma metastasis. Alternatively, inhibiting STAT5 expression significantly reduced the expression of Bcl-2 and decreased cell viability and increased apoptosis in the melanoma cell lines. In view of the critical role of Src in melanoma invasive proliferation, we further found that Src was negatively regulated by endogenous GM3 (Table.1). This result along with previous reports [51], [83]- [86] indicated that GM3 regulates melanoma invasive proliferation via Src at the early stage of melanoma or at the stage of transformation, but not in advanced stage of melanoma (Fig. 1). Although we haven't found detailed mechanism that GM3 regulates Src mRNA expression, which in turn resulting in melanoma metastasis, it is still noteworthy to emphasize that Src mediated melanoma invasive proliferation might be the pivotal mechanism, which mediates melanoma transformation or onset of disease at the early stage when GM3 expression is still relative low. Therefore, it is also important to elucidate the biological function of Src when the expression is still low at the early stage of melanoma progression. These future discoveries will make us understand which mechanism predominantly contributed to the metastasis progression of melanoma at different stages or at different steps of cancer metastasis.

3.8. Rho B

Recent studies confirmed the role of the Rho proteins in cancer by showing their involvement in cell transforamtion, invasion, metastasis and angiogenesis. The major members of the Rho subfamily comprise the Rho A, Rho B and Rho C proteins. Rho B is quite different from Rho A and Rho C in many aspects, although it shares 87% homology [20]. For example, Rho B has a tumor suppressive role, including inhibiting cell proliferation and inducing apoptosis in several human cancer cells, and inhibiting tumor growth in murine model, in contrast, activation of Rho A promotes cell malignant transformation, proliferation, invasion and metastasis, like other small GTPases such as Ras, Rac1 and Cdc42 [87] Moreover, Rho B, unlike the constitutively expressed Rho A, is inducible by genotoxic stress, such as U.V. light, growth factors (TGF-β1) and chemotherapeutic drugs (cisplatin and 5-FU). In our experimental system, we found that mRNA expression of Rho B is suppressed by Ly-GDI knocking down [5]. This observation partially implied that Rho B located downstream of Ly-GDI to mediate its inhibitory effects on melanoma invasive proliferation and would also exerts its effects at early stage of melanoma progression (Fig. 1).

http://dx.doi.org/10.5772/54941

3.9. Other genes

During the course of our investigation in melanoma metastasis, we also found the involvement of some pro-oncogenes or tumor suppressor genes, such as TGF-β1, N-Cam, integrin β5, PKN1 or E-cadherin *et al.*, (Table. 1) in GM3 biological functions to mediate melanoma cells invasive proliferation, adhesion, migration and invasion, which finally contribute to melanoma transformation and progression. Although these steps of melanoma metastasis are not separate, our *in vitro* experiments have partially revealed the mechanism of melanoma metastasis at different stages. More importantly, deciphering the mechanism of GM3 in mediating melanoma metastasis will help find new therapeutic strategies to treat melanoma disorders.

4. Conclusion

Metastasis, the spread of malignant tumor cells from a primary site to distant sites, is the most life-threatening complication of cancer and a major problem of cancer treatment [88], [89]. The metastatic process consists of multiple steps: 1) invasive proliferation as benign tumor at the primary site 2) dissociation of tumor cell(s) from the primary site with a concomitant loss of cell-cell and cell-ECM adhesions; 3) tumor-cell adhesion to and subsequent local digestion of basement membrane; 4) retraction of endothelial cells and subsequent intravasation; 5) survival within the vasculature; 6) extravasation from vasculature at a distinct site and 7) growth in a "foreign" or ectopic organ environment [90], [91]. In view of these prior theories, our data summarized here reinforce the notion that GM3 potentially plays a dual role in melanoma development, as has been described in our previously published works[4-6,] [39], [92]. At early stage of melanoma metastasis, lower level of GM3 induces melanoma invasive proliferation via Src, Rho B and Ly-GDI *et al.* Alternatively, higher levels of GM3 at the late stage of melanoma metastasis triggers cell migration and invasion via MMP-2, MMP-9 and Caveolin-1 etc. These *in vitro* observations not only decipher the codes of GM3 in regulating melanoma metastasis *in vivo*, but also help find new therapeutic strategies to treat melanoma disorders.

Nomenclature

GSLs, sialylated glycosphingolipids; RTK, receptor tyrosine kinase; PI3-K, phosphatidylinositol-3-kinase; Rb, retinoblastoma; PKN1, protein kinase 1; MMP-9, matrix matelloproteinase-9; MMP-2, matrix metalloproteinase-2; Apaf1, apoptotic protease activating factor 1; TNF-α, tumor necrosis factor-α; Plau, urokinase-type plasminogen activator; Plaur, urokinase-type plasminogen activator receptor; TGF-β1, transforming growth factor-β1; TGFBR2, transforming growth factor, beta receptor 2; RhoGDI, RhoGDP dissociation inhibitors; GAP, GTPase-activating proteins; Pdpk1, 3-phosphoinositide dependent protein kinase-1; mTOR, mammalian target of rapamycin; Raptor, regulatory associated protein of mTOR; ECM, extracellular matrix; d-GM3, De-N-acetyl GM3; IFNγ, interferon γ; SFKs, Src-family kinases; STAT3, signal transducer and activator of transcription 3; STAT5, signal transducer and activator of transcription 5; JAK1, Janus kinase 1.

Acknowledgements

This work was supported by funding from the Mizutani Foundation for Glycoscience 080029.

Author details

Pu Wang*[1,2,4], Feipei Guan*[1,2], Su Xu[3,4], Zhanyou Wang[2], Sadako Yamagata[4] and Tatsuya Yamagata[4]

1 Department of Chemical and Biomolecular Engineering, The Johns Hopkins University, Baltimore, Maryland, USA

2 College of Life and Health Sciences, Northeastern University, Shenyang, China

3 Department of Chemistry, University of Alabama at Birmingham, Birmingham, Alabama, USA

4 Laboratory of Tumor Biology and Glycobiology, Shenyang Pharmaceutical University, Shenyang, China

* contributed equally to this work

References

[1] Polsky D, Cordon-Cardo C. Oncogenes in melanoma. Oncogene. 2003; 22: 3087-91.

[2] Berger MF, Garraway LA. Applications of genomics in melanoma oncogene discovery. Hematol Oncol Clin North Am. 2009; 23: 397-414, vii.

[3] Flaherty KT, Fisher DE. New strategies in metastatic melanoma: oncogene-defined taxonomy leads to therapeutic advances. Clin Cancer Res. 2011; 17: 4922-8.

[4] Wang F, Wu P, Zhang J, Sato T, Yamagata S, Yamagata T. Positive regulation of tumor necrosis factor-alpha by ganglioside GM3 through Akt in mouse melanoma B16 cells. Biochem Biophys Res Commun. 2007; 356: 438-43.

[5] Wang P, Xu S, Wang Y, et al. GM3 suppresses anchorage-independent growth via Rho GDP dissociation inhibitor beta in melanoma B16 cells. Cancer Science. 2011: 1476-85.

[6] Wang P, Yamagata S, Yamagata T. Changing the nature of melanoma cells by manipulation of ganglioside expression. Breakthroughs in Melanoma Research Yohei Tanaka: InTech;. 2011: 77-102.

[7] Felicetti F, Parolini I, Bottero L, et al. Caveolin-1 tumor-promoting role in human melanoma. Int J Cancer. 2009; 125: 1514-22.

[8] Seftor EA, Meltzer PS, Kirschmann DA, et al. Molecular determinants of human uveal melanoma invasion and metastasis. Clin Exp Metastasis. 2002; 19: 233-46.

[9] Wang L, Takaku S, Wang P, et al. Ganglioside GD1a regulation of caveolin-1 and Stim1 expression in mouse FBJ cells: augmented expression of caveolin-1 and Stim1 in cells with increased GD1a content. Glycoconj J. 2006; 23: 303-15.

[10] Lau MT, Klausen C, Leung PC. E-cadherin inhibits tumor cell growth by suppressing PI3K/Akt signaling via beta-catenin-Egr1-mediated PTEN expression. Oncogene. 2011; 30: 2753-66.

[11] Tang A, Eller MS, Hara M, Yaar M, Hirohashi S, Gilchrest BA. E-cadherin is the major mediator of human melanocyte adhesion to keratinocytes in vitro. J Cell Sci. 1994; 107 (Pt 4): 983-92.

[12] Wong AS, Gumbiner BM. Adhesion-independent mechanism for suppression of tumor cell invasion by E-cadherin. J Cell Biol. 2003; 161: 1191-203.

[13] Semb H, Christofori G. The tumor-suppressor function of E-cadherin. Am J Hum Genet. 1998; 63: 1588-93.

[14] Fujita H, Okada F, Hamada J, et al. Gelsolin functions as a metastasis suppressor in B16-BL6 mouse melanoma cells and requirement of the carboxyl-terminus for its effect. Int J Cancer. 2001; 93: 773-80.

[15] Desai BS, Chellaiah M. Bisphosphonates inhibit osteopontin induced prostate cancer cell motility by attenuating MMP-9 activity. AACR Meeting Abstracts. 2006; 2006: 774-b.

[16] Wang X, Lu H, Urvalek AM, et al. KLF8 promotes human breast cancer cell invasion and metastasis by transcriptional activation of MMP9. Oncogene. 2011; 30: 1901-11.

[17] Leotlela PD, Wade MS, Duray PH, et al. Claudin-1 overexpression in melanoma is regulated by PKC and contributes to melanoma cell motility. Oncogene. 2007; 26: 3846-56.

[18] Denkert C, Siegert A, Leclere A, Turzynski A, Hauptmann S. An inhibitor of stress-activated MAP-kinases reduces invasion and MMP-2 expression of malignant melanoma cells. Clin Exp Metastasis. 2002; 19: 79-85.

[19] Rockmann H, Schadendorf D. Role of Apaf-1 in Melanoma Drug Resistance and Apoptosis. J Investig Dermatol. 2005; 125: 386-7.

[20] Jiang K, Sun J, Cheng J, Djeu JY, Wei S, Sebti S. Akt mediates Ras downregulation of RhoB, a suppressor of transformation, invasion, and metastasis. Mol Cell Biol. 2004; 24: 5565-76.

[21] Escalante CR, Aggarwal AK, Wilson PD, Burrow CR. Monomeric Midkine Induces Tumor Cell Proliferation in the Absence of Cell-Surface Proteoglycan Binding. Biochemistry. 2000; 39: 5977-87.

[22] Dobrzanski MJ, Reome JB, Hollenbaugh JA, Hylind JC, Dutton RW. Effector cell-derived lymphotoxin alpha and Fas ligand, but not perforin, promote Tc1 and Tc2 effector cell-mediated tumor therapy in established pulmonary metastases. Cancer Res. 2004; 64: 406-14.

[23] Katerinaki E, Evans GS, Lorigan PC, MacNeil S. TNF-alpha increases human melanoma cell invasion and migration in vitro: the role of proteolytic enzymes. Br J Cancer. 2003; 89: 1123-9.

[24] Lee J, Duk Jung I, Gyo Park C, Han JW, Young Lee H. Autotaxin stimulates urokinase-type plasminogen activator expression through phosphoinositide 3-kinase-Akt-nuclear [corrected] factor kappa B signaling cascade in human melanoma cells. Melanoma Res. 2006; 16: 445-52.

[25] Besch R, Berking C, Kammerbauer C, Degitz K. Inhibition of urokinase-type plasminogen activator receptor induces apoptosis in melanoma cells by activation of p53. Cell Death Differ. 2007; 14: 818-29.

[26] Taverna D, Crowley D, Connolly M, Bronson RT, Hynes RO. A direct test of potential roles for beta3 and beta5 integrins in growth and metastasis of murine mammary carcinomas. Cancer Res. 2005; 65: 10324-9.

[27] Taverna D, Moher H, Crowley D, Borsig L, Varki A, Hynes RO. Increased primary tumor growth in mice null for beta3- or beta3/beta5-integrins or selectins. Proc Natl Acad Sci U S A. 2004; 101: 763-8.

[28] Cardo-Vila M, Arap W, Pasqualini R. Alpha v beta 5 integrin-dependent programmed cell death triggered by a peptide mimic of annexin V. Mol Cell. 2003; 11: 1151-62.

[29] Niu JX, Zhang WJ, Ye LY, et al. The role of adhesion molecules, alpha v beta 3, alpha v beta 5 and their ligands in the tumor cell and endothelial cell adhesion. Eur J Cancer Prev. 2007; 16: 517-27.

[30] Zhang H, Li Z, Viklund EK, Stromblad S. P21-activated kinase 4 interacts with integrin alpha v beta 5 and regulates alpha v beta 5-mediated cell migration. J Cell Biol. 2002; 158: 1287-97.

[31] Leader M, Collins M, Patel J, Henry K. Vimentin: an evaluation of its role as a tumour marker. Histopathology. 1987; 11: 63-72.

[32] Paterson IC, Davies M, Stone A, et al. TGF-beta1 acts as a tumor suppressor of human malignant keratinocytes independently of Smad 4 expression and ligand-induced G(1) arrest. Oncogene. 2002; 21: 1616-24.

[33] Xu Z, Shen MX, Ma DZ, Wang LY, Zha XL. TGF-beta1-promoted epithelial-to-mesenchymal transformation and cell adhesion contribute to TGF-beta1-enhanced cell migration in SMMC-7721 cells. Cell Res. 2003; 13: 343-50.

[34] Li X, Placencio V, Iturregui JM, et al. Prostate tumor progression is mediated by a paracrine TGF-beta/Wnt3a signaling axis. Oncogene. 2008; 27: 7118-30.

[35] Anastassiou G, Schilling H, Stang A, Djakovic S, Heiligenhaus A, Bornfeld N. Expression of the cell adhesion molecules ICAM-1, VCAM-1 and NCAM in uveal melanoma: a clinicopathological study. Oncology. 2000; 58: 83-8.

[36] Frame MC. Src in cancer: deregulation and consequences for cell behaviour. Biochimica et Biophysica Acta (BBA) - Reviews on Cancer. 2002; 1602: 114-30.

[37] Bourguignon LY, Zhu H, Shao L, Chen YW. CD44 interaction with c-Src kinase promotes cortactin-mediated cytoskeleton function and hyaluronic acid-dependent ovarian tumor cell migration. J Biol Chem. 2001; 276: 7327-36.

[38] Hu D, Man Z, Wang P, et al. Ganglioside GD1a negatively regulates matrix metalloproteinase-9 expression in mouse FBJ cell lines at the transcriptional level. Connect Tissue Res. 2007; 48: 198-205.

[39] Wang P, Wang X, Wu P, et al. GM3 Upregulation of matrix metalloproteinase-9 possibly through PI3K, AKT, RICTOR, RHOGDI-2, and TNF-A pathways in mouse melanoma B16 cells. Adv Exp Med Biol. 2011; 705: 335-48.

[40] Wang P, Yang X, Wu P, et al. GM3 signals regulating TNF-alpha expression are mediated by Rictor and Arhgdib in mouse melanoma B16 cells. Oncology. 2007; 73: 430-8.

[41] Portoukalian J, Zwingelstein G, Dore JF. Lipid composition of human malignant melanoma tumors at various levels of malignant growth. Eur J Biochem. 1979; 94: 19-23.

[42] Hirabayashi Y, Hamaoka A, Matsumoto M, et al. Syngeneic monoclonal antibody against melanoma antigen with interspecies cross-reactivity recognizes GM3, a prominent ganglioside of B16 melanoma. J Biol Chem. 1985; 260: 13328-33.

[43] Hirabayashi Y, Sugimoto M, Ogawa T, Matsumoto M, Tagawa M, Taniguchi M. Reactivity of mouse monoclonal antibody M2590 against B16 melanoma cells with chemically synthesized GM3 ganglioside. Biochim Biophys Acta. 1986; 875: 126-8.

[44] Saha S, Mohanty KC. Enhancement of metastatic potential of mouse B16-melanoma cells to lung after treatment with gangliosides of B-16-melanoma cells of higher metastatic potential to lung. Indian J Exp Biol. 2003; 41: 1253-8.

[45] Saha S, Mohanty KC. Correlation of gangliosides GM2 and GM3 with metastatic potential to lungs of mouse B16 melanoma. J Exp Clin Cancer Res. 2003; 22: 125-34.

[46] Ueda T, Kikuchi A, Ohga N, Yamamoto J, Takai Y. Purification and characterization from bovine brain cytosol of a novel regulatory protein inhibiting the dissociation of GDP from and the subsequent binding of GTP to rhoB p20, a ras p21-like GTP-binding protein. J Biol Chem. 1990; 265: 9373-80.

[47] Gildea JJ, Seraj MJ, Oxford G, et al. RhoGDI2 is an invasion and metastasis suppressor gene in human cancer. Cancer Res. 2002; 62: 6418-23.

[48] Theodorescu D, Sapinoso LM, Conaway MR, Oxford G, Hampton GM, Frierson HF, Jr. Reduced expression of metastasis suppressor RhoGDI2 is associated with decreased survival for patients with bladder cancer. Clin Cancer Res. 2004; 10: 3800-6.

[49] Ota T, Maeda M, Suto S, Tatsuka M. LyGDI functions in cancer metastasis by anchoring Rho proteins to the cell membrane. Mol Carcinog. 2004; 39: 206-20.

[50] Maira SM, Furet P, Stauffer F. Discovery of novel anticancer therapeutics targeting the PI3K/Akt/mTOR pathway. Future Med Chem. 2009; 1: 137-55.

[51] Hersey P, Jamal O, Henderson C, Zardawi I, D'Alessandro G. Expression of the gangliosides GM3, GD3 and GD2 in tissue sections of normal skin, naevi, primary and metastatic melanoma. Int J Cancer. 1988; 41: 336-43.

[52] Bemelmans MH, van Tits LJ, Buurman WA. Tumor necrosis factor: function, release and clearance. Crit Rev Immunol. 1996; 16: 1-11.

[53] Balkwill F. Tumor necrosis factor or tumor promoting factor? Cytokine Growth Factor Rev. 2002; 13: 135-41.

[54] Dekker SK, Vink J, Vermeer BJ, Bruijn JA, Mihm MC, Jr., Byers HR. Differential effects of interleukin 1-alpha (IL-1 alpha) or tumor necrosis factor-alpha (TNF-alpha) on motility of human melanoma cell lines on fibronectin. J Invest Dermatol. 1994; 102: 898-905.

[55] Zhu N, Eves PC, Katerinaki E, et al. Melanoma cell attachment, invasion, and integrin expression is upregulated by tumor necrosis factor alpha and suppressed by alpha melanocyte stimulating hormone. J Invest Dermatol. 2002; 119: 1165-71.

[56] Gray-Schopfer VC, Karasarides M, Hayward R, Marais R. Tumor Necrosis Factor-alpha Blocks Apoptosis in Melanoma Cells when BRAF Signaling Is Inhibited. Cancer Research. 2007; 67: 122-9.

[57] Ladanyi A, Nagy JO, Jeney A, Timar J. Cytokine sensitivity of metastatic human melanoma cell lines-- simultaneous inhibition of proliferation and enhancement of gelatinase activity. Pathol Oncol Res. 1998; 4: 108-14.

[58] Hundsberger H, Verin A, Wiesner C, et al. TNF: a moonlighting protein at the interface between cancer and infection. Front Biosci. 2008; 13: 5374-86.

[59] Bianchini F, D'Alessio S, Fibbi G, Del Rosso M, Calorini L. Cytokine-dependent invasiveness in B16 murine melanoma cells: role of uPA system and MMP-9. Oncol Rep. 2006; 15: 709-14.

[60] Kim S, Choi JH, Kim JB, et al. Berberine suppresses TNF-alpha-induced MMP-9 and cell invasion through inhibition of AP-1 activity in MDA-MB-231 human breast cancer cells. Molecules. 2008; 13: 2975-85.

[61] Redondo P, Lloret P, Idoate M, Inoges S. Expression and serum levels of MMP-2 and MMP-9 during human melanoma progression. Clin Exp Dermatol. 2005; 30: 541-5.

[62] Liu JW, Sun P, Yan Q, et al. De-N-acetyl GM3 promotes melanoma cell migration and invasion through urokinase plasminogen activator receptor signaling-dependent MMP-2 activation. Cancer Res. 2009; 69: 8662-9.

[63] de Vries TJ, Quax PH, Denijn M, et al. Plasminogen activators, their inhibitors, and urokinase receptor emerge in late stages of melanocytic tumor progression. Am J Pathol. 1994; 144: 70-81.

[64] Yu W, Kim J, Ossowski L. Reduction in surface urokinase receptor forces malignant cells into a protracted state of dormancy. J Cell Biol. 1997; 137: 767-77.

[65] D'Alessio S, Margheri F, Pucci M, et al. Antisense oligodeoxynucleotides for urokinase-plasminogen activator receptor have anti-invasive and anti-proliferative effects in vitro and inhibit spontaneous metastases of human melanoma in mice. Int J Cancer. 2004; 110: 125-33.

[66] Almholt K, Lund LR, Rygaard J, et al. Reduced metastasis of transgenic mammary cancer in urokinase-deficient mice. Int J Cancer. 2005; 113: 525-32.

[67] Wang XQ, Sun P, Go L, Koti V, Fliman M, Paller AS. Ganglioside GM3 promotes carcinoma cell proliferation via urokinase plasminogen activator-induced extracellular signal-regulated kinase-independent p70S6 kinase signaling. J Invest Dermatol. 2006; 126: 2687-96.

[68] Kwiatkowski DJ, Mehl R, Izumo S, Nadal-Ginard B, Yin HL. Muscle is the major source of plasma gelsolin. J Biol Chem. 1988; 263: 8239-43.

[69] Lueck A, Brown D, Kwiatkowski DJ. The actin-binding proteins adseverin and gelsolin are both highly expressed but differentially localized in kidney and intestine. J Cell Sci. 1998; 111 (Pt 24): 3633-43.

[70] Stossel TP. The E. Donnall Thomas Lecture, 1993. The machinery of blood cell movements. Blood. 1994; 84: 367-79.

[71] Stossel TP, Hartwig JH, Janmey PA, Kwiatkowski DJ. Cell crawling two decades after Abercrombie. Biochem Soc Symp. 1999; 65: 267-80.

[72] Dosaka-Akita H, Hommura F, Fujita H, et al. Frequent loss of gelsolin expression in non-small cell lung cancers of heavy smokers. Cancer Res. 1998; 58: 322-7.

[73] Furuuchi K, Fujita H, Tanaka M, et al. Gelsolin as a suppressor of malignant phenotype in human colon cancer. Tumor Target. 1997; 2: 277-83.

[74] Moriya S, Yanagihara K, Fujita H, Kuzumaki N. Differential expression of hsp90, gelsolin and gst-pi in human gastric-carcinoma cell-lines. Int J Oncol. 1994; 5: 1347-51.

[75] Tanaka M, Mullauer L, Ogiso Y, et al. Gelsolin: a candidate for suppressor of human bladder cancer. Cancer Res. 1995; 55: 3228-32.

[76] Takada A, Ohmori K, Yoneda T, et al. Contribution of carbohydrate antigens sialyl Lewis A and sialyl Lewis X to adhesion of human cancer cells to vascular endothelium. Cancer Res. 1993; 53: 354-61.

[77] Furukawa H, Fujita H, Kokubu I, et al. Identification of a novel gelsolin truncate in the vertical and metastatic phase malignant melanomas. Melanoma Res. 2002; 12: 523-8.

[78] Litwin M, Nowak D, Mazur AJ, Baczynska D, Mannherz HG, Malicka-Blaszkiewicz M. Gelsolin affects the migratory ability of human colon adenocarcinoma and melanoma cells. Life Sci. 2012; 90: 851-61.

[79] Berta AI, Kiss AL, Kemeny-Beke A, Lukats A, Szabo A, Szel A. Different caveolin isoforms in the retina of melanoma malignum affected human eye. Mol Vis. 2007; 13: 881-6.

[80] Logozzi M, De Milito A, Lugini L, et al. High levels of exosomes expressing CD63 and caveolin-1 in plasma of melanoma patients. PLoS One. 2009; 4: e5219.

[81] Homsi J, Cubitt C, Daud A. The Src signaling pathway: a potential target in melanoma and other malignancies. Expert Opin Ther Targets. 2007; 11: 91-100.

[82] Budde RJ, Ke S, Levin VA. Activity of pp60c-src in 60 different cell lines derived from human tumors. Cancer Biochem Biophys. 1994; 14: 171-5.

[83] Mirmohammadsadegh A, Hassan M, Bardenheuer W, et al. STAT5 phosphorylation in malignant melanoma is important for survival and is mediated through SRC and JAK1 kinases. J Invest Dermatol. 2006; 126: 2272-80.

[84] Deconti RC, Messina J, Decker M, et al. Expression of STAT proteins and interferon receptors in benign and malignant melanocytic lesions: Correlation with recurrence. Journal of Clinical Oncology. 2004; 22: 7514.

[85] Niu G, Shain KH, Huang M, et al. Overexpression of a dominant-negative signal transducer and activator of transcription 3 variant in tumor cells leads to production of soluble factors that induce apoptosis and cell cycle arrest. Cancer Res. 2001; 61: 3276-80.

[86] Niu G, Heller R, Catlett-Falcone R, et al. Gene therapy with dominant-negative Stat3 suppresses growth of the murine melanoma B16 tumor in vivo. Cancer Res. 1999; 59: 5059-63.

[87] Du J, Jiang B, Coffey RJ, Barnard J. Raf and RhoA cooperate to transform intestinal epithelial cells and induce growth resistance to transforming growth factor beta. Mol Cancer Res. 2004; 2: 233-41.

[88] Dimitroff CJ, Sharma A, Bernacki RJ. Cancer metastasis: a search for therapeutic inhibition. Cancer Invest. 1998; 16: 279-90.

[89] Fidler IJ. Critical determinants of cancer metastasis: rationale for therapy. Cancer Chemother Pharmacol. 1999; 43 Suppl: S3-10.

[90] Meyer T, Hart IR. Mechanisms of tumour metastasis. Eur J Cancer. 1998; 34: 214-21.

[91] Woodhouse EC, Chuaqui RF, Liotta LA. General mechanisms of metastasis. Cancer. 1997; 80: 1529-37.

[92] Wang P, Wang X, Wu P, et al. GM3 upregulation of matrix metalloproteinase-9 possibly through PI3K, Akt, Rictor, RhoGDI2, and TNF-alpha pathways in mouse melanoma B16 cells. International Symposium on Molecular Immunology of Complex Carbonhydrate-3 (MICC-3). 2007: 369-86.

Chapter 15

After Surgery: Follow-Up Guidelines of Melanoma Patients

Paolo Fava, Pietro Quaglino,
Maria Grazia Bernengo and Paola Savoia

Additional information is available at the end of the chapter

http://dx.doi.org/10.5772/55335

1. Introduction

There are several main reasons to begin a follow-up schedule after surgical treatment of the primary cutaneous lesion in patients affected by melanoma.

The main goal is the early detection of disease recurrence, even if the impact of a prompt treatment on prognosis is still debated (Barth et al 1995, Atkins et al 2008, Garbe et al 2008). Several authors believe that early detection of asymptomatic metastases does not affect overall survival (Barth et al 1995, Atkins et al 2008). Others (Garbe et al 2008) showed a clear survival benefit for an early with respect to late metastases detection, with a 3-year survival rate of 76%, compared to the 38% of patients with late diagnosis. The early relapse recognition might lead to a more complete and less invasive surgical treatment, with potential benefits for the patient.

A loco-regional or distant spreading is a not uncommon event that arises in a percentage of patients varying from 15 to 35%. Indeed, in melanoma patients the risk of spreading is strictly related to the disease stage at diagnosis, and an effective follow-up program should taken in account both the AJCC classification (Balch et al 2009; Piris, Mihm & Duncan 2011) (Table 1) and the different patterns of metastatic dissemination related to site of primary, gender and age of patients (Quaglino et al 2007). On the basis of recently updated AJCC classification (Balch et al 2009), for patients affected by localized stage I or II melanomas, tumour thickness, mitotic rate and ulceration are considered the most relevant prognostic parameters; ulceration and thickness of primary tumour maintain a role as predictive independent factors on survival also in stage III patients, together to the number of involved lymph nodes, whereas for patients with distant metastases, elevated values of serum lactate dehydrogenase (LDH) define a category with poor prognosis. According to the primary location, no difference in the relapse rate was found for melanomas located on the head-neck, back, anterior trunk, upper limb and thigh-leg; conversely, a primary melanoma located to the foot was associated to a statistically significant higher relapse rate with respect to all the other sites (Quaglino et al 2007). As regard the first site of metastatic spreading, patients with a lower limb primary melanoma showed more frequently loco-regional metastases, whereas distant spreading was mainly observed in patients with melanoma located in the trunk (Savoia et al 2009). More in details, lower limb location showed a low incidence of visceral metastases as first site of relapse, irrespectively of the AJCC stage, compared to all other body sites (Quaglino et al 2007).

Clinical Staging				**Pathological Staging**			
0	Tis	N0	M0	0	Tis	N0	M0
IA	T1a	N0	M0	IA	T1a	N0	M0
IB	T1b	N0	M0	IB	T1b	N0	M0
	T2a	N0	M0		T2a	N0	M0
IIA	T2b	N0	M0	IIA	T2b	N0	M0
	T3a	N0	M0		T3a	N0	M0
IIB	T3b	N0	M0	IIB	T3b	N0	M0
	T4a	N0	M0		T4a	N0	M0
IIC	T4b	N0	M0	IIC	T4b	N0	M0
III	any T	N 1-3	M0	IIIA	T1-T4a	N1a/2a	M0
				IIIB	T1-T4b	N1a/2a	M0
					T1-T4a	N1b/2b	M0
					T1-T4a/b	N2c	M0
				IIIC	T1-T4b	N1b/2b/2c	M0
					any T	N3	M0
IV	any T	any N	M 1	IV	any T	any N	M 1

Table 1. Clinical and pathological staging, AJCC 2009.

The majority of guidelines encourage frequent clinical and radiological examination during the first 5 years from the diagnosis, due to the fact that almost 90% of all metastases occur during this period (Dummer et al 2011). However, it has been demonstrated that the time course of first relapse depend to the AJCC stage: the progressive decrease of relapse trend and the subsequent plateau is reached earlier in stage IA (after the second year) and later in stage IIB/IIC (from 5th to 8th year); moreover, distant relapses as first site of recurrences showed a low (<1.5%), but constant annual incidence, even beyond 10 years from diagnosis (Quaglino et al 2007); these data support the opinion of several authors who believe that a lifelong surveillance should be recommended (Garbe et al 2008, Dummer et al 2011).

http://dx.doi.org/10.5772/55335

The second reason to include melanoma patients in a follow-up program is the early identification of possible further primary melanomas or other skin tumours. Development of more than one primary melanoma in a sole patient is in fact a relatively common and well-recognized phenomenon; its frequency varies from 1.2 to 8.2% in the most recent published series (Savoia et al 2012) and it is probably due to a specific genetic background. In the majority of cases recently described (Bower et al 2010; Doubrowsky & Menzies 2003), there is a significant reduction in mean Breslow's thickness from the first to the second and successive primary melanomas, with a consequent favourable impact on prognosis. This is mainly resulting from well-timed diagnosis during follow-up programs.

Some melanoma patients also have an increased risk to develop non-melanoma skin tumours. In particular, 35% of patients affected by lentigo maligna melanomas develops others cutaneous malignancies within 5 years from the first diagnosis (Farshad et al 2002); this is probably related to the fact that this melanoma type prefers elderly patients with a chronic actinic skin damage. Also the relatively good prognosis of these patients may play a role.

Finally, a follow-up schedule should also perform an educational role, with the purpose of having a favourable impact on the population health and quality of life (Dummer et al 2010). Melanoma patients should be instructed not only in regular self-examination of the skin but also to avoid sunburns and prolonged unprotected solar or artificial ultraviolet exposure. Patients must also be aware that family members have an increased melanoma risk, consequent to both skin phototype and genetic background.

To date, even if these basic principles are approved, there is not a complete international agreement about the better follow-up schedule, with several differences in timing and duration between different Countries.

1.1. Imaging studies

Imaging studies can play a central role in the early detection of melanoma progression, allowing to a better treatment for patients. However, it is not generally accepted that the an early recognition of asymptomatic metastatic disease can affect the overall survival (Atkins et al 2008, Bichakjian et al 2011) and many imaging studies are considered uneconomical and not entirely risk-less for the patient. Thus, many international guidelines accept an imaging surveillance only in patients considered at higher risk of recurrence, as well stage IIIB and above, not approving the execution of instrumental tests in asymptomatic low risk patients (Marsden et al 2010, Bichakjian et al 2011). However, while ultrasonography is not harmful, relatively cheap and easy to perform, and can routinely be used not only in advanced, but also in stage I-II patients. In particular, even if sonography is operator-dependent, it remains more sensitive than clinical examination alone in the early identification of nodal metastases; sensitivity of ultrasound can be further improved by fine needle aspiration cytology, reaching the 80% in some selected series (Voit et al 2006, Negrier et al 2005). Higher sensitivity can be achieved only by sentinel node mapping. On the contrary, ultrasonography is relatively ineffective in detecting distant metastases: the calculated sensitivity for abdominal ultrasonography was only 53%, in comparison with 85% for CT scan (Forschner et al 2010). Similarly, traditional chest X-ray is less sensitive than CT-scan in the detection of lung metastases (Negrier et al 2005).

As a consequence of the high metabolic rate of melanoma cells, PET-CT can be useful to detect metastases in stage IIC or stage III patients, as well as in disease monitoring in stage IV patients (Bastiaannet et al 2009). This technique has a high sensitivity and allows an accurate study of the whole body, except the brain. The value of PET-CT in the follow-up of melanoma patients is supported by the recommendations from the update Swiss guidelines (Dummer et al 2011), that encourage the use of PET-CTC every 6-12 months for the first 5 years from diagnosis in stage IIC or stage III patients and by the fact that Swiss health insurances cover this imaging technique. However, PET-CT is not effective in the detection of positive sentinel lymph nodes in patients with primary melanomas (Negrier et al 2005, Clark et al 2006, Maubec et al 2007, Marsden et al 2011).

1.2. Screening blood tests

Routinely laboratory investigations have a relatively limited role in melanoma follow-up programs and are usually not recommended in asymptomatic patients affected by localized cutaneous melanoma of any thickness (Marsed et al 2010, Negrier et al 2005, Bichakjian et al 2011). However, recent advances in molecular biology techniques have permitted, in last years, the identification of several molecules with a potential prognostic and diagnostic role.

Melanoma patients with advanced disease share elevated lactate dehydrogenase (LDH) serum levels. Nevertheless, this marker act as an unfavourable prognostic factor only in stage IV disease and high LDH levels are also demonstrated in unspecific tissue necrosis conditions, such as haemolysis or myocardial infarction. So, the role of LDH in detection and monitoring of metastatic disease is still controversial (Wang et al 2004). As we mentioned in the previous paragraphs, in the updated AJCC classification (Balch et al 2009), for patients with distant metastases the presence of elevated lactate dehydrogenase serum levels define the M category, characterized by a poor prognosis.

Tyrosinase is the key enzyme responsible for the first two steps of melanin biosynthesis and is considered one of the most specific markers in melanocytic differentiation, as its expression is limited only to cells of neural crest derivation, such as melanocytes, melanoma cells and Schwann cells. Tyrosinase detection by reverse transcription-polymerase chain reaction (RT-PCR) analysis was initially applied to the detection of melanoma cells in SLN (Li et al 2000). More recently, the detection of tyrosinase transcripts using the nested RT-PCR has been proposed to identify the presence of melanoma cells in the peripheral blood in patients who have undergone radical surgery (Osella et al 2000), as well as a potential additional tool for the identification of melanoma cells in bone marrow and biological fluids other than blood (Gossein et al 1996, Hoon et al 1997, Osella et al 2003). However, the real diagnostic and prognostic relevance of this test is still controversial and its role in clinical practice is not yet fully defined.

The S-100 calcium binding protein represent an high-sensitive marker for melanocytic lesions, even if is no specific, since it stain either melanocytes or Langerhans and Schwann cells. In several studies it has been demonstrated to correlate with the tumour invasiveness in melanoma patients. Even if literature data about the melanoma–associated antigen S-100 are still controversial, the majority of published studies report that the percentage of patients with high S-100 levels increase progressively from stage I-II (0-12%) up to stage IV (Schultz et al 1998, Kaskel et al 1999, Jury et al 2000). The sensitivity and specificity of this marker in the identification of patients with a metastatic spread seems to be higher when compared with tyrosinase; the 64% of patients with serum S-100 levels exceeding 0.2mg/L showed distant metastases, confirmed by FDG-PET/CT scan (Forschner et al 2010). S-100 could play a role also in diagnosis of lymph node involvement: nodal metastases were identified in 19% of patients with high serum S-100 levels (Forschner et al 2010). Actually, S-100 is considered a good marker for melanoma relapse, especially for disease free stage III patients (Beyler et al 2006; Kruijff et al 2010), whereas in advanced stage patients, S-100 levels are related with treatment response and disease relapse (Garbe & Leiter 2003). The updated Swiss guidelines for the treatment and follow-up of cutaneous melanoma (Dummer et al 2011) suggest to monitorate S-100 levels every 6-12 months for the first 5 years from melanoma diagnosis in all stage II and III patients; for stage IV patients, timing of sampling for S-100 detection should be individualized for single patients.

Elevated serum levels of cytokines (IL-6, -8 and -10), soluble IL-2 receptor and soluble adhesion molecule (sICAM and sVCAM) (Eton et al 1998) has also been proposed as progression markers in melanoma patients; however, the relatively low sensibility and specificity of these molecules, together with their low cost-effectiveness ratio make them little used in clinical practice.

To date, others melanoma-associated antigens, such as melanoma inhibitory activity (MIA) and neuron-specific enolase (NSE) or molecular markers, including MART-1/Melan-A, gp100, TRP-1 and -2 showed a lower sensitivity and specificity and literature data regarding their potential role in the early detection of metastatic disease are still controversial. A multimarkers analysis appears to be associated with a sensitivity increase in the detection of circulating melanoma cells, but the impact of these data on patient's survival has not yet been conclusively defined.

2. Follow-up schedules according melanoma stage

2.1. In situ melanoma

Patients with a surgically treated in situ melanoma have no risk of metastases; so, the follow-up program should not include radiological examinations. It is also debated if clinical follow-up visits are needed. The 2010 UK guidelines of the British Association of Dermatologists recommend only a return visit after the complete excision to explain diagnosis and the education of patients to the self-examination for a new primary melanoma (Marseden et al 2010). Others authors recommend a closer follow up with a clinical check of the whole skin every 6-12 months (Dummer et al 2011). Even if the majority of multiple primary melanomas were identified within 1 year from the first diagnosis, a relevant percentage developed after 5 or also 10 year from the primary excision (Savoia et al 2012; van der Leest et al 2012), especially in younger patients. Consequently, in our opinion in consideration of the favourable prognosis of patients with a previous in situ melanoma, follow-up visits should be continuated, with the purpose of early diagnosis of possible further primary melanomas. Patients should also be instructed in avoidance of sunburn and informed that their consanguineous have an increased melanoma risk.

2.2. Stage IA melanoma

The 5-year overall survival of stage IA patients is over 90%, with virtually no risk of recurrences for patients with melanomas < 0.5 mm and a slightly worse prognosis for those with non-ulcerated 0.5-1 mm thick primary tumour (Einwachter-Thompson & MacKie 2008).

Considering this relatively low risk of disease progression, the revised UK guidelines for the management of melanoma (Marsden et al 2010) not recommended routinely imaging staging, due to the low true-positive rate and the high false-positive rate. According to the UK guidelines, patients should underwent to a series of two to four visits over the first years from the primary excision, in order to teach self-examination and then discharged from a regular follow-up. Similarly, the National French federation of cancer centres and the French society of dermatology suggest only periodical clinical examinations for patients in this clinical stage (Negrier et al 2005). Clinical follow-up at 6 monthly intervals, with the possible additional use of of ultrasonography, is considered appropriate by the majority of others groups (Quaglino et al 2007; Garbe et al 2010). Moreover, abdominal ultrasound imaging and chest x-ray are performed by many physicians to have baseline images for the further follow-up (Forschner et al 2010).

Routinely serological tests are not generally recommended in melanomas in the initial stage; however, the Catalan guidelines (Mangas et al 2010) suggest to perform at diagnosis complete blood count and biochemistry (including alkaline phosphatase, gamma-glutamyltransferase and lactate dehydrogenase) together with detection of molecular markers such as S-100, MIA and tyrosinase in all patients excepted those affected by melanoma in situ. Standard blood workup and LDH measurement should be repeated 6-monthly for the first 2 years and annualy for the following 2 years (Mangas et al 2010).

2.3. Stage IB and IIA melanoma

In this group of patients the risk of recurrence is of 15-35%, mainly within the first 5 years from diagnosis. A follow-up examination every 3 months at least for the first 5-years is recommended from the European consensus-based interdisciplinary guidelines (Garbe et al 2010), in order to detect early any loco-regional recurrences; a similar schedule is proposed also by Italian groups (Quaglino et al 2007). UK guidelines (Marsden et al 2010) admit checks every 3 months only for the first 3 years; then, patients should be instructed to self-examination also for loco regional metastases and visited only once every 6 months to 5 years. No routine instrumental investigations are required for this group of patients according UK follow-up schedule. Several studies demonstrated that ultrasonography of in-transit routes and regional lymph nodes are more sensitive than physical examination (89.2% vs. 71.4%) in the detection of nodal metastases in patients with an intermediate melanoma thickness (Blum et al 2000, Garbe et al 2003, Quaglino et al 2007). So, patients with a tumour thickness of 1 mm or more should be asked to undergo lymph node ultrasound imaging every 6 months (Forschner et al 2010). Ultrasonography of regional lymph node every 3-6 months within the first 5 years from diagnosis is suggested only for stage II patients also by French guidelines (Negrier et al 2005), whereas others imaging procedures are considered as optional. The clinical experience of major Italian referral centres for melanoma suggests performing a CT scan annually for the first 5 years also in stage IIA.

http://dx.doi.org/10.5772/55335

Screening blood tests are suggested only by Catalan guidelines, that propose standard blood workup and LDH detection 2 times a year for the first 5 years and then annually for the following 2 (Mangas et al 2010).

2.4. Stage IIB and IIC melanoma

UK guideline (Marsden et al 2010) did not recommend routine investigations also for stage IIB and IIC patients, despite the higher risk of recurrences (40-70%, above all in years 2-4); only self-examination and clinical visits 3-monthly for 3 years and 6-monthly to 5 years are suggested.

For stage IIC patients, as well for the more advanced stages, both Italian (Quaglino et al 2007) and French guidelines recommended not only a regional ultrasonography two times a year, but also brain, chest and abdomen CT scan that should be carried out annually for the first 5 years (Negrier et al 2005). Also for this group of patients, screening blood tests almost 2 times a years are recommended by Catalan authors (Mangas et al 2010).

Table 2 and 3 compare different follow-up visit schedules from European and US guidelines.

Clinical examination schedule (years 1-5 from diagnosis)						
Stage*	Dummer, 2011	Marsden, 2010	Mangas, 2010	Garbe, 2009	Quaglino, 2008	Négrier, 2005
In situ	f-u visit every 6-12 months	*no f-u visit required*	*f-u visit every 12 months*	*no f-u visit required*	*f-u visit every 12 months*	*NA*
IA	visit every 6 months	*visit every 3-4 months, then discharged*	visit every 3/6 months†	visit every 6 months	visit every 6 months	visit every 6 months
IB	visit every 3 months	visit every 3 months**	visit every 3/6 months†	visit every 3/6 months[1]	visit every 6 months	visit every 6 months
IIA	visit every 3 months	Visit every 3 months**	visit every 3/6 months†	visit every 3 months	visit every 4 months	visit every 3 months
IIB	visit every 3 months	visit every 3 months**	visit every 3 months†	visit every 3 months	visit every 4 months	visit every 3 months
IIC	visit every 3 months	visit every 3 months**	visit every 3 months†	visit every 3 months	visit every 4 months	visit every 3 months

* revised AJCC Classification.

** visit every 3 months for the first 3 years, then 6-monthly to 5 year.

[1] In consideration of Breslow thickness: for melanoma <1mm every 6 months; for melanoma >1 mm every 3 months.

† visit every 3 months for the first 2 years, then 6-monthly to 5 year.

Table 2. Clinical examination schedule (years 1-5 from diagnosis)

	Imaging examination schedule (years 1-5 from diagnosis)					
Stage*	Dummer, 2011	Marsden, 2010	Mangas, 2010	Garbe, 2009	Quaglino, 2008	Négrier, 2005
In situ	*Not required*	*Not required*	*Not required*	*Not required*	*Not required*	*NA*
IA	*Regional sonography every 6-12 months*	*No routine investigation required*	*Chest X-ray every 12 months; abdominal sonography every 12 months (optional)*	*No routine investigation required***	*Regional sonography every 12 months*	*No routine investigation required*
IB	*Regional sonography every 6-12 months*	*No routine investigation required*	*Chest X-ray every 6 months; abdominal sonography every 6 months (optional)*†	*No routine investigation required***	*Regional and abdomen sonography every 12 months; chest X-ray every 12 months*	*No routine investigation required*
IIA	*Regional sonography every 6-12 months. Abdominal sonography and chest X-ray individually*	*No routine investigation required*	*Chest X-ray every 6 months; abdominal sonography every 6 months (optional)*†	*No routine investigation required***	*Regional and abdomen sonography every 12 months; chest X-ray every 12 months; TC scan every 24 months*	Regional sonography every 3-6 months.
IIB	*Regional sonography every 6-12 months. Abdominal sonography and chest X-ray individually. CT scan every 6-12 mo*	*No routine investigation required*	*CT scan every 6/12 months*†	*No routine investigation required***	*Regional and abdomen sonography every 12 months; chest X-ray every 12 months; CT scan every 12 months*	Regional sonography every 3-6 months.
IIC	*Regional sonography every 6 months. Abdominal sonography and chest X-ray individually. CT scan every 6-12 mo*	*No routine investigation required*	*CT scan every 6/12 months*†	*No routine investigation required*	*Regional and abdomen sonography every 12 months; chest X-ray every 12 months*	Regional sonography every 3-6 months. PET-CT, and CT scan individually

* revised AJCC Classification.

** sonography individually

† every 6 months for the first 3 years, then annually to 5 year

Table 3. Imaging examination schedule (years 1-5 from diagnosis)

2.5. Stage III melanoma

At the initial visit prior to surgical treatment, brain, chest, abdominal and pelvic CT is recommended, in order to exclude visceral involvement; PET-CT and cranial MRI may be

http://dx.doi.org/10.5772/55335

proposed as alternative; Catalan guidelines suggest also a bone scintigraphy as optional (Mangas et al 2010).

Due to the high risk of visceral spreading in stage III patients, close follow-up and imaging investigations are accepted by almost all guidelines (Garbe et al 2010, Marseden et al 2010, Dummer et al 2010, Forschner et al 2010, Romano et al 2010). Head, chest and abdomen CT scan is normally useful to detect metastases, with higher sensitivity than ultrasound imaging; PET-CT can also be used alternatively (Negrier et al 2005). However, some other authors consider imaging investigation as optional in absence of specific sign or symptoms (Coit et al 2009).

Literature data reports also a wide range of follow-up approaches, without precise rules for timing and duration. A close follow-up regimen was proposed by Garbe et al (2003), with clinical visits every 3 months for the first 5 year and then every 6 months up to 10 years after lymph node dissection and instrumental examination (CT scan, PET-CT, chest x-ray or abdominal and lymph nodal ultrasound) every 6 months. In the sample of patients examined, a disease progression was detected by physical examination in almost the half of cases, and by imaging in more than one third of cases; on the contrary, relapses were rarely early discovered in patients outside of the scheduled follow-up. In this work, Garbe report a better 5-year survival in patients with early diagnosis of recurrences compared to that of patients with unresectable metastases, supporting the validity of a close follow-up program (Garbe et al 2003). Other similar follow-up programs (Hoffman et al 2002, Poo-Hwu 1999), with a relatively high frequency of visits (3-monthly for almost 3 years), come to similar results. The UK guidelines (Marsden et al 2010) suggest a 6-monthly follow-up to 5 years and then annually to 10 years, whereas regular follow-up every 6 months with whole body imaging is recommended by others (Forschner et al 2010).

The study recently published by Romano et al. (2010), focused on stage III patients, evaluate also the substage. For stage IIIA patients, the risk of loco-regional relapse was less than 5% after 3 years from stage IIIA diagnosis, suggesting that beyond this point of time clinical examinations may be referred. Similarly, the risk of loco-regional relapse dropped to less then 5% after 2 years from diagnosis for stage IIIB patients and after 7 months in stage IIIC. Stage IIIC patients are the subset with higher risk of visceral spreading, with a 36% of patients that develop the first relapse in the brain; so, this subgroup of patients should be subjected to imaging examination more fequently

Even if routinely blood tests usually fail in the early detection of metastases, in stage III melanoma patients tyrosinase (Osella- Abate et al 2003) or S100 (Dummer et al 2010, Forschner et al 2010) has been demonstrated good marker for relapse.

2.6. Stage IV melanoma

No international follow-up guidelines are available for patients with metastatic disease. The management strategy should be patient-taylored on the basis of primary melanoma characteristics, metastases site, age and general conditions.

The development in the last few years of a novel class of targeted drugs (such as ipilimumab, vemurafenib, imatinib) with an impact on survival, had an important effect on the management of these patients. C-kit and BRAF mutational state have to be evaluated in order to select patients who can underwent this targeted therapies; also the identification of subgroups of patients with different clinical behaviours is important for the right therapeutical choice, especially for the drugs that need time to act (e.g anti-CTLA-4).

3. Conclusions

The main follow-up goal is the early detection of disease recurrence, which can allow a prompt treatment with a potential prognostic benefit.

To date an international agreement about the most suitable follow-up guidelines for patients who underwent a surgical excision of a primary melanoma is still lacking. Several national guidelines are available, but the schedules differ as to the time frequency of both clinical visits and imaging. However it is generally accepted that the frequency of clinical examinations must to be decided on the basis of the AJCC stage at diagnosis and that a closer follow-up should required in the first five years from diagnosis due to the higher risk of recurrence observed in this time range. Regional node ultrasound is an useful tool for the detection of suspected superficial adenopathies.

On the other hand, the role of imaging for the detection of visceral metastases in asymptomatic patients is still a challenge: for low risk (IA) melanomas no routine investigations could be required; sonography is generally used in follow up of intermediate/high risk melanoma patients (IB to IIA), whereas the use of CT and PET scan is limited to patients with an higher relapse risk (stage IIC or higher). It is generally accepted that the follow up's strategy for disease-free stage III/IV patients, must to be tailored on the basis of clinical characteristics and general conditions.

Author details

Paolo Fava, Pietro Quaglino, Maria Grazia Bernengo and Paola Savoia*

University of Turin, Department of Medical Sciences, Turin, Italy

References

[1] Atkins MB, Hsu J, Lee S, Cohen GI, Flaherty LE, Sosman JA, Sondak VK &. Kirkwood JM. Phase III trial comparing concurrent biochemotherapy with cisplatin, vinblastine, dacarbazine, interleukin-2, and interferon alfa-2b with cisplatin, vinblastine,

and dacarbazine alone in patients with metastatic malignant melanoma (E3695): a trial coordinated by the Eastern Cooperative Oncology Group. J Clin Oncol 2008; 26:5748-54.

[2] Balch CM, Gershenwald JE, Soong SJ, Thompson JF, Atkins MB, Byrd DR, Buzaid AC, Cochran AJ, Coit DG, Ding S, Eggermont AM, Flaherty KT, Gimotty PA, Kirkwood JM, McMasters KM, Mihm MC Jr, Morton DL, Ross MI, Sober AJ & Sondak VK. Final version of 2009 AJCC melanoma staging and classification. J Clin Oncol. 2009; 27: 6199-6206.

[3] Barth A, Wanek LA & Morton DL. Prognostic factors in 1,521 melanoma patients with distant metastases. J Am Coll Surg 1995; 181:193-201.

[4] Bastiaannet E, Wobbes T, Hoekstra OS, van der Jagt EJ, Brouwers AH, Koelemij R, de Klerk JM, Oyen WJ, Meijer S, & Hoekstra HJ. Prospective comparison of [18f]fluorodeoxyglucose positron emission tomography and computed tomography in patients with melanoma with palpable lymph node metastases: Diagnostic accuracy and impact on treatment. J Clin Oncol. 2009; 27:4774–80.

[5] Beyeler M, Waldispuhl S, Strobel K, Joller-Jemelka HI, Burg G & Dummer R. Detection of melanoma relapse: First comparative analysis on imaging techniques versus s100 protein. Dermatology. 2006; 213:187–91.

[6] Bichakjian C K, Halpern AC , Johnson TM, Foote Hood A , Grichnik JM., Swetter SM., Tsao H , Holloway Barbosa V, Chuang TY, Duvic M, Ho VC, Sober AJ, Beutner KR, Bhushan R & Smith Begolka K. Guidelines of care for the management of primary cutaneous melanoma. J Am Acad Dermatol 2011; 1032-1047.

[7] Blum A, Schlagenhauff B, StroebelW, Breuninger H, Rassner G & Garbe C. Ultrasound examination of regional lymph nodes significantly improves early detection of locoregional metastases during the follow-up of patients with cutaneous melanoma: results of a prospective study of 1288 patients. Cancer 2000; 88:2534-9.

[8] Bower MR, Scoggins CR, Martin RC 2nd, Mays MP, Edwards MJ, Reintgen DS, Ross MI, Urist MM, Noyes RD, Sussman JJ, Hagendoorn LJ, Stromberg AJ & McMasters K .Second primary melanomas: incidence and outcome. Am Surg. 2010; 76(7):675-81.

[9] Clark PB, Soo V, Kraas J, Shen P & Levine EA. Futility of fluorodeoxyglucose F 18 positron emission tomography in initial evaluation of patients with T2 to T4 melanoma. Arch Surg 2006;141:284e8.

[10] Coit DG, Andtbacka R, Anker CJ, Bichakjian CK, Carson WE 3rd, Daud A, Dilawari RA, Dimaio D, Guild V, Halpern AC, Hodi FS Jr, Kelley MC, Khushalani NI, Kudchadkar RR, Lange JR, Lind A, Martini MC, Olszanski AJ, Pruitt SK, Ross MI, Swetter SM, Tanabe KK, Thompson JA, Trisal V & Urist MM; National Comprehensive Cancer Network : Melanoma. J Natl Compr Canc Netw 2009 7:250-275.

[11] Doubrovsky A & Menzies SW. Enhanced survival in patients with multiple primary melanoma.Arch Dermatol. 2003;139(8):1013-8.

[12] Dummer R, Guggenheim M, Arnold WA, Braun R & von Moos R. Updated Swiss guidelines for the treatment and follow-up of cutaneous melanoma. Eu J Med Sci 2011; 141:w13320.

[13] Einwachter-Thompson J & MacKie RM. An evidence base for reconsidering current follow-up guidelines for patients with cutaneous melanoma less than 0.5 mm thick at diagnosis. Br J Dermatol 2008;159:337e41.

[14] Eton O, Legha SS, Moon TE, Buzaid AC, Papadopoulos NE, Plager C, Burgess AM, Bedikian AY, Ring S, Dong Q, Glassman AB, Balch CM & Benjamin RS. Prognostic factors for survival of patients treated systemically for disseminated melanoma. J. Clin. Oncol. 1998; 16(3), 1103–1111.

[15] Farshad A, Burg G, Panizzon R & Dummer R. A retrospective study of 150 patients with lentigo maligna and lentigo maligna melanoma and the efficacy of radiotherapy using grenz or soft x-rays. Br J Dermatol.2002; 146:1042–1046.

[16] Forschner A, Eigentler TK, Pflugfelder A, Leiter U, Weide B, Held L, Meier F & Garbe C. Melanoma staging: facts and controversies. Clin Dermatol. 2010;28(3): 275-80.

[17] Garbe C, Leiter U, Ellwanger U, Blaheta HJ, Meier F & Schittek B. Diagnostic value and prognostic significance of protein S-100β, melanomainhibitory activity, and tyrosinase/MART-1 reverse transcription-polymerase chain reaction in the follow-up of high-risk melanoma patients. Cancer 2003; 97(7), 1737–1745.

[18] Garbe C, & Leiter U. In reply: Prospective evaluation of a follow-up schedule in 2,008 patients with cutaneous melanoma: recommendations for an effective follow-up strategy. J Clin Oncol 2003; 21:3706-7.

[19] Garbe C, Schadendorf D, Stolz W, Volkenandt M, Reinhold U, Kortmann RD, Kettelhack C, Frerich B, Keilholz U, Dummer R, Sebastian G, Tilgen W, Schuler G, Mackensen A, Kaufmann R & Hauschild A. Short german guidelines: Malignant melanoma. J Dtsch Dermatol Ges. 2008; 6(Suppl 1):S9–S14.

[20] Ghossein RA, Coit D, Brennan M, Zhang ZF, Wang Y, Bhattacharya S, Houghton A & Rosai J. Prognostic significance of peripheral blood and bone marrow tyrosinase messenger RNA in malignant melanoma. Clin Canc Res 1998; 4, 419-428.

[21] Hofmann U, Szedlak M, Rittgen W, Jung EG, Schadendorf D : Primary staging and follow-up in melanoma patients: Monocenter evaluation of methods, costs and patient survival. Br J Cancer 2002; 87:151-157.

[22] Hoon DS, Wang Y, Dale PS, Conrad AJ, Schmid P, Garrison D, Kuo C, Foshag LJ, Nizze AJ & Morton DL. Detection of occult melanoma cells in blood with a multiple-marker polymerase chain reaction assay. J Clin. Oncol 1995; 13, 2109-2116.

[23] Kaskel P, Berking C, Sander S, Volkenandt M, Peter RU & Krahn G. S-100 protein in peripheral blood: a marker for melanoma metastases: a prospective 2- center study of 570 patients with melanoma. J Am Acad Dermatol. 1999; 41(6), 962–969.

[24] Kruijff S, Bastiaannet E, Muller Kobold AC, van Ginkel RJ, Suurmeijer AJ & Hoekstra HJ. Erratum to: S-100b concentrations predict disease free survival in stage iii melanoma patients. Ann Surg Oncol. 2010; 16(12):3455-62.

[25] Jury CS, McAllister EJ & MacKie RM. Rising levels of serum S100 protein precede other evidence of disease progression in patients with malignant melanoma. Br. J. Dermatol. 2000; 143(2), 269–274.

[26] Li W, Stall A, Shivers SC, Lin J, Haddad F, Messina J, Glass LF, Lyman G, Reintgen DS: Clinical relevance of molecular staging for melanoma: comparison of RT-PCR and immunohistochemistry staining in sentinel lymph nodes of patients with melanoma. Ann. Surg. 2000; 231, 795–803.

[27] Mangas C, Paradelo C, Puig S, Gallardo F, Marcoval J, Azon A, Bartralot R, Bel S, Bigatà X, Curcó N, Dalmau J, del Pozo LJ, Ferrándiz C, Formigón M, González A, Just M, Llambrich A, Llistosella E, Malvehy J, Martí RM, Nogués ME, Pedragosa R, Rocamora V, Sàbat M & Salleras M. Initial evaluation, diagnosis, staging, treatment, and follow-up of patients with primary cutaneous malignant melanoma. Consensus statement of the Network of Catalan and Balearic Melanoma Centers Actas Dermosifiliogr. 2010;101(2):129-42.

[28] Maubec E, Lumbroso J, Masson F, Suciu V, Kolb F, Mamelle G, Cavalcanti A, Boitier F, Spatz A, Aupérin A, Leboulleux S & Avril MF. F-18 fluorodeoxy-Dglucose positron emission tomography scan in the initial evaluation of patients with a primary melanoma thicker than 4 mm. Melanoma Res 2007;17:147e54.

[29] Marsden JR, Newton-Bishop JA, Burrows L, Cook M, Corrie PG, Cox NH, Gore ME, Lorigan P, Mackie R, Nathan P, Peach H, Powell B & Walker C. Revised UK guidelines for the management of cutaneous melanoma 2010. J Plast Reconstr Aesthet Surg. 2010;63(9):1401-19.

[30] Négrier S, Saiag P, Guillot B, Verola O, Avril MF, Bailly C, Cupissol D, Dalac S, Danino A, Dreno B, Grob JJ, Leccia MT, Renaud-Vilmer C &Bosquet L. Guidelines for clinical practice: Standards, Options and Recommendations 2005 for the management of adult patients exhibiting an M0 cutaneous melanoma, full report. National Federation of Cancer Campaign Centers. French Dermatology Society. Update of the 1995 Consensus Conference and the 1998 Standards, Options, and Recommendations. Ann Dermatol Venereol. 2005;132(12 Pt 2):10S3-10S85.

[31] Osella Abate S, Savoia P, Cambieri I, Salomone B, Quaglino P & Bernengo MG. Role of RT-PCR tyrosinase detection in the monitoring of patients with advanced metastatic melanoma. Melanoma Res 2000; 10(6), 545-555.

[32] Osella-Abate S, Quaglino P, Savoia P, Leporati C, Comessatti A & Bernengo MG. VEGF-165 serum levels and tyrosinase expression in melanoma patients: correlation with the clinical course. Melanoma Res 2002; 12(4), 325-334.

[33] Osella-Abate S, Savoia P, Quaglino P, Fierro MT, Leporati C, Ortoncelli M & Bernengo MG. Tyrosinase expression in the peripheral blood of stage III melanoma patients is associated with a poor prognosis: a clinical follow-up study of 110 patients. Br J Cancer 2003; 89(8), 1457-1462.

[34] Piris A, Mihm MC Jr & Duncan LM. AJCC melanoma staging update: impact on dermatopathology practice and patient management. J Cutan Pathol. 2011; 38(5):394-400.

[35] Poo-Hwu WJ, Ariyan S, Lamb L, Papac R, Zelterman D, Hu GL, Brown J, Fischer D, Bolognia J & Buzaid AC. Follow-up recommendations for patients with American Joint Committee on Cancer Stages I-III malignant melanoma. Cancer 1999; 86:2252-2258.

[36] Quaglino P, Borgognoni L, Bottoni U, Calvieri S, Carli P, Catricalà C, Eibenschutz L, Manganoni A, Moretti S, Pellacani G, Pimpinelli N, Seidenari S, Bernengo MG. Italian guidelines for staging and follw-up of stage I-I cutaneous melanoma patients. G Ital Dermatol Venereol 2007; 142: 41-47.

[37] Romano E, Scordo M, Dusza SW, Coit DG & Chapman PBSite and timing of first relapse in stage III melanoma patients: implications for follow-up guidelines. J Clin Oncol. 2010;28(18):3042-7.

[38] Savoia P, Fava P, Nardò T, Osella-Abate S, Quaglino P & Bernengo MG. Skin metastases of malignant melanoma: a clinical and prognostic survey. Melanoma Res. 2009; 19(5):321-6.

[39] Savoia P, Osella-Abate S, Deboli T, Marenco F, Stroppiana E, Novelli M, Fierro MT & Bernengo MG. Clinical and prognostic reports from 270 patients with multiple primary melanomas: a 34-year single-institution study. J Eur Acad Dermatol Venereol. 2012; 26(7):882-8.

[40] Schultz ES, Diepgen TL & Von Den Driesch P. Clinical and prognostic relevance of serum S-100 β protein in malignant melanoma. Br. J. Dermatol. 1998; 138(3), 426–430.

[41] Van der Leest RJ, Liu L, Coebergh JW, Neumann HA, Mooi WJ, Nijsten T, de Vries E.Risk of second primary in situ and invasive melanoma in Dutch population-based cohort: 1989 – 2008. Br J Dermatol. 2012; Jul 3.

[42] Voit C, Kron M, Schäfer G, Schoengen A, Audring H, Lukowsky A, Schwürzer-Voit M, Sterry W, Winter H & Rademaker J.Ultrasound-guided fine needle aspiration cytology prior to sentinel lymph node biopsy in melanoma patients..Ann Surg Oncol. 2006;13(12):1682-9.

http://dx.doi.org/10.5772/55335

[43] Wang TS, Johnson TM, Cascade PN, Redman BG, Sondak VK & Schwartz JL. Evaluation of staging chest radiographs and serum lactate dehydrogenase for localized melanoma. J Am Acad Dermatol 2004;51:399-405.